T0229007

Management of Metastatic Liver Tumors

Editor

MICHAEL D'ANGELICA

SURGICAL ONCOLOGY CLINICS OF NORTH AMERICA

www.surgonc.theclinics.com

Consulting Editor
TIMOTHY M. PAWLIK

January 2021 • Volume 30 • Number 1

ELSEVIER

1600 John F. Kennedy Boulevard • Suite 1800 • Philadelphia, Pennsylvania, 19103-2899

http://www.theclinics.com

SURGICAL ONCOLOGY CLINICS OF NORTH AMERICA Volume 30, Number 1
January 2021 ISSN 1055-3207, ISBN-13: 978-0-323-76449-0

Editor: John Vassallo (j.vassallo@elsevier.com)
Developmental Editor: Julia Mckenzie

Surgical Oncology Clinics of North America (ISSN 1055-3207) is published quarterly by Elsevier Inc., 360 Park Avenue South, New York, NY 10010-1710. Months of publication are January, April, July, and October. Business and Editorial Offices: 1600 John F. Kennedy Blvd., Ste. 1800, Philadelphia, PA 19103-2899. Customer Service Office: 3251 Riverport Lane, Maryland Heights, MO 63043. Periodicals postage paid at New York, NY and additional mailing offices. Subscription prices are $315.00 per year (US individuals), $750.00 (US institutions) $100.00 (US student/resident), $352.00 (Canadian individuals), $784.00 (Canadian institutions), $100.00 (Canadian student/resident), $456.00 (foreign individuals), $784.00 (foreign institutions), and $205.00 (foreign student/resident). Foreign air speed delivery is included in all *Clinics* subscription prices. All prices are subject to change without notice. **POSTMASTER**: Send address changes to *Surgical Oncology Clinics of North America*, Elsevier Health Science Division, Subscription Customer Service, 3251 Riverport Lane, Maryland Heights, MO 63043. **Customer Service: 1-800-654-2452 (US and Canada). 314-447-8871 (outside US and Canada). Fax: 314-447-8029. E-mail: journalscustomerservice-usa@elsevier.com (for print support); journalsonline support-usa@elsevier.com (for online support)**.

Reprints. For copies of 100 or more, of articles in this publication, please contact the Commercial Reprints Department, Elsevier Inc., 360 Park Avenue South, New York, New York 10010-1710. Tel. 212-633-3874; Fax: 212-633-3820; E-mail: reprints@elsevier.com.

Surgical Oncology Clinics of North America is covered in *MEDLINE/PubMed (Index Medicus)* and *EMBASE/ Excerpta Medica, Current Contents/Clinical Medicine, and ISI/BIOMED.*

Contributors

CONSULTING EDITOR

TIMOTHY M. PAWLIK, MD, MPH, PhD, FACS, FRACS (Hon)
Professor and Chair, Department of Surgery, The Urban Meyer III and Shelley Meyer Chair for Cancer Research, Professor of Surgery, Oncology, and Health Services Management and Policy, Surgeon in Chief, The Ohio State University Wexner Medical Center, Columbus, Ohio, USA

EDITOR

MICHAEL D'ANGELICA, MD, FACS
Vice Chair for Education, Enid A. Haupt Chair in Surgery, Memorial Sloan Kettering Cancer Center, Attending Surgeon, Hepatopancreatobiliary Service, Memorial Sloan Kettering Cancer Center, Program Director, Complex Surgical Oncology and HPB Fellowship, Professor of Surgery, Cornell University, Weill Medical College, New York, New York, USA

AUTHORS

MICHAEL D'ANGELICA, MD, FACS
Vice Chair for Education, Enid A. Haupt Chair in Surgery, Memorial Sloan Kettering Cancer Center, Attending Surgeon, Hepatopancreatobiliary Service, Memorial Sloan Kettering Cancer Center, Program Director, Complex Surgical Oncology and HPB Fellowship, Professor of Surgery, Cornell University, Weill Medical College, New York, New York, USA

RONALD P. DeMATTEO, MD
Department of Surgery, University of Pennsylvania, Philadelphia, Pennsylvania, USA

H. RICHARD ALEXANDER Jr. MD
Head, Department of Surgery, Division of Surgical Oncology, Chief Surgical Officer, Rutgers Cancer Institute of New Jersey, Rutgers Robert Wood Johnson Medical School, New Brunswick, New Jersey, USA

JORDAN BERLIN, MD
Professor, Department of Medicine, Division of Hematology Oncology, Vanderbilt University Medical Center, Nashville, Tennessee, USA

KIMBERLY A. BERTENS, MD, MPH, FRCSC, FACS
Liver and Pancreas Unit, Department of Surgery, Division of Medical Oncology, Department of Medicine, The Ottawa Hospital, University of Ottawa, Ottawa, Ontario, Canada

MARIA IGNEZ FREITAS MELRO BRAGHIROLI, MD
Medical Oncologist, Instituto do Cancer do Estado de Sao Paulo (ICESP), University of Sao Paulo, and Rede D'Or Sao Paulo

ROBERT E. BRISTOW, MD
Chair, Department of Obstetrics and Gynecology, University of California, Orange, California, USA

CHRISTINA CANIL, MD, FRCPC
Division of Medical Oncology, Department of Medicine, The Ottawa Hospital, University of Ottawa, Ottawa, Ontario, Canada

MICHAEL J. CAVNAR, MD
Department of Surgery, University of Kentucky, Lexington, Kentucky, USA

CHANDRIKHA CHANDRASEKHARAN, MBBS
Clinical Assistant Professor, Department of Internal Medicine, Division of Hematology, Oncology and Blood and Marrow Transplantation, University of Iowa Carver College of Medicine, Iowa City, Iowa, USA

KIRAN H. CLAIR, MD
Fellow, Division of Gynecologic Oncology, University of California, Orange, California, USA

FABRICIO FERREIRA COELHO, MD, PhD
Digestive Surgery Division, Liver Surgery Unit, Department of Gastroenterology, University of Sao Paulo Medical School, São Paulo, São Paulo, Brazil

LOUISE C. CONNELL, MB BCH, BAO, BMedSc
Assistant Attending Physician, Gastrointestinal Oncology Service, Division of Solid Tumor Oncology, Department of Medicine, Memorial Sloan Kettering Cancer Center, New York, New York, USA

CHRISTOPHER H. CRANE, MD
Department of Radiation Oncology, Memorial Sloan Kettering Cancer Center, New York, New York, USA

SATYA DAS, MD, MSCI
Assistant Professor, Department of Medicine, Division of Hematology Oncology, Vanderbilt University Medical Center, Nashville, Tennessee, USA

MARIO DE BELLIS, MD
Department of Surgical Oncology, The University of Texas MD Anderson Cancer Center, Houston, Texas, USA

VIRGINIA DEVI-CHOU, BA, MA
Division of Surgical Oncology, Rutgers Cancer Institute of New Jersey, Rutgers Robert Wood Johnson Medical School, New Brunswick, New Jersey, USA

GREGOR DUWE, MD
Department of Surgical Oncology, The University of Texas MD Anderson Cancer Center, Houston, Texas, USA

BRETT L. ECKER, MD
Department of Surgery, University of Pennsylvania, Philadelphia, Pennsylvania, USA

ALEXANDER M.M. EGGERMONT, MD, PhD
Princess Máxima Center for Pediatric Oncology, Utrecht, the Netherlands

GILTON MARQUES FONSECA, MD, PhD
Digestive Surgery Division, Liver Surgery Unit, Department of Gastroenterology, University of Sao Paulo Medical School, São Paulo, São Paulo, Brazil

DIRK J. GRÜNHAGEN, MD, PhD
Department of Surgical Oncology and Gastrointestinal Surgery, Erasmus MC Cancer Institute, Rotterdam, the Netherlands

DIEDERIK J. HÖPPENER, MD
Department of Surgical Oncology and Gastrointestinal Surgery, Erasmus MC Cancer Institute, Rotterdam, the Netherlands

PAULO HERMAN, MD, PhD
Digestive Surgery Division, Liver Surgery Unit, Department of Gastroenterology, University of Sao Paulo Medical School, São Paulo, São Paulo, Brazil

JAMES R. HOWE, MD
Professor, Department of Surgery, Division of Surgical Oncology and Endocrine Surgery, University of Iowa Carver College of Medicine, Iowa City, Iowa, USA

YOSHIKUNI KAWAGUCHI, MD, PhD
Department of Surgical Oncology, The University of Texas MD Anderson Cancer Center, Houston, Texas, USA; Hepato-Biliary-Pancreatic Surgery Division, Department of Surgery, Graduate School of Medicine, The University of Tokyo, Tokyo, Japan

NANCY E. KEMENY, MD
Attending Physician, Gastrointestinal Oncology Service, Division of Solid Tumor Oncology, Department of Medicine, Memorial Sloan Kettering Cancer Center, New York, New York, USA

MARYAM B. LUSTBERG, MD, MPH
Associate Professor, Department of Medicine, Division of Medical Oncology, The Ohio State University Medical School, Columbus, Ohio, USA

ROBERT G. MAKI, MD, PhD
Department of Medicine, University of Pennsylvania, Philadelphia, Pennsylvania, USA

GUILLAUME MARTEL, MD, MSc, FRCSC, FACS
Liver and Pancreas Unit, Department of Surgery, The Ottawa Hospital, University of Ottawa, Ottawa, Ontario, Canada

BRIAN P. NEAL, PhD
Medical Physics, ProCure Proton Therapy Center, Somerset, New Jersey, USA

DANIEL P. NUSSBAUM, MD
Department of Surgery, Memorial Sloan Kettering Cancer Center, New York, New York, USA

CHANDRASEKHAR PADMANABHAN, MD
Department of Surgery, Memorial Sloan Kettering Cancer Center, New York, New York, USA

ELENA PANETTIERI, MD
Department of Surgical Oncology, The University of Texas MD Anderson Cancer Center, Houston, Texas, USA

TIMOTHY M. PAWLIK, MD, MPH, PhD, FACS, FRACS (Hon)
Professor and Chair, Department of Surgery, The Urban Meyer III and Shelley Meyer Chair for Cancer Research, Professor of Surgery, Oncology, and Health Services Management and Policy, Surgeon in Chief, The Ohio State University Wexner Medical Center, Columbus, Ohio, USA

JAIME ARTHUR PIROLA KRUGER, MD, PhD
Digestive Surgery Division, Liver Surgery Unit, Department of Gastroenterology,
University of Sao Paulo Medical School, São Paulo, São Paulo, Brazil

AMIR A. RAHNEMAI-AZAR, MD
Assistant Professor, Department of Surgery, Division of Surgical Oncology, California
University of Science and Medicine, Colton, California, USA

PAUL B. ROMESSER, MD
Department of Radiation Oncology, Memorial Sloan Kettering Cancer Center, Early Drug
Development Service, Department of Medicine, Memorial Sloan Kettering Cancer Center,
New York, New York, USA

LUKE V. SELBY, MD, MS
Fellow, Department of Surgery, Division of Surgical Oncology, The Ohio State University
Medical School, Columbus, Ohio, USA

SCOTT K. SHERMAN, MD
Assistant Professor, Department of Surgery, Division of Surgical Oncology and Endocrine
Surgery, University of Iowa Carver College of Medicine, Iowa City, Iowa, USA

CATHERINE G. TRAN, MD
General Surgery Resident, Department of Surgery, University of Iowa Hospitals & Clinics,
Iowa City, Iowa, USA

ASTRID A.M. van der VELDT, MD, PhD
Department of Medical Oncology, Erasmus MC Cancer Institute, Rotterdam, the
Netherlands

JEAN-NICOLAS VAUTHEY, MD, FACS
Department of Surgical Oncology, The University of Texas MD Anderson Cancer Center,
Houston, Texas, USA

CORNELIS VERHOEF, MD, PhD, FEBS
Department of Surgical Oncology and Gastrointestinal Surgery, Erasmus MC Cancer
Institute, Rotterdam, the Netherlands

JULIET WOLFORD, MD
Fellow, Division of Gynecologic Oncology, University of California, Orange, California,
USA

JASON A. ZELL, DO
Associate Professor, Division of Hematology/Oncology, Department of Medicine,
University of California, Orange, California, USA

Contents

Approximately 50% of colorectal cancer patients develop liver metastases. Hepatic metastases represent the most common cause of colorectal cancer-related mortality. Metastasectomy, if possible, represents the most effective treatment strategy; 20% of patients will be cured and more than 50% survive at least 5 years. Nuances to treatment planning hinge on whether patients present with resectable disease upfront, whether the future liver remnant is adequate, and whether the primary tumor, if present, is colon versus rectal in origin. This article discusses considerations impacting our approach to patients with colorectal liver metastases and the role for various multimodal treatment options.

Hepatic resection for patients with isolated breast cancer liver metastases (BCLM) is associated with prolonged disease-free interval and better overall survival in highly selected patients. Patients with limited disease who are not candidates for surgery benefit from ablative therapies for isolated breast cancer metastasis in addition to systemic chemotherapy. In the era of modern effective systemic chemotherapy for BCLM, local regional therapies are warranted, yet only in well-selected patients following discussion in a multidisciplinary setting. This article reviews data related to hepatic resection and ablative therapies of BCLM, as well as long-term outcomes of women treated with these approaches.

Patients with neuroendocrine tumor liver metastases (NETLMs) may develop carcinoid syndrome, carcinoid heart disease, or other symptoms from overproduction of hormones. Hepatic resection and cytoreduction is the most direct treatment of NETLMs in eligible patients, and cytoreduction improves symptoms, may reduce the sequelae of carcinoid syndrome, and extends survival. Parenchymal-sparing procedures, such as ablation and enucleation, should be considered during cytoreduction to maximize treatment of multifocal tumors while preserving healthy liver tissue. For patients with large hepatic tumor burdens, high-grade disease, or comorbidities precluding surgery, liver-directed and systemic therapies can be used to palliate symptoms and improve progression-free survival.

MLM patients are divided by their primary melanoma location; cutaneous, uvea (eye), and mucosal melanoma. If patients with isolated cutaneous MLMs are considered for surgical resection, treatment with systemic therapy should be part of the treatment course. For uveal MLMs, complete surgical or ablative treatment of all MLMs suggests superior results compared with other liver-directed or systemic therapies. Based on current evidence, no recommendations for any liver-directed regional therapy in the treatment of mucosal MLMs can be made.

The liver is the most common site of metastases from solid gastrointestinal tract tumors. Over the past few decades, the role of locoregional therapies, resection and thermal ablation, for neuroendocrine and colorectal liver metastases has been widely studied. However, for liver metastases originating from other gastrointestinal organs, the role of locoregional treatment remains unclear. This review summarizes and discusses the available evidence regarding benefits, risks, and indications for locoregional therapies for non-colorectal and non-neuroendocrine gastrointestinal liver metastases, highlighting the importance of multidisciplinary approach and patient selection.

Colorectal cancer (CRC) is one of the leading cancers globally in terms of both incidence and cancer-related mortality. Liver metastatic disease is the main prognostic driver for patients with CRC. The management options for liver metastatic CRC continue to evolve, particularly with the incorporation of locoregional therapies into the treatment paradigm. Hepatic arterial infusion (HAI) chemotherapy is one such liver directed approach used with the goal of converting patients to liver resection, reducing the risk of recurrence, treating recurrent disease, and most importantly improving overall survival. This article summarizes the role of HAI chemotherapy in the treatment of liver metastatic CRC.

Stereotactic ablative radiotherapy (SABR) commonly is used for small liver metastases. Modern conformal radiotherapy techniques, including 3-dimensional conformal radiotherapy and intensity-modulated radiation therapy, enable the safe delivery of SABR to small liver volumes. For larger tumors, the safe delivery of SABR can be challenging due to a more limited volume of healthy normal liver parenchyma and the proximity of the tumor to radiosensitive organs, such as the stomach, duodenum, and large intestine. Controlling respiratory motion, the use of image guidance, and increasing the number of radiation fractions sometimes are necessary for the safe delivery of SABR in these situations.

The management of patients with diffuse liver metastases remains a significant clinical challenge. In many cancer patients, metastatic disease may be isolated to the liver or the liver may be the dominant site of progressive metastatic cancer. In this setting, progression of disease in the liver generally is the most significant cause of morbidity and mortality.

Hepatic metastases are a major cause of morbidity and mortality for patients with cancer. Apart from curative resection, which offers patients the potential for long-term survival, an array of locoregional therapies, with limited evidence of improving survival, are used to treat them. The authors use examples from the realm of gastrointestinal cancer, largely focusing on the experience of patients with neuroendocrine cancer, hepatobiliary cancer, and colorectal cancer, to suggest that current systemic therapies offer, at minimum, similar survival outcomes for patients compared with these locoregional approaches.

The benefit of resection of liver metastases depends on primary diseases. Neuroendocrine tumors are associated with favorable prognosis after resection of liver metastases. Gastric cancer has worse tumor biology, and resection of gastric liver metastases should be performed in selected patients. A multidisciplinary approach is well established for colorectal liver metastases (CLMs). Resection remains the only curative treatment of CLM. Chemotherapy and molecular-targeted therapy have improved survival in unresectable metastatic colorectal cancer. Understanding of the following two strategies, conversion therapy and two-stage hepatectomy, are important to make this patient group to be candidates for curative-intent surgery.

SURGICAL ONCOLOGY
CLINICS OF NORTH AMERICA

SERIES OF RELATED INTEREST

Surgical Clinics of North America
http://www.surgical.theclinics.com
Thoracic Surgery Clinics
http://www.thoracic.theclinics.com
Advances in Surgery
http://www.advancessurgery.com

THE CLINICS ARE AVAILABLE ONLINE!
Access your subscription at:
www.theclinics.com

Foreword

Management of Metastatic Liver Tumors

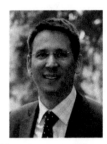

Timothy M. Pawlik, MD, MPH, PhD, FACS, FRACS (Hon.)
Consulting Editor

This issue of the *Surgical Oncology Clinics of North America* focuses on the Management of Metastatic Liver Tumors. Over the last several decades, as systemic and targeted agents have become more effective in treating and prolonging the life of patients with a wide range of malignancies, indications for treatment of metastatic disease have broadened. Perhaps this point is best illustrated among patients with colorectal liver metastasis. In particular, while 20 or 30 years ago colorectal liver metastasis size and number, as well as CEA level, "dictated" operability, surgeons now focus less on these morphologic and laboratory factors. Rather, operability of colorectal liver metastasis is currently predicated on being able to extirpate all disease sites in the liver while maintaining an adequate future liver remnant. While perhaps not as dramatic, there has been a corresponding paradigm shift in the approach to noncolorectal liver metastasis. Specifically, while resection of liver metastasis from noncolorectal, non-neuroendocrine primary tumors was traditionally not widely considered, now with appropriate use of preoperative chemotherapy, as well as rigorous patient selection by a multidisciplinary team, a subset of these patients is indeed candidates for surgical resection. In addition to resection, other local modalities to treat liver metastasis, including interarterial therapy and radiotherapy, have become increasingly utilized.

Management of liver metastasis therefore requires a well-informed multidisciplinary approach that often incorporates medical oncology, radiation oncology, and surgery. In turn, surgeons must be familiar with current knowledge regarding selection and treatment options for patients with liver metastasis. In light of this need, I am grateful to have Dr Michael D'Angelica be the guest editor of this important issue of *Surgical Oncology Clinics of North America*. Dr D'Angelica is Professor of Surgery at Memorial Sloan Kettering Cancer Center, where he holds the Enid A. Haupt Chair in Surgery. In addition to being the Vice Chair of Education and the Program Director for the Complex Surgical Oncology and Hepato-Pancreato-Biliary Fellowships at

Surg Oncol Clin N Am 30 (2021) xiii–xiv
https://doi.org/10.1016/j.soc.2020.09.006
1055-3207/21/© 2020 Published by Elsevier Inc.

Memorial Sloan Kettering, Dr D'Angelica is an international expert on the management of liver metastasis. Dr D'Angelica is currently the President-Elect of the Association of Hepato-Pancreato-Biliary Association, an international association of over 1000 hepato-pancreato-biliary surgeons. Dr D'Angelica has conducted substantial research toward the understanding of managing liver metastasis with over 100 articles in peer-reviewed journals. Given Dr D'Angelica's stature as an international leader in the management of liver metastasis, there is no one more suited to be the guest editor of this important issue of the *Surgical Oncology Clinics of North America*.

The issue covers a number of important topics, including the selection as well as medical and surgical management of patients with a wide range of liver metastases from different types of primary tumors. In particular, experts from around the globe define state-of-the-art management of liver metastasis from colorectal, neuroendocrine, breast, sarcoma, gynecologic, as well as other types, of primary tumors. Other clinical modalities, such as locoregional interarterial therapy, perfusion, as well as radiation therapy of liver metastasis, are also covered. Furthermore, the medical management and the key importance of patient selection are delineated. In addition, the perspective of medical oncology is emphasized, as the incorporation of these team members is so critical when addressing the systemic aspects of stage IV disease. I want to thank Dr D'Angelica for his assistance in identifying a fantastic group of authors who are leaders in the field of liver metastasis. This amazing team of authors has done an expert job in highlighting the important and relevant aspects of caring for patients with liver metastasis. The information contained in this issue of *Surgical Oncology Clinics of North America* will assist both faculty and trainees in understanding best practices related to the care of patients with liver metastasis. I would like to thank Dr D'Angelica and all the contributing authors for an excellent issue of the *Surgical Oncology Clinics of North America*.

Timothy M. Pawlik, MD, MPH, PhD, FACS, FRACS (Hon.)
Department of Surgery
Surgery, Oncology, Health Services Management and Policy
The Ohio State University
Wexner Medical Center
395 West 12th Avenue, Suite 670
Columbus, OH 43210, USA

E-mail address:
tim.pawlik@osumc.edu

Preface

Metastatic Liver Tumors: The Path to Disease-Free Survival

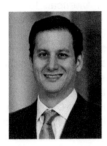

Michael D'Angelica, MD, FACS
Editor

It has been a great honor to edit this issue of *Surgical Oncology Clinics of North America* addressing the role of resection for liver metastases. It is a topic that has dominated my clinical and academic career for nearly 2 decades, and it is therefore near and dear to my heart. While the role of surgery for metastatic colorectal cancer has been well validated, the role of hepatic resection for other malignancies is less well studied. The lack of data is mostly due to the rarity of patients presenting with a pattern of disease that would even be considered for surgery and the diffuse systemic nature of most metastatic cancer. There are no prospective randomized trials that serve to justify the role of surgery for liver metastases, and thus, all the pieces of data we analyze on the topic are observational and inherently subject to the powerful effects of selection bias.

How then has surgery become so well accepted for oligometastatic colorectal cancer confined to the liver? A simple observation that does not require randomization is all it takes. With surgery, approximately 25% of well-imaged and well-selected patients are cured, and without surgery, that number is as close to zero as you can get. To steal a concept that others have used, would you perform a randomized trial of whether to deploy a parachute when jumping out of an airplane at high altitudes? While the selection of the appropriate candidates remains a critical issue, this simple observation solidified the role of hepatic resection for metastatic colorectal cancer. The larger question, which most of the other articles in this issue attempt to address, is how do we select patients for hepatic resection in other diseases where the data are lacking? A few concepts arise. The clinical scenario of "oligometastatic disease" is real and may be better treated with the judicious use of combined chemotherapy and surgery rather than chronic systemic therapy alone.

Indolent cancer that recurs at long time intervals with low-volume disease (isolated liver tumors being a common example) can be treated with surgery with clinically

Surg Oncol Clin N Am 30 (2021) xv–xvi
https://doi.org/10.1016/j.soc.2020.09.005
1055-3207/21/© 2020 Published by Elsevier Inc.

surgonc.theclinics.com

relevant periods of disease-free survival as well as prolonged overall survival. Furthermore, the use of surgery can result in long periods of time off toxic systemic therapies, which can improve the quality of life of these chronic cancer patients. This scenario of indolent oligometastatic disease, albeit uncommon, seems to exist among nearly all solid tumor malignancies, and I hope that these reviews serve to raise awareness of this concept. Indeed, in many of the articles, we asked the surgical authors to have a medical oncologist provide a short perspective. In all cases, this served to support the role of surgery combined with effective systemic therapies for limited metastatic disease. It is critical that decision making about the use of surgery for metastatic disease be multidisciplinary.

When we consider the outcomes of surgery for liver metastases, we must be critical of the data and always consider alternative hypotheses. In case series reporting outcomes after liver resection for metastases, a brief review of the publications typically reveals small numbers of patients representing a tiny proportion of all patients and overall survival outcomes that do not address recurrence. Selection bias and operating on young healthy patients who have withstood substantial tests of time can result in prolonged overall survival; however, prolonged (however defined) disease-free survival in which patients remain free of any detectable cancer is probably the best measure of a successful treatment. There is frequently a very small proportion of patients treated without surgery that survive long term, and with thoughtful selection, these patients end up in surgical series with a dramatically reduced denominator. Never underestimate the power of selection! Manipulation of the denominator is a very effective method of improving overall survival rates. Recurrence-free survival is probably a better measure of the impact of surgery and may be less susceptible to selection bias. There are also arguments that regional control of disease in the liver can prolong survival by protecting a susceptible organ despite active disease in other organs. This is a valid point that likely has some merit but is quite hard to prove.

While the excellent writing of the authors we have selected for this issue made my job as an editor easy, the one task I found myself executing throughout the editing process was changing definitive statements claiming benefit to sentences that more accurately describe associations. Retrospective associations must always be viewed with extreme caution and honestly interpreted. One pertinent question is whether improvements in systemic treatment will result in an increased role of surgery for metastatic disease or will surgery be rendered unnecessary? I think eventually surgery for cancer will go away, but I suspect that will be a long time from now. We ended this issue with this debate, and I suspect you know which way I would vote for the foreseeable future.

Michael D'Angelica, MD, FACS
Memorial Sloan Kettering Cancer Center
Hepatopancreatobiliary Service
Cornell University
Weill Medical College
New York, NY 10065, USA

E-mail address:
dangelim@MSKCC.ORG

Surgical Management of Colorectal Cancer Liver Metastases

Chandrasekhar Padmanabhan, MD[a], Daniel P. Nussbaum, MD[a],
Michael D'Angelica, MD[b],*

KEYWORDS

- Liver metastases • Colon cancer • Rectal cancer • Colorectal cancer

KEY POINTS

- Multiple randomized controlled trials have demonstrated that neoadjuvant or perioperative chemotherapy does not improve survival in patients with low-volume colorectal liver metastases and may, in fact, result in increased perioperative morbidity.
- Resection of colorectal liver metastases is associated with cure rates of approximately 20% and 5-year survival rates greater that 50%.
- For initially resectable colorectal liver metastases, treatment strategies are determined based on whether patients present with simultaneous or metachronous lesions and whether the primary tumor is of colon or rectal origin.
- For initially unresectable colorectal liver metastases, multimodal treatment plans may include strategies to improve the future liver remnant or to convert tumors to a resectable state with chemotherapy.
- Hepatic artery infusion pump chemotherapy is an attractive option in the management of colorectal liver metastases both for adjuvant treatment after liver resection and for conversion therapy in patients with initially unresectable disease.

INTRODUCTION

Colorectal cancer is the second most common cancer diagnosis in women and the third most common cancer diagnosis in men worldwide.[1] Approximately 1.8 million cases of colorectal cancer were newly diagnosed worldwide with 880,000 deaths in 2018.[2] The majority of colorectal cancer-related mortality is due to metastatic disease.[3] The liver is the most common site (80%–85%) of metastatic disease and up to 50% of patients with colorectal cancer present with liver metastases.[4] Although a majority of these liver metastases are unresectable, metastatectomy of resectable

a Department of Surgery, Memorial Sloan Kettering Cancer Center, 1275 York Avenue, C-1272, New York, NY 10065, USA; b Memorial Sloan Kettering Cancer Center, 1275 York Avenue, C-898, New York, NY 10065, USA
* Corresponding author.
E-mail address: DangeliM@mskcc.org

Surg Oncol Clin N Am 30 (2021) 1–25
https://doi.org/10.1016/j.soc.2020.09.002   surgonc.theclinics.com

colorectal liver metastases (CRLM) has been associated with improvements in 5-year overall survival from 25% to 30% in the 1980s to as high as 50% to 60% in recent years.[5–8] Moreover, approximately 20% of patients are cured of their disease altogether after hepatic resection.[9] This review highlights the pertinent aspects of the surgical management of CRLM. Much of this article focuses on the treatment of CRLM in the absence of extrahepatic disease, but there is a brief discussion of the role of hepatic resection for CRLM in the setting of extrahepatic disease at the end of this article.

LONG-TERM OUTCOMES

There are sporadic reports of successful liver resections before the 1950s, but most were for benign indications. One of the first reported successful liver resections in the United States for metastatic colorectal cancer was performed in 1940 by Dr Richard Cattell at the Lahey Clinic and the patient was reportedly alive and well 12 months postoperatively. Over the next 30 years, there was increased interest in liver resection for metastatic tumors and initial analyses focused on patient selection and who might benefit from what, at the time, was a morbid operation. Dr George T. Pack of Memorial Cancer Hospital in New York wrote that "perhaps the strongest indication for [hepatic] metastatectomy occurs when a very long latent period (1 to 5 or more years) intervenes between the treatment of the original cancer and the discovery of hepatic metastases."[10] Interestingly, this sentiment was not universal at the time. Dr Julian K. Quattlebaum, of Savannah, Georgia, wrote of his experiences with major liver resection and suggested that, "if resection of the involved liver was possible, the patient was probably better off with this focus of malignancy removed."[11] He went on to propose hepatic metastatectomy for all tumor types unless the patient was deemed "incurable" but did not elaborate on what actually defined cure. Determining which patients with metastases confined to the liver are incurable is something surgeons and oncologists still struggle with today.

Short-term morbidity and mortality after liver resection had a major impact on long-term survival in the early experience after liver resection. Posthepatectomy liver failure was reported as high as 30% in the early literature.[12,13] More recently, however, the incidence of posthepatectomy liver failure has decreased to as low as 1% to 2% in some studies.[13,14] Advances in liver imaging have had a great impact in reducing posthepatectomy liver failure by allowing for improved preoperative planning and patient selection. High resolution computed tomography (CT) scans, contrast-enhanced MRI, and multiphase imaging have allowed for preoperative prediction of future liver remnants.[15] This imaging allows for adjunct procedures such as portal vein and/or hepatic vein embolization to be performed before liver resection to allow for adequate volume of remining liver parenchyma after resection.[15] In essence, patients with inadequate liver growth are spared from a potentially lethal liver resection in the modern era, something that could not be predicted in the past.

Historically, in the absence of complete resection, the median survival for unresected CRLM ranged from 5 to 9 months with no 5-year survivors.[16] As resection for CRLM became more common, improvements in surgical technique and perioperative management were associated with improved perioperative outcomes. Scheele and colleagues[17] reported on 1209 patients with CRLM in 1990 and noted a median survival of 6.9 months for unresectable CRLM, 14.9 months for resectable CRLM that were not resected, and 30 months for CRLM resected with negative margins. 5-year survival was noted to be 38% in the resected patients.

Over the last 20 years, there have been improvements in systemic chemotherapy for CRLM, especially with the use of oxaliplatin and irinotecan. Targeted therapies against the endothelial growth factor and vascular endothelial growth factor pathways have also been introduced into treatment regimens with some success. Despite these advances, however, the median overall survival is at best 2 years with no long-term survivors in the absence of complete resection.[18]

With improvements in surgical technique and chemotherapeutics, there has been much interest in identifying factors associated with long-term survival and cure after hepatic resection. The Clinical Risk Score (CRS), initially published by Fong and colleagues,[19] identified 5 independently prognostic clinical factors (nodal status of the primary tumor, disease-free interval from the primary to the discovery of liver metastases <12 months, number of tumors >1, preoperative carcinoembryonic antigen [CEA] >200 ng/mL, and size of the largest tumor >5 cm) and attributed 1 point to each such that a patient could have a CRS ranging from 0 to 5. In the initial series of 1001 consecutive liver resections for CRLM, patients with a CRS of 0 to 2 were found to have 5-year survivals of 40% or greater, whereas patients with CRS of 3 to 5 were found to have 5-year survivals of 25% or less.[19] Although Fong and colleagues had success using the CRS as a prognostic tool, it is important to note that it has not been validated at other institutions and may have limited value across institutions.[20,21]

In the modern era, 5-year survival after complete resection of CRLM has been reported to be in the 50% to 60% range.[5] In a series of 1211 patients with resection of CRLM between 1992 and 2004, Creasy and colleagues[9] reported a median disease-specific survival of 4.9 years (95% confidence interval [CI], 4.4–5.3). The estimated 10-year disease-specific survival was 34% (95% CI, 31%–37%) with 193 patients censored at 10 years (**Fig. 1**). Twenty-four percent of patients in the cohort survived at least 10 years with a majority (77%) harboring no evidence of disease. The observed cure rate was 20.6% with cure defined as free of any disease at 10 years. This definition included patients with a resected recurrence after 10 years with at least 3 years of disease-free survival. Factors associated with the highest likelihood of cure included node negative primary tumors (30% probability of cure), perioperative hepatic arterial infusion pump chemotherapy (30% probability of cure), metachronous liver metastases (28% probability of cure), CRS of 2 or lower (27% probability of cure), and

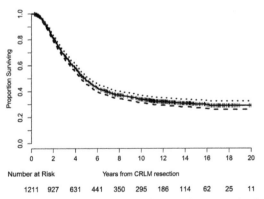

Fig. 1. Disease-specific survival after resection of CRLM (n = 1211). The median disease-specific survival was 4.9 years. The 10-year disease-specific survival estimated at 34%. There were 295 (24.4%) actual 10-year survivors with 220 (77%) harboring no evidence of disease. Two hundred fifty patients (20.6%) of patients were cured of their disease. (*From* Creasy JM, Sadot E, Koerkamp BG et al. Actual 10-year survival after hepatic resection of colorectal liver metastases: what factors preclude cure? Surgery 2018;163:1238-1244; with permission.)

margin negative resection (27% probability of cure). Factors associated with the lowest probability of cure were extrahepatic disease (8% probability of cure), margin positive resection (8% probability of cure), CEA of greater than 200 ng/mL (9% probability of cure), and the presence of more than 10 tumors (3% probability of cure).

Recent efforts have attempted to determine the impact of somatic mutations on outcomes after liver resection of CRLM. Margonis and colleagues[22] reported their finding that *KRAS* mutations were an independent predictor of worse overall survival (hazard ratio, 1.65; 95% CI, 1.07–2.54; $P = .02$). In a follow-up study, it was noted that mutations of codon 12 were independent predictors of worse overall survival.[23] A recent report proposed modifying the Fong CRS by replacing disease-free interval, number of tumors, and CEA level with *RAS* mutation status.[21] They found that their modified CRS outperformed the Fong CRS in both an investigational cohort as well as a multi-center validation cohort.

More recent data suggest that, although *KRAS* mutations are associated with poorer survival, this result may be due to the presence of concomitant *TP53* mutations.[24,25] Chun and colleagues[24] reported on 401 patients with CRLM who underwent resection and found that, although *KRAS* mutations were associated with poorer overall survival in the cohort, this negative prognostic effect persisted only in patients with coaltered *TP53* mutations when stratified by both mutations. Similarly, Datta and colleagues[25] reported on 609 patients with CRLM who underwent resection and found that *KRAS* mutations were associated with poorer survival only in patients with coaltered *TP53* mutations when stratified by both mutations.

In addition to *RAS* mutations, *BRAF* mutations in CRLM, although rare among resectable patients, have also been shown to be prognostic of outcome after hepatic resection. Gagnière and colleagues[26] recently reported a multi-institutional series of 1497 patients who underwent hepatectomy for CRLM, of whom 2% of patients were found to have *BRAF* mutations. Median overall survival in the *BRAF* wild-type patients was 81 months versus 40 months for *BRAF* mutated patients ($P<.001$). The median disease-free survival was 22 months in the wild-type patients versus 10 months in the mutated patients ($P<.001$). In addition, *BRAF*-mutated patients were found to present more frequently with multiple, synchronous tumors with a bilobar distribution.

In summary, improvements in survival over the last 40 years have largely been driven by advances in surgical technique, better imaging, improved patient selection, improvements in intraoperative and perioperative management, and the introduction of newer systemic chemotherapeutic agents. Clinical risk scores have allowed for the identification of prognostic factors that most impact survival and outcome, but have not gained universal applicability given the lack of clinical usefulness. The identification of prognostic gene mutations and gene signatures has gained interest in recent years but has not had any major clinical impact as of yet, given that these mutations and signatures have not been validated in a prospective fashion.

GENERAL PRINCIPLES OF LIVER RESECTION FOR RESECTABLE COLORECTAL LIVER METASTASES

Given that complete resection offers the greatest opportunity for long-term survival, assessment at the time liver metastases are diagnosed must initially focus on whether a margin negative resection is possible and, if so, whether there are additional factors (eg, extrahepatic metastases) that would render resection ineffective at prolonging survival. In general, the principles of resectability involve medical, biologic, and technical assessments. For patients with CRLM, medical fitness typically depends on performance status and any cardiopulmonary comorbidities that would preclude safe recovery. Underlying liver dysfunction that puts the patient at risk for postoperative liver failure, although common in primary liver cancers, is rare in this patient population. If present, it is typically secondary to prolonged preoperative chemotherapy. Biologic criteria, based on tumor and other disease characteristics, assess whether a margin-negative resection would effectively offer the chance for cure or prolong survival. As mentioned elsewhere in this article, multiple clinical risk scores have been developed to predict recurrence and longer term outcomes after resection of colorectal cancer liver metastases.[19,21,27–29] Larger tumors, a greater number of metastatic lesions, shorter disease-free interval, and lymph node-positive primary tumors all portend inferior outcomes that in some cases may be noninferior to systemic chemotherapy alone. That said, all clinical risk scores are imperfect, and there are no absolute biologic contraindications to resection if a patient can be rendered disease free, because even a small percentage of high-risk individuals may experience cure.[30] Finally, technical resectability is defined as the ability to achieve a margin-negative resection with an adequate volume of the future liver remnant, while preserving vascular inflow, outflow, and biliary drainage. The volume of liver that can safely be resected—typically less than 70% to 80% standardized volume of an otherwise healthy liver[31]—is heavily influenced by underlying liver dysfunction and duration of prior chemotherapy. Technical resectability can thus only be assessed with high-quality, liver-specific imaging.

Preoperative imaging should assess the number of liver metastases, delineate their anatomic relationship to neighboring vascular/biliary structures, and quantify the volumetric ratio of the future liver remnant to the preoperative total liver volume (subtracting tumor volume) or total body weight.[32] Thus, it should also assess for signs of any underlying liver dysfunction, including cirrhosis, steatosis, and parenchymal atrophy. A CT scan is frequently the first study obtained, because it can also be used to evaluate for extrahepatic abdominal/thoracic metastases, and reconstructions can be generated to perform volumetric assessment. In modern series, a CT scan has a diagnostic sensitivity of 75% and specificity greater than 95% for CRLM,[33] and is best performed using thin slices including noncontrast, arterial, venous, and delayed contrast phases. Although traditionally MRI has been considered superior to a CT scan in detecting subcentimeter lesions, with modern CT techniques it is most useful in patients with significant steatosis, which makes lesion detection challenging with a CT scan.[34] In the absence of significant steatosis, a high-quality CT scan is typically adequate for determining technical resectability. Recently, the use of hepatocyte-specific MRI contrast agents such as gadoxetate disodium (Eovist) has been evaluated in several meta-analyses.[35–37] Although small improvements in sensitivity have been reported, whether these modalities change patient management remains controversial. Finally, PET with a CT scan was initially reported as a useful adjunct to cross-sectional imaging[38] because of its potential to detect otherwise occult metastatic lesions. A randomized trial evaluating the routine use of preoperative PET CT scan demonstrated that its use altered management in 8% of patients, including both aborted procedures and more extensive resections; however, false-positive results were also common (8%), and no difference in survival or resectability was observed between groups. PET CT scan is most useful if there is a high suspicion for extrahepatic metastasis, or for indeterminate lesions identified on other cross-sectional imaging.

Once resectability has been established, operative considerations unique to CRLM include the need for diagnostic laparoscopy, the use of intraoperative ultrasound for restaging and transection planning, and the extent of intended margins. Before modern cross-sectional imaging, diagnostic laparoscopy proved useful at detecting locally unresectable and occult extrahepatic metastases, thus preventing unnecessary laparotomy.[39] Improved sensitivity of both CT scan and MRI have minimized the yield of diagnostic laparoscopy, and it is now typically reserved for those patients with imaging suggestive of, but not diagnostic of, unresectable disease.[40] Similarly, intraoperative liver ultrasound examination now has a more limited role for identifying subcentimeter lesions but remains invaluable for intraoperative anatomic guidance.

Historically, a margin of at least 1 cm was encouraged for colorectal cancer liver metastases. Subsequent studies suggested that that any negative margins provided improved and equivalent survival relative to R1 resection, and that observed differences in margin width of less than 1 cm, likely reflected confounding from nonanatomic factors such as the extent of disease.[41–43] More recently, using a large series with the ability to appropriately adjust for established confounders, it was shown that, although even submillimeter-negative margins were superior to microscopically positive margins, increasing margin widths resulted in modest but statistically significant improvements in survival.[41] This same study, however, demonstrated the challenge of predicting final margin status when a subcentimeter margin is anticipated. Therefore, trying to obtain a wider margin may result in the unnecessary resection of excess healthy liver and an increased risk of postoperative morbidity and liver insufficiency.

Over the past decade, a parenchymal sparing approach has proven equivalent to anatomic resection in terms of final margin status, recurrence, and overall survival, while decreasing the risk of postoperative liver failure.[44–46] Data suggest that the optimal strategy is to minimize parenchymal resection while ensuring a microscopically negative margin. In some cases, this process may mean combining anatomic or large nonanatomic resections with additional smaller wedge resections. Ablative techniques can also be selectively used for smaller metastases when their anatomic location would require additional resection that would threaten the adequacy of the future liver remnant.[47]

The morbidity and mortality associated with liver resection has been extensively described across disease types, and includes bile leak, hemorrhage, cardiopulmonary events, venous thromboembolism, and liver failure. In noncirrhotic patients, who make up the vast majority of patients undergoing resection of CRLM, morbidity is proportional to the extent of liver resection, with extended and major hepatectomies carrying a higher risk than more limited resections; other factors associated with complications include older age, male sex, preexisting cardiopulmonary comorbidities, obesity, and the presence of ascites.[48] Postoperative liver failure and mortality are strongly associated with the extent of resection and this finding further supports the use of parenchymal-sparing approaches.[49,50] For patients who require preoperative chemotherapy, resultant sinusoidal obstruction and steatosis can increase perioperative morbidity and mortality.[51] In general, similar outcomes for simultaneous versus staged resections have been reported and these nuances are discussed in detail elsewhere in this article (see Strategies for Initially Resectable Colorectal Liver Metastases).

STRATEGIES FOR INITIALLY UNRESECTABLE RESECTABLE COLORECTAL LIVER METASTASES

Among all patients that ultimately develop CRLM, fewer than 20% will be candidates for resection at the time of initial diagnosis.[52,53] As discussed elsewhere in this article, patients may be deemed initially unresectable owing to technical limitations imposed by the tumor(s) or biologic features that would render an otherwise optimal resection unlikely to improve long-term outcomes. To some extent, these definitions overlap. In all cases of unresectable disease, the first consideration must be whether adjunctive treatment options could potentially render the patient suitable for resection, either by improving the future liver remnant, or by shrinking 1 or more tumors such that a more limited hepatectomy can be performed or a margin-negative resection becomes technically feasible.

Options to improve the future liver remnant include venous embolization as well as associating liver partition and portal vein ligation for staged hepatectomy (ALPPS). Less common options include hepatic venous and arterial embolization procedures. Collectively, these strategies are typically used either when an anatomic major hepatectomy would result in an inadequate liver remnant (typically <30% of the standardized volume of an otherwise healthy liver,[31] almost always in the setting of a right or extended right hepatectomy).

Portal vein embolization shunts inflow away from the embolized branch(es) feeding the diseased liver, resulting in atrophy of that territory and compensatory hypertrophy of the future remnant. Although there are multiple methods for volumetric assessment based off of three-dimensional CT reconstruction, the future liver remnant should be defined as the volume of functional liver that will remain after resection (ie, adequate perfusion and venous/biliary drainage). This assessment is then compared with the preoperative total liver volume (subtracting tumor volume and atrophic, nonfunctional parenchyma secondary to vascular/biliary compromise) or total body weight.[32] Beyond achieving an adequate future liver remnant, both rate and degree of hypertrophy are important predictors of posthepatectomy liver failure.[54–56] In fact, the kinetic growth rate, using a cutoff of 2% per week after portal vein embolization, may be a more accurate predictor of postoperative hepatic insufficiency and liver-related mortality than conventional volumetric parameters, especially in the case of small remnant livers.[57] Importantly, patients who have been treated with prolonged chemotherapy require a larger future liver remnant owing to chemotherapy-induced liver injury (typically >30%), as do patients with intrinsic liver dysfunction (typically >40%).[31,58] In retrospective series, patients who undergo portal vein embolization followed by resection have a marked improvement in survival relative to patients whose remnants preclude hepatectomy.[59] Portal vein embolization can safely be combined with preoperative chemotherapy to optimize outcomes.[60] In select cases where an adequate liver remnant is not achieved initially, repeat selective portal vein embolization (eg, segment IV branches if right trisegmentectomy is planned) or combination with hepatic vein embolization can be used to further augment the anticipated remnant liver.

ALPPS involves operative ligation of the right portal vein and division of the right and left hemilivers to disrupt collateral vascular supply between lobes, followed by a second surgery (typically 1 week later) for resection after a brief period of rapid liver hypertrophy.[61] Relative to portal vein embolization, hypertrophy of the future liver remnant occurs at a faster rate[62]; however, morbidity and mortality have been reported as high as 40% and 22%, respectively, after resection.[63]

The initial retrospective series comparing portal vein embolization with ALPPS suggested that portal vein embolization provided equivalent oncologic outcomes with a decreased risk of perioperative morbidity.[63] A recent randomized trial directly compared ALPPS with a 2-stage hepatectomy with portal vein embolization or ligation in patients with CLRM.[64] All patients had also received systemic chemotherapy. After a 4-week interval, nearly twice as many patients in the ALPPS group had reached a future liver remnant of greater than 30% (92 vs 47%; $P<.0001$), and both resection rates (92 vs 57%; $P<.0001$) and time to resection (11 vs 43 days; $P<.0001$) were superior in patients randomized to the ALPPS arm. No differences were observed in perioperative morbidity or mortality rates; however, both were markedly higher than observed in most modern series. Moreover, at a median follow-up time of 38 months, the overall median survival was 46 months among patients randomized to ALPPS, and 26 months among patients randomized to portal vein embolization ($P = .026$).[65] At present, it seems that ALPPS results in a greater degree and rate of hypertrophy relative to portal vein embolization, and this factor may increase resection rates based on current radiographic criteria. Whether this finding translates to improvements in longer term oncologic outcomes that continue to compensate for higher rates of perioperative morbidity remains to be seen, and thus ALPPS is an option that can be considered selectively at high-volume centers.

In addition to securing an adequate future liver remnant, it is also necessary at times to shrink the size of tumors so as to allow complete resection. Conversion therapy refers to chemotherapy administered to patients with initially unresectable disease, with the intent of downsizing tumors to facilitate a margin-negative resection. It can be used alone or in combination with strategies aimed to improve the future liver remnant. The effectiveness of multiple systemic regimens—typically 5-fluoracil (5-FU)/leucovorin combined with either oxaliplatin or irinotecan—have been reported.[66–70] To date, the largest study describes 1104 consecutive patients with initially unresectable CRLM treated at a single institution, predominantly with either FOLFOX (70%), FOLFIRI (7%), or FOLFOXIRI (4%).[66] Ultimately, 11.6% of patients were able to undergo complete resection, among whom 5-year disease-free and overall survival were 22% and 33%, respectively. Patients at the highest risk for long-term mortality included patients with rectal cancer, 3 or more metastases, any tumor greater than 10 cm, and a CA 19-9 of greater than 100 UI/L. Patients without any of these features had a 5-year overall survival of 59%, although there were no long-term survivors among patients with all 4 of these disease characteristics. Longer term follow-up suggests that a cure can be achieved in 16% of patients who ultimately undergo resection.[71]

Other studies have reported rates of complete resection (including extrahepatic disease) of 3% to 19%, with resected patients demonstrating a median overall survival of 16.7 to 42.2 months.[67–70] Two randomized trials have specifically evaluated FOLFOXIRI versus FOLFIRI as conversion therapy.[69,72] In both trials, although FOLFOXIRI was associated with increased toxicity, it also resulted in higher rates of complete resection. An improvement in overall survival associated with FOLFOXIRI, however, was only observed in 1 trial (22.6 months vs 16.7 months; $P = .032$).[69] In general, this regimen is reserved for young, healthy patients who are likely to tolerate the associated toxicity. The addition of biologic agents to these regimens in appropriately selected patients may also improve conversion rates and outcomes for patients with initially unresectable CLRM.[73–77] Given the known challenges in predicting final margin status before surgery,[41] the subjective and nonstandardized nature of this end point is a limitation to all studies evaluating conversion rates. Moreover, retrospective series evaluating conversion chemotherapy may be biased toward excluding patients thought to be at very low likelihood of successful conversion. Thus, among all initially unresectable patients, the likelihood of successful conversion to a disease-free state is likely reflected within the lower end of these reported estimates.

Although chemotherapy may allow initially unresectable patients to ultimately undergo surgery, oxaliplatin- and irinotecan-containing regimens are associated with significant liver toxicity—related to both the regimen and duration of therapy—which may increase the risk of postoperative liver failure and other perioperative morbidity.[51,78–80] Sinusoidal obstruction and steatohepatitis associated with oxaliplatin and irinotecan, respectively, can cause an in increase in postoperative morbidity and mortality.[51,78,81–84] The risk of chemotherapy-induced morbidity and mortality is related not only to agent, but also to duration of therapy.[80,85] This is given that the most pronounced volumetric response to chemotherapy occurs during the first 2 months of systemic treatment, and after 4 months of treatment, no further decrease in tumor response should be expected.[86] Thus, the National Comprehensive Cancer Network recommends frequent restaging during chemotherapy, with cross-sectional imaging performed bimonthly while on treatment. Chemotherapy should be terminated and resection should be attempted as soon as technical resectability becomes possible to decrease the effects of chemotherapy-induced liver injury on outcomes.

Finally, hepatic artery infusion chemotherapy (HAIC) has emerged as an attractive adjunct to systemic chemotherapy to improve conversion rates. Although there is no randomized trial specific to this patient population evaluating modern combination systemic therapy alone versus in combination with HAIC, single-arm prospective trials demonstrate impressive conversion rates and overall survival. In an early phase I trial of 49 patients with unresectable colorectal cancer metastases treated with floxuridine HAIC in addition to systemic chemotherapy, 92% of patients had at least a partial response, and 47% were able to undergo resection, despite substantial disease burden.[87] Among 23 patients who had not previously received chemotherapy, the median overall survival from the start of pump therapy was 51 months. More recently, in a phase II trial of 64 patients with unresectable colorectal cancer liver metastases, 52% of patients treated with floxuridine via HAIC were converted to resection. Nearly all patients (95%) had bilobar metastases with a median of 13 tumors and 67% had received prior systemic chemotherapy. Among all patients, the median overall survival from the time of diagnosis was 46 months and among treatment naïve patients, the median overall survival was 76.6 months.[88] A significant difference in survival was observed for patients who were able to undergo margin negative resection compared with those were never resected (5-year overall survival of 63.3% vs 12.5%; $P<.001$), and among the 9 patients who remained without evidence of disease for a median 96 months, 8 had undergone resection. Encouraging results have also been observed when other chemotherapeutic agents are used as HAIC, such as oxaliplatin and 5-FU with or without the addition of irinotecan.[89–101] Despite the lack of randomized evidence, studies to date suggest that the addition of HAIC to systemic chemotherapy provides treatment responses and conversion rates that are superior to chemotherapy alone.

STRATEGIES FOR INITIALLY RESECTABLE COLORECTAL LIVER METASTASES

As described elsewhere in this article, the definition of resectable CRLM has typically revolved around achieving a margin negative resection while leaving an adequate volume of functioning liver in situ. In addition to these technical considerations, the presence of extrahepatic disease, high CEA (>200 ng/mL), and greater than 10 tumors in the liver negatively affect the possibility of achieving long-term survival and/or cure and therefore must also be taken into consideration when planning liver resection for CRLM.[9] Once a patient is determined to have resectable disease, both from a technical and oncologic standpoint, a surgeon must then decide whether to proceed with resection or treat with neoadjuvant chemotherapy. Some centers will administer neoadjuvant chemotherapy for nearly all patients with resectable CRLM to select patients who will most benefit from resection.[102] It is important to note here, however, that there is no Level 1 evidence that demonstrates improved survival with upfront chemotherapy in patients with initially resectable CRLM. Indeed, the European Organization for Research and Treatment of Cancer 40983 trial compared perioperative FOLFOX (6 cycles preoperatively and 6 cycles postoperatively) with surgery alone for patients with resectable CRLM and found no improvement in overall survival (5-year overall survival, 51% vs 48%; P = .34) or progression-free survival (3-year progression-free survival, 38% vs 30%; P = .068).[103] In addition, of the 151 patients randomized to the perioperative chemotherapy arm who underwent resection, only 11 patients (7%) of the patients progressed while receiving chemotherapy and only 8 patients (4%) were found to have unresectable disease at the time of surgery.[104] This result suggests that neoadjuvant chemotherapy is, in fact, not an effective tool to select patients who would benefit from resection.

In addition to the lack of survival benefit, there is some evidence that preoperative chemotherapy increases operative morbidity. As mentioned elsewhere in this article, preoperative oxaliplatin has been shown to cause hepatic sinusoidal obstruction in patients with CRLM.[81–83] There are also data to suggest that preoperative irinotecan increases the degree of steatohepatitis in patients undergoing liver resection for CRLM.[78,84] Both hepatic sinusoidal obstruction and steatohepatitis have been shown to be associated with increased perioperative morbidity.[51] In a series of 406 patients who underwent hepatic resection for CRLM, Vauthey and colleagues[78] also reported an increase in perioperative mortality in the setting of preoperative steatohepatitis (14.7% vs 1.6%; P = .001; odds ratio, 10.5; 95% CI, 2.0–36.4). Given the absence of a survival benefit, increased perioperative morbidity and possibly mortality, and minimal impact on patient selection associated with neoadjuvant chemotherapy, it is the authors' preference to proceed straight to resection in patients with initially resectable disease.

Although the majority of patients with initially resectable CRLM should proceed to resection as just discussed, there are select scenarios in which neoadjuvant chemotherapy can be considered. First, patients with simultaneous liver metastases from rectal primary tumors will often require neoadjuvant chemoradiation to the pelvis to decrease local recurrence rates after resection. Concomitant systemic chemotherapy in this setting is reasonable if a combined liver and rectal resection is planned in the future to minimize the risk of hepatic progression while treating the pelvis. Second, neoadjuvant chemotherapy is reasonable in patients with larger tumors that could be spared a larger liver resection if their tumors were to recede away from a major vascular pedicle or draining vein. As discussed elsewhere in this article, it is imperative that the duration of neoadjuvant chemotherapy be as brief as possible, given that there is little volumetric response beyond 2 months (4 cycles) and the increased perioperative morbidity and mortality associated with neoadjuvant chemotherapy.[51,78,86]

Resectable CRLM are often classified as either synchronous or metachronous based on the timing of their diagnosis in relation to the diagnosis of the primary tumor. The authors prefer using the term simultaneous, instead of synchronous, for CRLM that are diagnosed before or at the time of diagnosis of the primary tumor and metachronous for CRLM are those that are diagnosed after a certain amount of time has elapsed since the diagnosis of the primary tumor. In the authors' opinion, the management of metachronous CRLM is relatively straightforward; if the patient is medically fit and would tolerate a liver resection, has no evidence of unresectable extrahepatic disease, has an adequate future liver remnant, and is willing, resection should be offered. Simultaneous CRLM, on the other hand, pose several unique challenges.

Simultaneous CRLM have historically been considered a sign of poor prognosis. Indeed, in a recent study analyzing the LiverMetSurvey international registry of patients undergoing liver resection for CRLM, Adam and colleagues[105] demonstrated a significant difference in survival after liver resection when CRLM were detected before versus after the diagnosis of the primary tumor. As such, there has been much debate surrounding the sequence and timing of resection in patients who present with simultaneous CRLM. Historically, patients with simultaneous CRLM would have their primary tumor removed first and then treated with chemotherapy. If the liver metastases did not progress on treatment, then patients would then be considered for liver resection.[17] Unfortunately, only 30% of patients would actually undergo hepatectomy.[106] A liver-first approach has been proposed, especially for patients who require a major hepatectomy with asymptomatic primary tumors and patients with primary rectal tumors to allow for adequate time to treat with chemotherapy and/or radiation. Simultaneous resections gained favor in lieu of staged resections, however, after it was shown to have no difference in perioperative mortality and perhaps a decrease in perioperative morbidity by avoiding a second laparotomy.[107–109] This result was confirmed in a meta-analysis of 24 nonrandomized studies that demonstrated no difference in postoperative complications, overall survival, or disease-free survival in patients undergoing simultaneous resections.[110] In light of this evidence and the experience at our institution, the authors prefer simultaneous resection for most synchronous CRLM. Certain situations do, however, call for a staged approach, including bowel obstruction and intractable bleeding from the primary tumor. In these scenarios, dealing with the primary tumor first and delaying hepatectomy is appropriate.

As alluded to elsewhere in this article, simultaneous liver metastases from rectal primary tumors provide a unique challenge. Historically, concurrent major hepatectomy and rectal resection was controversial owing to the increased morbidity and mortality reported in early experiences.[111] More recently, similar outcomes were seen with simultaneous liver and rectal resection as compared with staged resections; therefore, combined resections increased in popularity.[112] In the modern era, there has been an increased interest in nonoperative management, or "watch and wait," for rectal cancer.[113–115] In these unique scenarios, the timing of chemotherapy is often decided in a multidisciplinary fashion. Patients with resectable liver metastases will typically undergo hepatectomy first followed by chemotherapy and/or chemoradiation to treat the rectal tumor.

Bilobar CRLM also provide a unique challenge and can be managed in many different ways. At the authors' institution, patients are typically treated with systemic chemotherapy first. If there is no progression of disease after 4 to 6 months, and the left hemiliver can be cleared of metastatic disease, a combination of ablation and wedge resections is used with the goal of parenchymal preservation because the left liver is typically the future liver remnant. The disease in the right liver is left in situ. The patient is then treated with postoperative chemotherapy and at our institution, we typically offer hepatic arterial infusion pump chemotherapy (for reasons described elsewhere in this article) in addition to systemic chemotherapy. If the predicted future liver remnant remains inadequate after surgery, portal vein embolization can be performed during the latter cycles of adjuvant chemotherapy to allow for left hemiliver hypertrophy. If there is no progression of disease and there is an adequate future liver remnant, a the right hemiliver will be cleared of disease or resected at a later date.

If the left liver is unable to be cleared at the initial operation, the authors will consider placement of a hepatic arterial infusion pump alone and treat the patient with hepatic arterial infusion with fluorodeoxyuridine and systemic chemotherapy for up to 6 months. If there is adequate response, we then proceed with staged or synchronous liver resections to clear the liver as described elsewhere in this article.

The timing of chemotherapy is also a point of debate in the management of simultaneous, resectable CRLM. As discussed elsewhere in this article, some centers prefer a neoadjuvant approach in nearly all patients.[102] A recent international consensus also promoted the use of neoadjuvant chemotherapy, but acknowledged the lack of compelling evidence for this recommendation.[105] One retrospective, multi-institutional, study demonstrated a statistically significant association between at least 6 months of postoperative chemotherapy and improved recurrence-free survival and overall survival.[116] Given the lack of Level 1 evidence, the authors opt to proceed with simultaneous resection of synchronous CRLM if initially resectable. The authors do note the ongoing CHARISMA trial[117] that has randomized high-risk patients (CRS of >3) with initially resectable CRLM to surgery alone versus neoadjuvant XELOX chemotherapy followed by surgery with overall survival as a primary end point, and we eagerly await these results.

ADJUVANT CHEMOTHERAPY

The benefits of adjuvant chemotherapy after resection of node positive colorectal cancer are well known and have been studied extensively.[118–121] The use of adjuvant chemotherapy after resection of CRLM has been extrapolated from these studies. It seems logical that the benefits of adjuvant chemotherapy would carry over, but this has not been demonstrable in randomized trials (**Table 1**). In 2006, Portier and colleagues[122] reported on a series of 173 patients who were randomized to resection of CRLM alone versus resection and adjuvant 5-FU/leucovorin between 1991 and 2001. Adjuvant chemotherapy had no significant effect on overall survival in this study (5-year overall survival of 51% vs 42%; $P = .13$) but had a modest effect on disease-free survival (5-year disease-free survival, 34% vs 27%; $P = .028$). The median disease-free survival was increased by a meager 6 months. This study was plagued with slow accrual and criticized for its use of an inferior chemotherapeutic regimen (which was standard therapy at the start of the study). In 2008, Mitry and colleagues[123] pooled patients from Portier and colleagues and another similar clinical trial that also struggled with accrual problems. Three hundred two patients were randomized to resection alone versus resection and adjuvant 5-FU/leucovorin. Despite pooling and increasing sample size, adjuvant 5-FU/leucovorin had no significant effect on overall survival (5-year overall survival, 53% vs 40%; $P = .095$) and had no significant effect on progression-free survival (5-year progression-free survival, 37% vs 28%; $P = .058$). With the advent of more modern chemotherapeutics, Ychou and colleagues[124] randomized 306 patients with CRLM to either 5-FU/leucovorin or FOLFIRI after liver resection. FOLFIRI had no significant impact on 3-year overall survival (73% vs 72%; $P = .69$) and no significant impact on 2-year disease-free survival (51% vs 46%; $P = .44$). There were more grade 3 and 4 toxicities reported in the FOLFIRI group (47%) versus the 5-FU/leucovorin group (30%). In the last decade, targeted therapies have been investigated in the adjuvant setting after resection of CRLM. The EPOC randomized controlled trial randomized patients with *KRAS* wild-type, resectable, CRLM to receive perioperative chemotherapy with or without cetuximab (**Table 2**). Adjuvant cetuximab was associated with worse progression-free survival (14 months vs 20 months; hazard ratio, 1.48; 95% CI, 1.04–2.12; $P = .03$) at the interim analysis and the trial was therefore terminated.[125] On final analysis, the reduced progression-free survival translated into worse overall-survival (55 months vs 81 months; hazard ratio, 1.45; 95% CI, 1.02–2.05; $P = .036$).[126] Despite these negative trials, adjuvant chemotherapy after resection of CRLM is commonly used in the United States. Further studies should focus on identifying which patients would benefit from adjuvant chemotherapy after resection.

Table 1
Randomized prospective clinical trials of hepatic resection of CRLM with or without chemotherapy

Author	Arm	n	5-Year Overall Survival (%)	P (Overall Survival)	5-Year Disease-Free Survival (%)	P (Disease-Free Survival)
Portier et al,[122] 2006	Surgery	85	42	.13	27	.028
	surgery → 5FU + leucovorin	86	51		34	
Mitry et al,[123] 2008	Surgery	140	40	.095	28	.058
	surgery → 5FU + Leucovorin	138	53		37	
Ychou et al,[124] 2009	Surgery → 5FU + leucovorin	153	72*	.69	46#	.44
	surgery FOLFIRI	153	73*		51#	
Nordlinger et al	Surgery	182	48	.34	30**	.068
	FOLFOX → surgery → FOLFOX	182	51		38**	

* 3-year OS; # 2-year DFS; ** 3-year PFS.
None of the trials demonstrated an overall survival benefit. Only Portier et al. demonstrated a statistically significant benefit in progression-free survival that amounted to a 6-month increase in median survival.

Table 2
Randomized trial of perioperative chemotherapy versus perioperative chemotherapy and Cetuximab

Author	Arm	n	Median Overall Survival (mo)	P	Median Progression-Free Survival (mo)	P
Bridgewater et al,[126] 2020	Chemo → surgery → chemo chemo/Cetux → surgery → chemo/Cetux	128 129	81 55.4	.036	22.2 15.5	.304

Bridgewater et al.[126] demonstrated a reduced overall survival when Cetuximab was added to chemotherapy with a reduction of median overall survival by 25 months.

Adjuvant hepatic arterial infusion pump chemotherapy is another option for patients undergoing hepatic resection of CRLM. Although this topic is extensively discussed later in this issue, adjuvant hepatic arterial infusion pump chemotherapy in addition to systemic chemotherapy has been shown to impact hepatic progression-free survival,[127–129] systemic progression-free survival,[127–130] and overall survival.[127,128] The greatest effect can be seen in hepatic progression-free survival, which may lead to the overall survival benefit. It is the authors' preference to offer adjuvant hepatic arterial infusion pump chemotherapy after curative liver resection given the familiarity with the procedure, its complications, and the administration of the chemotherapy itself.

HEPATECTOMY IN THE SETTING OF EXTRAHEPATIC METASTASES

Extrahepatic metastases were traditionally considered a contraindication to hepatectomy[131]; however, over the past 2 decades, eligibility for liver resection has expanded to patients with low-volume pulmonary metastases and even peritoneal disease suitable for debulking. Low-volume pulmonary metastases, particularly subcentimeter nodules, do not seem to substantially affect outcomes after hepatectomy,[132–134] and liver resection can be performed with or without concomitant pulmonary resection. Optimal outcomes have been reported when the patient can be rendered disease free via concomitant resection of pulmonary metastases,[134] and thus this strategy is preferred in appropriately selected patients.

For patients with peritoneal carcinomatosis, hepatectomy can be performed as a part of optimal debulking strategies intended to render the patient disease-free. In large series of patients treated with debulking with or without heated intraperitoneal peritoneal chemotherapy, overall survival after surgery has been reported at approximately 30 to 40 months,[135] and the need for concomitant liver resection does not seem to negatively impact survival outcomes. Ongoing studies are investigating debulking and heated intraperitoneal peritoneal chemotherapy compared with debulking alone to better understand the contribution of intraperitoneal chemotherapy. In general, these procedures should be performed only at highly experienced centers within a clinical trial setting.

The impact of hepatectomy combined with metastatectomy in other locations, such as the adrenal glands, ovaries, or retroperitoneal lymph nodes, has been not been well-defined.[135,136] Involvement of the portal, celiac, and paraaortic lymph nodes portends a dismal prognosis, and has in some cases been considered a relative contraindication to hepatectomy.[136,137]

POSTHEPATECTOMY SURVEILLANCE AND SALVAGE TREATMENTS

The goal of surveillance after resection of CRLM is to identify recurrences that are potentially amenable to curative salvage therapy or allow for the earlier initiation of palliative treatments aimed at prolonging life. The vast majority (75%) of recurrences occur within 2 years of initial hepatectomy and close to 90% occur within 3 years.[138] For a subset of patients (approximately 25%), salvage surgery is associated with long-term survival and cure.[139] Thus, the National Comprehensive Cancer Network recommends contrast-enhanced CT of the chest, abdomen, and pelvis with CEA measurement every 3 to 6 months for the first 2 years, and then every 6 to 12 months for up to 5 years. False-positive elevations in CEA are not uncommon, representing approximately 50% of elevated values.[140] False-positive results tend to be modestly elevated (<35 ng/mL), and approximately one-third return to normal levels on follow-up testing. Using a threshold of 10 ng/mL, the sensitivity and specificity of CEA for diagnosing recurrence are 68% and 97%, respectively. The usefulness of PET CT in surveillance has not been well-validated.

Among patients who develop recurrences, the median disease-free interval in 1 large series has been reported at 13 months, and 27% of patients were able to undergo at least 1 attempt at salvage resection after recurrence.[139] Not surprisingly, patients who underwent salvage surgery had markedly improved survival compared with patients treated with palliative therapy alone (median disease-specific survival of 87 months vs 34 months from the time of initial liver resection), although selection bias for patients fit enough to undergo re-resection likely contributes to this survival difference. Factors associated with the use of salvage surgery included younger age, margin-negative resection of the initial hepatectomy, smaller tumor size, and site of recurrence, with liver-only and lung-only recurrences being more amenable to salvage than multiple-site recurrences. Although the intensity of surveillance strategies has not demonstrated an association with long-term survival outcomes,[141] and to date randomized studies have not been performed, retrospective data indicate that select patients can clearly be benefit from 1 or more attempts at salvage resection in the appropriate clinical context.

THE MEDICAL ONCOLOGIST'S PERSPECTIVE

In patients with colorectal cancer, the liver is the preferred site of metastases and remains the main prognostic driver.[3,4] The traditional approach to CRLM was somewhat nihilistic in nature. With more modern systemic chemotherapy regimens, better understanding of the molecular profiling of tumors and its implications, and the evolution of the multidisciplinary team, there has been a substantial step forward in the management of such patients. However, despite the advancements in chemotherapy, surgery remains the only individual approach that offers patients the chance of cure.[7]

Systemic chemotherapy alone, even using modern combinations including biologics, is noncurative, with 2-year survival rates of approximately 40%. In routine clinical practice, many patients with CRLM never meet with a hepatobiliary surgeon, and the sole intent of treatment becomes palliative in nature. However, selected patients with CLRM can be cured, but this can only occur with the incorporation of surgery in the treatment paradigm.

Historically, liver surgery was a rare occurrence and was considered only for those with low-volume metastatic disease to the liver that met strict criteria. However, this represented just 10% of all patients who developed CRLM. The boundaries of surgical resection are being pushed persistently. Liver resection is now routinely considered for patients with higher volumes of metastatic disease confined to the liver. The key to determining suitability for liver resection no longer focuses on the burden of liver involvement but more on whether the future liver remnant after surgery is sufficient to maintain adequate liver function. The synergistic combination of modern systemic chemotherapy with safe resection can lead to cure in patients. Furthermore, the use of novel therapies such as hepatic arterial infusion chemotherapy with systemic chemo-therapy after liver resection is associated with lower intrahepatic recurrence rates and better disease-free survival and overall survival.[128–130]

As a practicing oncologist, the early involvement of a hepatobiliary surgeon in the management of a patient with CRLM is crucial to best determine the timing and sequence of chemotherapy with surgery, and hence improve patient outcomes and survival. More effective systemic chemotherapy regimens allow for the selection of pa-tients with a more favorable biology, as well as downstaging of some patients, to facil-itate more effective surgical approaches. For a patient who responds well to chemotherapy with good tolerance, there may be a temptation to continue systemic treatment and spare the patient a surgery. However, it is impractical to continue sys-temic therapy indefinitely. In addition to selecting patients for a curative-intent resec-tion of CRLM, it is important for a surgeon to identify those who are not, and who are unlikely to become, surgical candidates, so that other liver-directed therapies including hepatic arterial infusion chemotherapy, ablation, and chemoembolization can be considered to positively impact survival.

SUMMARY

In the modern era, the treatment of CRLM has certainly become more challenging and, at the same time, rewarding. Moving forward, we need to integrate the medical and surgical advances in the treatment of metastatic colorectal cancer by establishing a standard of care that insists on true multidisciplinary evaluation of every patient with CLRM.

DISCLOSURE

The authors have nothing to disclose.

REFERENCES

1. American Cancer Society. Global cancer facts & figures. 4th edition. Atlanta, Georgia: American Cancer Society; 2018. p. 1–76.
2. Bray F, Ferlay J, Soerjomataram I, et al. Global cancer statistics 2018: GLOBO-CAN estimates of incidence and mortality worldwide for 36 cancers in 185 coun-tries. CA Cancer J Clin 2018;68(6):394–424.
3. American Cancer Society. Colorectal cancer facts & figures 2017-2019. Atlanta, Georgia: American Cancer Society; 2017. p. 1–40.
4. Siegel R, Naishadham D, Jemal A. Cancer statistics, 2012. CA Cancer J Clin 2012;62(1):10–29.
5. Choti MA, Sitzmann JV, Tiburi MF, et al. Trends in long-term survival following liver resection for hepatic colorectal metastases. Ann Surg 2002;235(6):759–66.
6. de Haas RJ, Wicherts DA, Salloum C, et al. Long-term outcomes after hepatic resection for colorectal metastases in young patients. Cancer 2009;116(3): 647–58.

7. Tomlinson JS, Jarnagin WR, DeMatteo RP, et al. Actual 10-Year Survival After Resection of Colorectal Liver Metastases Defines Cure. J Clin Oncol 2007; 25(29):4575–80.

8. Frankel TL, D'Angelica MI. Hepatic resection for colorectal metastases. J Surg Oncol 2013;109(1):2–7.

9. Creasy JM, Sadot E, Koerkamp BG, et al. Actual 10-year survival after hepatic resection of colorectal liver metastases: what factors preclude cure? Surgery 2018;163(6):1238–44.

10. Pack GT, Brasfield RD. Metastatic cancer of the liver: the clinical problem and its management. Am J Surg 1955;90(5):704–16.

11. Quattlebaum JK. Massive Resection of the Liver. Ann Surg 1953;137(6):787–95.

12. Rahbari NN, Garden OJ, Padbury R, et al. Posthepatectomy liver failure: a definition and grading by the International Study Group of Liver Surgery (ISGLS). Surgery 2011;149(5):713–24.

13. Kauffmann R, Fong Y. Post-hepatectomy liver failure. Hepatobiliary Surg Nutr 2014;3(5):238–46.

14. Ren Z, Xu Y, Zhu S. Indocyanine green retention test avoiding liver failure after hepatectomy for hepatolithiasis. Hepatogastroenterology 2012;59(115):782–4.

15. Shoup M, Gonen M, D'Angelica M, et al. Volumetric analysis predicts hepatic dysfunction in patients undergoing major liver resection. J Gastrointest Surg 2003;7(3):325–30.

16. Foster JH, Berman MM. Solid liver tumors; 1977. Philadelphia: W.B Saunders Company.

17. Scheele J, Stangl R, Altendorf-Hofmann A. Hepatic metastases from colorectal carcinoma: impact of surgical resection on the natural history. Br J Surg 1990; 77(11):1241–6.

18. Gallagher DJ, Kemeny N. Metastatic colorectal cancer: from improved survival to potential cure. Oncology 2010;78(3–4):237–48.

19. Fong Y, Fortner J, Sun RL, et al. Clinical score for predicting recurrence after hepatic resection for metastatic colorectal cancer: analysis of 1001 consecutive cases. Ann Surg 1999;230(3):309–18 [discussion: 318–21].

20. Zakaria S, Donohue JH, Que FG, et al. Hepatic resection for colorectal metastases. Ann Surg 2007;246(2):183–91.

21. Brudvik KW, Jones RP, Giuliante F, et al. RAS mutation clinical risk score to predict survival after resection of colorectal liver metastases. Ann Surg 2019; 269(1):120–6.

22. Margonis GA, Spolverato G, Kim Y, et al. Effect of KRAS mutation on long-term outcomes of patients undergoing hepatic resection for colorectal liver metastases. Ann Surg Oncol 2015;1–8. https://doi.org/10.1245/s10434-015-4587-z.

23. Margonis GA, Kim Y, Spolverato G, et al. Association between specific mutations in KRASCodon 12 and colorectal liver metastasis. JAMA Surg 2015; 150(8):722–8.

24. Chun YS, Passot G, Yamashita S, et al. Deleterious effect of RAS and evolutionary high-risk TP53 double mutation in colorectal liver metastases. Ann Surg 2019;269(5):917–23.

25. Datta J, Smith JJ, Chatila WK, et al. Coaltered Ras/B-raf and TP53 Is associated with extremes of survivorship and distinct patterns of metastasis in patients with metastatic colorectal cancer. Clin Cancer Res 2020;26(5):1077–85.

26. Gagnière J, Dupré A, Gholami SS, et al. Is hepatectomy justified for BRAF mutant colorectal liver metastases? Ann Surg 2020;271(1):147–54.

27. Nordlinger B, Guiguet M, Vaillant JC, et al. Surgical resection of colorectal carcinoma metastases to the liver. A prognostic scoring system to improve case selection, based on 1568 patients. Association Française de Chirurgie. Cancer 1996;77(7):1254–62.
28. Nagashima I, Takada T, Adachi M, et al. Proposal of criteria to select candidates with colorectal liver metastases for hepatic resection: comparison of our scoring system to the positive number of risk factors. World J Gastroenterol 2006;12(39): 6305–9.
29. Konopke R, Kersting S, Distler M, et al. Prognostic factors and evaluation of a clinical score for predicting survival after resection of colorectal liver metastases. Liver Int 2009;29(1):89–102.
30. Roberts KJ, White A, Cockbain A, et al. Performance of prognostic scores in predicting long-term outcome following resection of colorectal liver metastases. Br J Surg 2014;101(7):856–66.
31. Kishi Y, Abdalla EK, Chun YS, et al. Three hundred and one consecutive extended right hepatectomies: evaluation of outcome based on systematic liver volumetry. Ann Surg 2009;250(4):540–8.
32. Chun YS, Ribero D, Abdalla EK, et al. Comparison of two methods of future liver remnant volume measurement. J Gastrointest Surg 2008;12(1):123–8.
33. Floriani I, Torri V, Rulli E, et al. Performance of imaging modalities in diagnosis of liver metastases from colorectal cancer: a systematic review and meta-analysis. J Magn Reson Imaging 2010;31(1):19–31.
34. Fernandez FG, Ritter J, Goodwin JW, et al. Effect of steatohepatitis associated with irinotecan or oxaliplatin pretreatment on resectability of hepatic colorectal metastases. J Am Coll Surg 2005;200(6):845–53.
35. Vreugdenburg TD, Ma N, Duncan JK, et al. Comparative diagnostic accuracy of hepatocyte-specific gadoxetic acid (Gd-EOB-DTPA) enhanced MR imaging and contrast enhanced CT for the detection of liver metastases: a systematic review and meta-analysis. Int J Colorectal Dis 2016;31(11):1739–49.
36. Vilgrain V, Esvan M, Ronot M, et al. A meta-analysis of diffusion-weighted and gadoxetic acid-enhanced MR imaging for the detection of liver metastases. Eur Radiol 2016;26(12):4595–615.
37. Chen L, Zhang J, Zhang L, et al. Meta-analysis of gadoxetic acid disodium (Gd-EOB-DTPA)-enhanced magnetic resonance imaging for the detection of liver metastases. PLoS One 2012;7(11):e48681.
38. Moulton C-A, Gu C-S, Law CH, et al. Effect of PET before liver resection on surgical management for colorectal adenocarcinoma metastases. JAMA 2014; 311(18):1863–7.
39. Jarnagin WR, Bodniewicz J, Dougherty E, et al. A prospective analysis of staging laparoscopy in patients with primary and secondary hepatobiliary malignancies. J Gastrointest Surg 2000;4(1):34–43.
40. Bickenbach KA, DeMatteo RP, Fong Y, et al. Risk of occult irresectable disease at liver resection for hepatic colorectal cancer metastases: a contemporary analysis. Ann Surg Oncol 2013;20(6):2029–34.
41. Sadot E, Groot Koerkamp B, Leal JN, et al. Resection margin and survival in 2368 patients undergoing hepatic resection for metastatic colorectal cancer: surgical technique or biologic surrogate? Ann Surg 2015;262(3):476–85 [discussion: 483–5].
42. Pawlik TM, Scoggins CR, Zorzi D, et al. Effect of surgical margin status on survival and site of recurrence after hepatic resection for colorectal metastases. Ann Surg 2005;241(5):715–22 [discussion: 722–4].

43. Miller CL, Taylor MS, Qadan M, et al. Prognostic significance of surgical margin size after neoadjuvant FOLFOX and/or FOLFIRI for colorectal liver metastases. J Gastrointest Surg 2017;21(11):1831–40.
44. Sarpel U, Bonavia AS, Grucela A, et al. Does anatomic versus nonanatomic resection affect recurrence and survival in patients undergoing surgery for colorectal liver metastasis? Ann Surg Oncol 2009;16(2):379–84.
45. Moris D, Ronnekleiv-Kelly S, Rahnemai-Azar AA, et al. Parenchymal-sparing versus anatomic liver resection for colorectal liver metastases: a systematic review. J Gastrointest Surg 2017;21(6):1076–85.
46. Deng G, Li H, Jia G-Q, et al. Parenchymal-sparing versus extended hepatectomy for colorectal liver metastases: a systematic review and meta-analysis. Cancer Med 2019;8(14):6165–75.
47. Kingham TP, Tanoue M, Eaton A, et al. Patterns of recurrence after ablation of colorectal cancer liver metastases. Ann Surg Oncol 2012;19(3):834–41.
48. Kneuertz PJ, Pitt HA, Bilimoria KY, et al. Risk of morbidity and mortality following hepato-pancreato-biliary surgery. J Gastrointest Surg 2012;16(9):1727–35.
49. Jarnagin WR, Gonen M, Fong Y, et al. Improvement in perioperative outcome after hepatic resection: analysis of 1,803 consecutive cases over the past decade. Ann Surg 2002;236(4):397–406 [discussion: 406–7].
50. Balzan S, Belghiti J, Farges O, et al. The "50-50 criteria" on postoperative day 5: an accurate predictor of liver failure and death after hepatectomy. Ann Surg 2005;242(6):824–8 [discussion: 828–9].
51. Zhao J, van Mierlo KMC, Gómez-Ramírez J, et al. Systematic review of the influence of chemotherapy-associated liver injury on outcome after partial hepatectomy for colorectal liver metastases. Br J Surg 2017;104(8):990–1002.
52. Tzeng C-WD, Aloia TA. Colorectal liver metastases. J Gastrointest Surg 2013;17(1):195–201 [quiz: 201–2].
53. Smith JJ, D'Angelica MI. Surgical management of hepatic metastases of colorectal cancer. Hematol Oncol Clin North Am 2015;29(1):61–84.
54. Corrêa D, Schwartz L, Jarnagin WR, et al. Kinetics of liver volume changes in the first year after portal vein embolization. Arch Surg 2010;145(4):351–4 [discussion: 354–5].
55. Leung U, Simpson AL, Araujo RLC, et al. Remnant growth rate after portal vein embolization is a good early predictor of post-hepatectomy liver failure. J Am Coll Surg 2014;219(4):620–30.
56. Ribero D, Abdalla EK, Madoff DC, et al. Portal vein embolization before major hepatectomy and its effects on regeneration, resectability and outcome. Br J Surg 2007;94(11):1386–94.
57. Shindoh J, Truty MJ, Aloia TA, et al. Kinetic growth rate after portal vein embolization predicts posthepatectomy outcomes: toward zero liver-related mortality in patients with colorectal liver metastases and small future liver remnant. J Am Coll Surg 2013;216(2):201–9.
58. Shindoh J, Tzeng C-WD, Aloia TA, et al. Optimal future liver remnant in patients treated with extensive preoperative chemotherapy for colorectal liver metastases. Ann Surg Oncol 2013;20(8):2493–500.
59. Wicherts DA, de Haas RJ, Andreani P, et al. Impact of portal vein embolization on long-term survival of patients with primarily unresectable colorectal liver metastases. Br J Surg 2010;97(2):240–50.
60. Covey AM, Brown KT, Jarnagin WR, et al. Combined portal vein embolization and neoadjuvant chemotherapy as a treatment strategy for resectable hepatic colorectal metastases. Ann Surg 2008;247(3):451–5.

61. Schnitzbauer AA, Lang SA, Goessmann H, et al. Right portal vein ligation combined with in situ splitting induces rapid left lateral liver lobe hypertrophy enabling 2-staged extended right hepatic resection in small-for-size settings. Ann Surg 2012;255(3):405–14.

62. Schadde E, Ardiles V, Slankamenac K, et al. ALPPS offers a better chance of complete resection in patients with primarily unresectable liver tumors compared with conventional-staged hepatectomies: results of a multicenter analysis. World J Surg 2014;38(6):1510–9.

63. Shindoh J, Vauthey J-N, Zimmitti G, et al. Analysis of the efficacy of portal vein embolization for patients with extensive liver malignancy and very low future liver remnant volume, including a comparison with the associating liver partition with portal vein ligation for staged hepatectomy approach. J Am Coll Surg 2013; 217(1):126–33 [discussion: 133–4].

64. Sandström P, Røsok BI, Sparrelid E, et al. ALPPS improves resectability compared with conventional two-stage hepatectomy in patients with advanced colorectal liver metastasis: results from a Scandinavian multicenter randomized controlled trial (LIGRO trial). Ann Surg 2018;267(5):833–40.

65. Hasselgren K, Røsok BI, Larsen PN, et al. ALPPS improves survival compared with TSH in patients affected of CRLM: survival analysis from the randomized controlled trial LIGRO. Ann Surg 2019. https://doi.org/10.1097/SLA. 0000000000003701.

66. Adam R, Delvart VR, Pascal GR, et al. Rescue surgery for unresectable colorectal liver metastases downstaged by chemotherapy. Ann Surg 2004;240(4): 644–58.

67. Giacchetti S, Itzhaki M, Gruia G, et al. Long-term survival of patients with unresectable colorectal cancer liver metastases following infusional chemotherapy with 5-fluorouracil, leucovorin, oxaliplatin and surgery. Ann Oncol 1999;10(6): 663–9.

68. Delaunoit T, Alberts SR, Sargent DJ, et al. Chemotherapy permits resection of metastatic colorectal cancer: experience from Intergroup N9741. Ann Oncol 2005;16(3):425–9.

69. Falcone A, Ricci S, Brunetti I, et al. Phase III trial of infusional fluorouracil, leucovorin, oxaliplatin, and irinotecan (FOLFOXIRI) compared with infusional fluorouracil, leucovorin, and irinotecan (FOLFIRI) as first-line treatment for metastatic colorectal cancer: the Gruppo Oncologico Nord Ovest. J Clin Oncol 2007;25(13):1670–6.

70. Masi G, Loupakis F, Pollina L, et al. Long-term outcome of initially unresectable metastatic colorectal cancer patients treated with 5-fluorouracil/leucovorin, oxaliplatin, and irinotecan (FOLFOXIRI) followed by radical surgery of metastases. Ann Surg 2009;249(3):420–5.

71. Adam R, Wicherts DA, de Haas RJ, et al. Patients with initially unresectable colorectal liver metastases: is there a possibility of cure? J Clin Oncol 2009;27(11): 1829–35.

72. Souglakos J, Androulakis N, Syrigos K, et al. FOLFOXIRI (folinic acid, 5-fluorouracil, oxaliplatin and irinotecan) vs FOLFIRI (folinic acid, 5-fluorouracil and irinotecan) as first-line treatment in metastatic colorectal cancer (MCC): a multicentre randomised phase III trial from the Hellenic Oncology Research Group (HORG). Br J Cancer 2006;94(6):798–805.

73. Van Cutsem E, Köhne C-H, Hitre E, et al. Cetuximab and chemotherapy as initial treatment for metastatic colorectal cancer. N Engl J Med 2009;360(14):1408–17.

74. Bokemeyer C, Bondarenko I, Makhson A, et al. Fluorouracil, leucovorin, and oxaliplatin with and without cetuximab in the first-line treatment of metastatic colorectal cancer. J Clin Oncol 2009;27(5):663–71.
75. Modest DP, Martens UM, Riera-Knorrenschild J, et al. FOLFOXIRI Plus panitumumab as first-line treatment of RAS wild-type metastatic colorectal cancer: the randomized, open-label, phase II VOLFI Study (AIO KRK0109). J Clin Oncol 2019;37(35):3401–11.
76. Saltz LB, Clarke S, Díaz-Rubio E, et al. Bevacizumab in combination with oxaliplatin-based chemotherapy as first-line therapy in metastatic colorectal cancer: a randomized phase III study. J Clin Oncol 2008;26(12):2013–9.
77. Ye L-C, Liu T-S, Ren L, et al. Randomized controlled trial of cetuximab plus chemotherapy for patients with KRAS wild-type unresectable colorectal liver-limited metastases. J Clin Oncol 2013;31(16):1931–8.
78. Vauthey J-N, Pawlik TM, Ribero D, et al. Chemotherapy regimen predicts steatohepatitis and an increase in 90-day mortality after surgery for hepatic colorectal metastases. J Clin Oncol 2006;24(13):2065–72.
79. Wolf PS, Park JO, Bao F, et al. Preoperative chemotherapy and the risk of hepatotoxicity and morbidity after liver resection for metastatic colorectal cancer: a single institution experience. J Am Coll Surg 2013;216(1):41–9.
80. Karoui M, Penna C, Amin-Hashem M, et al. Influence of preoperative chemotherapy on the risk of major hepatectomy for colorectal liver metastases. Ann Surg 2006;243(1):1–7.
81. Rubbia-Brandt L, Audard V, Sartoretti P, et al. Severe hepatic sinusoidal obstruction associated with oxaliplatin-based chemotherapy in patients with metastatic colorectal cancer. Ann Oncol 2004;15(3):460–6.
82. Aloia T, Sebagh M, Plasse M, et al. Liver histology and surgical outcomes after preoperative chemotherapy with fluorouracil plus oxaliplatin in colorectal cancer liver metastases. J Clin Oncol 2006;24(31):4983–90.
83. Robinson SM, Wilson CH, Burt AD, et al. Chemotherapy-associated liver injury in patients with colorectal liver metastases: a systematic review and meta-analysis. Ann Surg Oncol 2012;19(13):4287–99.
84. Kooby DA, Fong Y, Suriawinata A, et al. Impact of steatosis on perioperative outcome following hepatic resection. J Gastrointest Surg 2003;7(8):1034–44.
85. Kneuertz PJ, Maithel SK, Staley CA, et al. Chemotherapy-associated liver injury: impact on surgical management of colorectal cancer liver metastases. Ann Surg Oncol 2011;18(1):181–90.
86. White RR, Schwartz LH, Munoz JA, et al. Assessing the optimal duration of chemotherapy in patients with colorectal liver metastases. J Surg Oncol 2008; 97(7):601–4.
87. Kemeny NE, Melendez FDH, Capanu M, et al. Conversion to resectability using hepatic artery infusion plus systemic chemotherapy for the treatment of unresectable liver metastases from colorectal carcinoma. J Clin Oncol 2009; 27(21):3465–71.
88. Pak LM, Kemeny NE, Capanu M, et al. Prospective phase II trial of combination hepatic artery infusion and systemic chemotherapy for unresectable colorectal liver metastases: long term results and curative potential. J Surg Oncol 2018; 117(4):634–43.
89. Kern W, Beckert B, Lang N, et al. Phase I and pharmacokinetic study of hepatic arterial infusion with oxaliplatin in combination with folinic acid and 5-fluorouracil in patients with hepatic metastases from colorectal cancer. Ann Oncol 2001; 12(5):599–603.

90. Mancuso A, Giuliani R, Accettura C, et al. Hepatic arterial continuous infusion (HACI) of oxaliplatin in patients with unresectable liver metastases from colorectal cancer. Anticancer Res 2003;23(2C):1917–22.

91. Fiorentini G, Rossi S, Dentico P, et al. Oxaliplatin hepatic arterial infusion chemotherapy for hepatic metastases from colorectal cancer: a phase I-II clinical study. Anticancer Res 2004;24(3b):2093–6.

92. Ducreux M, Ychou M, Laplanche A, et al. Hepatic arterial oxaliplatin infusion plus intravenous chemotherapy in colorectal cancer with inoperable hepatic metastases: a trial of the Gastrointestinal Group of the Fédération Nationale des Centres de Lutte Contre le Cancer. J Clin Oncol 2005;23(22):4881–7.

93. Boige V, Malka D, Elias D, et al. Hepatic Arterial Infusion of Oxaliplatin and Intravenous LV5FU2 in Unresectable Liver Metastases from Colorectal Cancer after Systemic Chemotherapy Failure. Ann Surg Oncol 2007;15(1):219–26.

94. Goéré D, Deshaies I, De Baere T, et al. Prolonged survival of initially unresectable hepatic colorectal cancer patients treated with hepatic arterial infusion of oxaliplatin followed by radical surgery of metastases. Ann Surg 2010;251(4):686–91.

95. Tsimberidou AM, Fu S, Ng C, et al. A phase 1 study of hepatic arterial infusion of oxaliplatin in combination with systemic 5-fluorouracil, leucovorin, and bevacizumab in patients with advanced solid tumors metastatic to the liver. Cancer 2010;116(17):4086–94.

96. Tsimberidou AM, Leick MB, Lim J, et al. Dose-finding study of hepatic arterial infusion of oxaliplatin-based treatment in patients with advanced solid tumors metastatic to the liver. Cancer Chemother Pharmacol 2012;71(2):389–97.

97. Allard MA, Sebagh M, Baillie G, et al. Comparison of complete pathologic response and hepatic injuries between hepatic arterial infusion and systemic administration of oxaliplatin in patients with colorectal liver metastases. Ann Surg Oncol 2015;22(6):1925–32.

98. Volovat SR, Volovat C, Negru SM, et al. The efficacy and safety of hepatic arterial infusion of oxaliplatin plus intravenous irinotecan, leucovorin and fluorouracil in colorectal cancer with inoperable hepatic metastasis. J Chemother 2016;28(3):235–41.

99. Lévi FA, Boige V, Hebbar M, et al. Conversion to resection of liver metastases from colorectal cancer with hepatic artery infusion of combined chemotherapy and systemic cetuximab in multicenter trial OPTILIV. Ann Oncol 2016;27(2):267–74.

100. Lim A, Le Sourd S, Senellart H, et al. Hepatic arterial infusion chemotherapy for unresectable liver metastases of colorectal cancer: a multicenter retrospective study. Clin Colorectal Cancer 2017;16(4):308–15.

101. Sato Y, Inaba Y, Ura T, et al. Outcomes of a phase I/II trial of hepatic arterial infusion of oxaliplatin combined with intravenous 5-fluorouracil and l-leucovorin in patients with unresectable liver metastases from colorectal cancer after systemic chemotherapy failure. J Gastrointest Cancer 2017;49(2):132–7.

102. Kopetz S, Vauthey J-N. Perioperative chemotherapy for resectable hepatic metastases. Lancet 2008;371(9617):963–5.

103. Nordlinger B, Sorbye H, Glimelius B, et al. Perioperative FOLFOX4 chemotherapy and surgery versus surgery alone for resectable liver metastases from colorectal cancer (EORTC 40983): long-term results of a randomised, controlled, phase 3 trial. Lancet Oncol 2013;14(12):1208–15.

104. Nordlinger B, Sorbye H, Glimelius B, et al. Perioperative chemotherapy with FOLFOX4 and surgery versus surgery alone for resectable liver metastases

from colorectal cancer (EORTC Intergroup trial 40983): a randomised controlled trial. Lancet 2008;371(9617):1007–16.

105. Adam R, de Gramont A, Figueras J, et al. Managing synchronous liver metastases from colorectal cancer: a multidisciplinary international consensus. Cancer Treat Rev 2015;41(9):729–41.

106. Andres A, Toso C, Adam R, et al. A survival analysis of the liver-first reversed management of advanced simultaneous colorectal liver metastases: a LiverMetSurvey-based study. Ann Surg 2012;256(5):772–8 [discussion: 778–9].

107. Elias D, Detroz B, Lasser P, et al. Is simultaneous hepatectomy and intestinal anastomosis safe? Am J Surg 1995;169(2):254–60.

108. Lyass S, Zamir G, Matot I, et al. Combined colon and hepatic resection for synchronous colorectal liver metastases. J Surg Oncol 2001;78(1):17–21.

109. Martin R, Paty P, Fong Y, et al. Simultaneous liver and colorectal resections are safe for synchronous colorectal liver metastasis. J Am Coll Surg 2003;197(2):233–41.

110. Slesser AAP, Simillis C, Goldin R, et al. A meta-analysis comparing simultaneous versus delayed resections in patients with synchronous colorectal liver metastases. Surg Oncol 2013;22(1):36–47.

111. Reddy SK, Pawlik TM, Zorzi D, et al. Simultaneous resections of colorectal cancer and synchronous liver metastases: a multi-institutional analysis. Ann Surg Oncol 2007;14(12):3481–91.

112. Silberhumer GR, Paty PB, Temple LK, et al. Simultaneous resection for rectal cancer with synchronous liver metastasis is a safe procedure. Am J Surg 2015;209(6):935–42.

113. Habr-Gama A, Perez RO, Nadalin W, et al. Operative versus nonoperative treatment for stage 0 distal rectal cancer following chemoradiation therapy: long-term results. Ann Surg 2004;240(4):711–7 [discussion: 717–8].

114. Habr-Gama A, Gama-Rodrigues J, São Julião GP, et al. Local recurrence after complete clinical response and watch and wait in rectal cancer after neoadjuvant chemoradiation: impact of salvage therapy on local disease control. Int J Radiat Oncol Biol Phys 2014;88(4):822–8.

115. Smith JJ, Strombom P, Chow OS, et al. Assessment of a watch-and-wait strategy for rectal cancer in patients with a complete response after neoadjuvant therapy. JAMA Oncol 2019;5(4):e185896.

116. Reddy SK, Zorzi D, Lum YW, et al. Timing of multimodality therapy for resectable synchronous colorectal liver metastases: a retrospective multi-institutional analysis. Ann Surg Oncol 2008;16(7):1809–19.

117. Ayez N, van der Stok EP, de Wilt H, et al. Neo-adjuvant chemotherapy followed by surgery versus surgery alone in high-risk patients with resectable colorectal liver metastases: the CHARISMA randomized multicenter clinical trial. BMC Cancer 2015;15(1):180–7.

118. Wolmark N, Rockette H, Fisher B, et al. The benefit of leucovorin-modulated fluorouracil as postoperative adjuvant therapy for primary colon cancer: results from National Surgical Adjuvant Breast and Bowel Project protocol C-03. J Clin Oncol 1993;11(10):1879–87.

119. André T, Boni C, Mounedji-Boudiaf L, et al. Oxaliplatin, fluorouracil, and leucovorin as adjuvant treatment for colon cancer. N Engl J Med 2004;350(23):2343–51.

120. André T, Boni C, Navarro M, et al. Improved overall survival with oxaliplatin, fluorouracil, and leucovorin as adjuvant treatment in stage II or III colon cancer in the MOSAIC trial. J Clin Oncol 2009;27(19):3109–16.

121. Haller DG, Tabernero J, Maroun J, et al. Capecitabine plus oxaliplatin compared with fluorouracil and folinic acid as adjuvant therapy for stage III colon cancer. J Clin Oncol 2011;29(11):1465–71.

122. Portier G, Elias D, Bouche O, et al. Multicenter randomized trial of adjuvant fluorouracil and folinic acid compared with surgery alone after resection of colorectal liver metastases: FFCD ACHBTH AURC 9002 trial. J Clin Oncol 2006; 24(31):4976–82.

123. Mitry E, Fields ALA, Bleiberg H, et al. Adjuvant chemotherapy after potentially curative resection of metastases from colorectal cancer: a pooled analysis of two randomized trials. J Clin Oncol 2008;26(30):4906–11.

124. Ychou M, Hohenberger W, Thezenas S, et al. A randomized phase III study comparing adjuvant 5-fluorouracil/folinic acid with FOLFIRI in patients following complete resection of liver metastasis from colorectal cancer. Ann Oncol 2009; 20(12):1964–70.

125. Primrose J, Falk S, Finch-Jones M, et al. Systemic chemotherapy with or without cetuximab in patients with resectable colorectal liver metastasis: the New EPOC randomised controlled trial. Lancet Oncol 2014;15(6):601–11.

126. Bridgewater JA, Pugh SA, Maishman T, et al. Systemic chemotherapy with or without cetuximab in patients with resectable colorectal liver metastasis (New EPOC): long-term results of a multicentre, randomised, controlled, phase 3 trial. Lancet Oncol 2020;21(3):398–411.

127. Lygidakis NJ, Sgourakis G, Vlachos L, et al. Metastatic liver disease of colorectal origin: the value of locoregional immunochemotherapy combined with systemic chemotherapy following liver resection. Results of a prospective randomized study. Hepatogastroenterology 2001;48(42):1685–91.

128. Kemeny N, Huang Y, Cohen AM, et al. Hepatic arterial infusion of chemotherapy after resection of hepatic metastases from colorectal cancer. N Engl J Med 1999;341(27):2039–48.

129. Kemeny MM, Adak S, Gray B, et al. Combined-modality treatment for resectable metastatic colorectal carcinoma to the liver: surgical resection of hepatic metastases in combination with continuous infusion of chemotherapy–an intergroup study. J Clin Oncol 2002;20(6):1499–505.

130. Kemeny NE, Gonen M. Hepatic arterial infusion after liver resection. N Engl J Med 2005;352(7):734–5.

131. Fong Y, Cohen AM, Fortner JG, et al. Liver resection for colorectal metastases. J Clin Oncol 1997;15(3):938–46.

132. Maithel SK, Ginsberg MS, D'Amico F, et al. Natural history of patients with subcentimeter pulmonary nodules undergoing hepatic resection for metastatic colorectal cancer. J Am Coll Surg 2010;210(1):31–8.

133. Miller G, Biernacki P, Kemeny NE, et al. Outcomes after resection of synchronous or metachronous hepatic and pulmonary colorectal metastases. J Am Coll Surg 2007;205(2):231–8.

134. Mise Y, Kopetz S, Mehran RJ, et al. Is complete liver resection without resection of synchronous lung metastases justified? Ann Surg Oncol 2015;22(5):1585–92.

135. Elias D, Ouellet J-F, Bellon N, et al. Extrahepatic disease does not contraindicate hepatectomy for colorectal liver metastases. Br J Surg 2003;90(5):567–74.

136. Carpizo DR, Are C, Jarnagin W, et al. Liver resection for metastatic colorectal cancer in patients with concurrent extrahepatic disease: results in 127 patients treated at a single center. Ann Surg Oncol 2009;16(8):2138–46.

137. Adam R, de Haas RJ, Wicherts DA, et al. Is hepatic resection justified after chemotherapy in patients with colorectal liver metastases and lymph node involvement? J Clin Oncol 2008;26(22):3672–80.
138. D'Angelica M, Kornprat P, Gonen M, et al. Effect on outcome of recurrence patterns after hepatectomy for colorectal metastases. Ann Surg Oncol 2011;18(4): 1096–103.
139. Butte JM, Gonen M, Allen PJ, et al. Recurrence after partial hepatectomy for metastatic colorectal cancer: potentially curative role of salvage repeat resection. Ann Surg Oncol 2015;22(8):2761–71.
140. Litvak A, Cercek A, Segal N, et al. False-positive elevations of carcinoembryonic antigen in patients with a history of resected colorectal cancer. J Natl Compr Canc Netw 2014;12(6):907–13.
141. Hyder O, Dodson RM, Mayo SC, et al. Post-treatment surveillance of patients with colorectal cancer with surgically treated liver metastases. Surgery 2013; 154(2):256–65.

Surgical Management of Breast Cancer Liver Metastasis

Amir A. Rahnemai-Azar, MD[a], Luke V. Selby, MD, MS[b],
Maryam B. Lustberg, MD, MPH[c], Timothy M. Pawlik, MD, MPH, PhD[b],*

KEYWORDS

- Metastatic breast cancer • Liver resection • Breast cancer liver metastasis
- Liver metastasectomy

KEY POINTS

- Hepatic metastasectomy is safe and effective in well-selected patients with isolated BCLM.
- Appropriate patient selection before proceeding with hepatic metastasectomy is vital.
- Percutaneous ablative therapies are effective at extending life in patients not eligible for hepatic metastasectomy.

INTRODUCTION

Breast cancer is the second most commonly diagnosed cancer and second leading cause of cancer death among women after skin and lung cancers, respectively. An estimated 279,100 new cases of invasive breast cancer with about 42,690 deaths are expected in the United States in 2020.[1] The mortality of breast cancer, now at approximately 19.8 deaths per 100,000 cases, is roughly 40% of the 1989 peak of 33.2 people per 100,000 cases.[2] This dramatic change reflects the combination of early detection and improved treatments. Almost 6% to 10% of women still present with distant metastasis at the time of diagnoses with a reported 5-year survival of 27%, which is markedly lower than women who have earlier stages of disease.[3] Involvement of different organs may occur during the course of the disease with a

[a] Department of Surgery, Division of Surgical Oncology, California University of Science and Medicine, Colton, CA 92324, USA; [b] Department of Surgery, Division of Surgical Oncology, The Ohio State University Medical School, Columbus, OH 43210, USA; [c] Department of Medicine, Division of Medical Oncology, The Ohio State University Medical School, Columbus, OH 43210, USA
* Corresponding author. Department of Surgery, The Ohio State University Wexner Medical Center, 395 West. 12th Avenue, Suite 670, Columbus, OH 43210, USA
E-mail address: tim.pawlik@osumc.edu

Surg Oncol Clin N Am 30 (2021) 27–37
https://doi.org/10.1016/j.soc.2020.09.003
surgonc.theclinics.com

predominance of bone and lung metastasis, followed by liver.[4] More than one-half of patients with metastatic breast cancer develop liver involvement at some point, with the liver being the only site of metastatic disease in 5% of patients.[5,6]

The outcome of women with metastatic breast cancer is generally poor with a reported median survival of 18 to 24 months. Patients with breast cancer liver metastasis (BCLM) have the worst prognosis, with historic median survival ranging from 14 to 16 months.[7] However, these data have been largely derived from an era with less-effective systemic therapy, and lack of locoregional therapies, such as resection and ablative therapies for BCLM.[8] In view of disseminated disease, systemic therapy is the cornerstone of treatment of patients with BCLM. However, noting the curative potential of liver resection in management of some other metastatic diseases, such as colorectal and neuroendocrine liver metastasis, some surgeons have advocated for liver resection for BCLM. With recent improvements in the effectiveness of systemic therapy, and the decreased morbidity and mortality of partial hepatectomy, resection has been increasingly considered for a select group of patients with BCLM. In the absence of clinical trials with large number of patients, there is no definitive consensus accepted among experts. To this point, although the National Comprehensive Cancer Network guidelines do not recommend liver resection as an option for BCLM, the 4th ESO–ESMO International Consensus Guidelines for Advanced Breast Cancer (ABC 4) note that liver resection for BCLM is considered in select patients. We herein review data related to hepatic resection and ablative therapies of BCLM, and review data on the long-term outcomes of women treated with these approaches.[9]

HEPATIC RESECTION OF BREAST CANCER LIVER METASTASES

In 1997, Pocard and Salmon[10] introduced the notion of "adjuvant surgery" for BCLM in a series of 21 patients who underwent hepatic resection for BCLM. In this highly selected group of patients, the 5-year survival following resection of BCLM was 60%. One-half of patients did not receive any additional postoperative chemotherapy.[10] In a subsequent series of 52 patients with BCLM who underwent liver resection, the disease-free interval between the time of the primary breast cancer diagnosis and BCLM was noted to be one of the strongest factors associated with prolonged survival.[9] Specifically, the reported postoperative 3-year survival of patients who developed BCLM within 48 months of the primary breast cancer was significantly lower than the group who had a longer disease-free time interval (45% vs 82%, respectively; $P = .023$). Higher lymph node disease (N1b-N2) burden at the time of original diagnosis was also associated with higher 3-year intrahepatic recurrence with 83% among patients with N1b-N2 disease compared with 41% among individuals with N0 or N1 disease ($P = .021$).[9] Both of these findings highlighted the importance of patient selection for hepatic resection of BCLM. Of note, almost 46% of patient in this series did not receive any additional chemotherapy.

In a case-control study of patients with isolated BCLM who underwent surgery and/or ablation (n = 69) versus a group who received systemic medical therapy alone (n = 98), the surgery group had a lower hepatic disease burden, a longer disease-free interval before BCLM diagnosis (53 vs 30 months; $P<.001$), and were more likely to have estrogen receptor (ER)-positive tumors (78% vs 59%).[11] In the surgery group, the median recurrence-free interval was 28.5 months (95% confidence interval [CI], 19–38 months) and 10 patients (15%) were recurrence-free at 5-year. However, despite favorable disease characteristics in the surgical group, median overall survival (OS) was not significantly different between the two cohorts, with median OS and 5-year survival of 50 months and 38% in surgery group versus 45 months and 39% in the nonsurgical cohort, respectively. Of note, many patients in the nonsurgical cohort had long-term disease stability with a progression-free interval of 28.5 months and a median chemotherapy-free interval of 25 months.[11]

Margonis and colleagues[12] published a multi-institutional study of 131 patients who underwent an operation for BCLM between 1980 and 2014. The reported median disease-free interval was 34 months. Most patients (n = 81; 89%) had either T1 or T2 primary breast tumors, more than one-half (n = 58; 59.8%) had nodal metastasis at the time of diagnosis, and most (n = 90; 85.7%) received adjuvant therapy following the index breast surgery. Median size of the BCLM was 3 cm and 13% of patients (n = 16) had extrahepatic disease. Following hepatic resection, virtually all women either had cytotoxic chemotherapy (n = 41; 51.9%) or hormonal therapy (n = 43; 47.8%) in the adjuvant setting. During follow-up, 61 patients (51.7%) experienced recurrence with a median recurrence-free interval of 24 months. Among women who recurred, 33% had an intrahepatic recurrence, 52.6% had an extrahepatic recurrence, and 14% recurred at an intrahepatic and extrahepatic site. On multivariate analysis, tumor size less than 3 cm and resection with microscopic negative margins (R0 resection) were associated with improved survival. There was no statistically significant correlation between extrahepatic disease or ER status with survival.

In another series of 67 patients with BCLM who underwent partial hepatectomy, He and colleagues[13] reported a median survival time and 5-year OS of 57.6 months and 32.2%, respectively. The 3-year intrahepatic recurrence-free was 10.9%, with a median recurrence-free time of 13.5 months. An interval between breast surgery and BCLM diagnosis of more than 2 years (hazard ratio [HR], 0.178; 95% CI, 0.037–0.869) and hepatic portal triad clamping during surgery (HR, 0.117; 95% CI, 0.015–0.942) were independent predictors of OS. A longer interval between breast surgery and BCLM diagnosis, in addition to the tumor pathologic differentiation, were also associated with a lower incidence of intrahepatic recurrence.

Ercolani and colleagues[14] reported an institutional experience of 184 patients who underwent liver resection for noncolorectal nonneuroendocrine liver metastasis. Among 55 patients with BCLM, all but two patients had four or fewer metastasis and no patient had extrahepatic disease. The median time interval between primary treatment of the breast cancer and hepatic resection was 51 months. Most patients (n = 31; 61%) underwent major hepatectomy, and adjuvant chemotherapy was administered to all patients in the postoperative period. On multivariable analysis, BCLM size greater than 5 cm, R1 resection, and triple negative primary breast tumor status were associated with poor long-term outcomes. In a different multicenter retrospective series of resection for noncolorectal nonneuroendocrine tumors, among 59 patients with BCLM, most patients presented with metachronous disease (n = 49; 89%), unilateral liver disease (n = 41; 75%), and underwent a major hepatic resection (n = 34; 58%).[15] Because short- or long-term outcomes were not reported separately in the subgroup of patients with BCLM, and because of the absence of a control group, a survival advantage related to hepatectomy in BCLM could not be determined.

In a review of 25 papers published between 1999 and 2010, Bergenfeldt and colleagues[16] reported that postoperative median survival following hepatic resection of BCLM ranged from 20 to 67 months with 2-, 3-, and 5-year survival ranging from 58% to 86%, 35% to 79%, and 21% to 61%, respectively. These findings were generally consistent with data from other studies (**Table 1**). Specifically, there was no consistent association between characteristics of the primary breast tumor and index breast surgery with postresection survival of BCLM. Although several studies have noted that a longer interval between primary breast cancer diagnosis and BCLM was associated with prolonged survival, this finding has not been universal. Moreover,

Table 1
Recent studies investigating the clinical impact of hepatic metastasectomy for BCLM

Study, Year	Design	Extent of Hepatectomy		Timing of Systemic Therapy		Median Survival (mo)	Improved Survival Prognostic Factors
Pocard et al,[9] 2000	Retrospective single institution, n = 52	Major resection	n = 24 (46%)	Adjuvant chemotherapy	28%, 53.8%	42	Interval between primary diagnosis and diagnosis of liver metastasis (≤48 mo vs >48 mo)
		Minor resection	n = 28 (54%)	Adjuvant endocrine therapy	31%, 59.6%		
Margonis et al,[12] 2016	Retrospective multi-institutional, n = 131	Major resection	n = 43 (37.1%)	Adjuvant chemotherapy	41 (51.9%)	53.4	Negative surgical margin Diameter of BCLM (≤3 cm vs >3 cm)
		Minor resection	n = 73 (62.9%)	Adjuvant hormonal treatment	43 (47.8%)		
				Adjuvant biologic therapy	21 (27.3%)		
Sadot et al,[11] 2016	Retrospective single institution, n = 69	Major resection	n = 24 (47%)	Not reported		50	No survival benefit
		Minor resection	n = 27 (53%)				
Ercolani et al,[14] 2018	Retrospective single institution, n = 51	Minor resection	n = 20 (39%)	Adjuvant chemotherapy	n = 51 (100%)	51	Tumor diameter (≤5 cm) R0 resection Triple-negative tumor (negative association)
		Major resection	n = 31 (61%)				
Labgaa et al,[15] 2018	Retrospective multi-institutional, n = 59	Minor resection	n = 25 (42.4%)	Not reported		97.6	Age <60 y
		Major resection	n = 34 (57.6%)				

| He et al,[13] 2020 | Prospective multi-institutional, n = 67 | Minor resection Major resection | n = 35 n = 32 | Neoadjuvant treatment n = 26 (38%) | 57.59 | Pringle maneuver Increased interval between breast surgery and BCLM diagnosis |
| Chun et al,[18] 2020 | Prospective, n = 136 | Minor resection Major resection | n = 79 (58%) n = 57 (42%) | All patients received different types of adjuvant therapy based on receptor status | 81 mo in best group (varied based on receptor status) | Breast cancer receptor status |

Major hepatectomy: resection of ≥3 segment.
Data from Refs.[9,11–15,18]

the hepatic volume of disease, primary breast tumor hormone status, and extent of resection all have been variably associated with outcomes following surgery for BCLM. The reason for these disparate results is undoubtedly multifactorial. In particular, most studies on BCLM have involved a small sample size (eg, <100 patients) and represent a small fraction of patients with breast cancer. Furthermore, statistical analyses were limited and most studies suffered from inability to perform robust multivariable analyses, underpowered analyses (type II error), and inappropriate overfitted statistical models. In addition, the data have been retrospective in nature and therefore were subject to selection bias, confounding by indication, and other types of causal inference shortcomings.

To overcome some of these shortcomings, a few authors have reported propensity-matched studies.[17,18] In a study of 384 patients with BCLM, Feng and colleagues[17] used propensity score matching to compare the clinical outcomes of patients (n = 65) who underwent hepatic resection with individuals who received systemic treatment only (n = 319). After propensity score matching, the mean OS and 3- and 5-year OS among patients who underwent hepatic resection were significantly better than the nonresection cohort with 61.8 versus 38.6 months, 54.7% versus 45.6%, and 54.7% versus 21.9%, respectively (P<.007). Hepatic resection was also associated with improved intrahepatic progression-free survival (PFS) with a 5-year PFS of 41% versus 3.8% in the nonsurgical group. Multivariate analysis identified hormonal receptor status and hepatic resection as independent prognostic factors. The authors concluded that hepatic resection might offer a survival benefit compared with systemic treatment alone, especially among patients with positive hormonal receptors. In a separate trial, Chun and colleagues[18] reported a propensity-matched analysis of 136 patients who underwent hepatectomy plus systemic therapy versus 763 patients who received systemic therapy alone. Intrinsic subtypes were defined as luminal A (ER+ and/or progesterone receptor [PR]+, human epidermal growth factor receptor 2 [HER2]-), luminal B (ER and/or PR+, HER2+), HER2-enriched (ER and PR-, HER2+), and basal-like (ER, PR, HER2-). After hepatectomy, independent predictors of poor OS were number and size of liver metastases, and intrinsic subtype (HR, 1.11, 1.16, and 4.28, respectively). Postresection median OS among patients with luminal B, HER2-enriched, basal-like, and luminal A subtypes were 75, 81, 17, and 53 months, respectively (P<.001). Similarly, median PFS among patients with the HER2-enriched subtype with 60 months, was significantly better than the 17, 16, and 5 months reported in luminal A, luminal B, and basal-like subtypes, respectively (P<.001). After propensity score matching, 5-year OS in the surgery group was significantly better than systemic therapy alone cohort (56% vs 40%, respectively; P = .018). In turn, the authors suggest that hepatic resection of BCLM was associated with higher OS compared with systemic therapy alone and may have prolonged PFS among patients with the HER2-enriched subtype.[18] These findings support the use of surgical therapy in appropriately selected patients based on intrinsic subtypes.

In addition to being associated with better long-term outcomes, at least one group has suggested that hepatic resection of BCLM may also be associated with cost-savings. Spolverato and colleagues[19] estimated the cost-effectiveness of liver resection followed by adjuvant systemic therapy relative to systemic therapy alone for patients with BCLM. A decision-analytic Markov model was constructed to evaluate the cost-effectiveness of liver resection followed by postoperative conventional systemic therapy (strategy A) versus conventional therapy alone (strategy B) versus newer targeted therapy alone (strategy C). The implications of using different chemotherapeutic regimens based on ER and HER-2 status was also assessed. Outcomes included quality-adjusted life months (QALMs), incremental cost-effectiveness ratio, and net health benefit (NHB). The authors noted that NHB of strategy A was 10.9 QALMs compared with strategy B when letrozole was used as systemic therapy, whereas it was only 0.3 QALMs when docetaxel + trastuzumab was used as a systemic therapy. The addition of newer biologic agents (strategy C) significantly decreased the cost-effectiveness of strategy B (conventional systemic therapy alone). The NHB of strategy A was 31.6 QALMs versus strategy C when palbociclib was included in strategy C; similarly, strategy A had an NHB of 13.8 QALMs versus strategy C when pertuzumab was included in strategy C. Monte Carlo simulation demonstrated that the main factor influencing NHB of strategy A over strategy C was the cost of systemic therapy. As such, liver resection for BCLM may be cost-effective compared with systemic therapy alone, particularly in ER+ tumors or when newer more expensive agents were used.[19]

NONSURGICAL LOCOREGIONAL THERAPY FOR BREAST CANCER LIVER METASTASES

In addition to hepatic resection, there has been increased interest in other locoregional therapies, such as thermal ablation and intra-arterial therapies for BCLM. Bergenfeldt and coworkers[16] reviewed the results of seven studies that applied radiofrequency ablation (RFA) (n = 6) or laser-induced interstitial thermotherapy (n = 1) in the management of patients with BCLM. Post-treatment OS ranged from 30 to 60 months with 3- and 5-year survival ranging from 43% to 75% and 27% to 41%, respectively. Of note, disease burden and comorbidity status among patients who underwent local ablative therapy was generally worse than patients who underwent hepatic resection. Vogl and colleagues[20] reported a review of nine articles that specifically used thermal ablative therapies for patients with BCLM, yet the indication was largely palliative. Thermal ablation for BCLM was associated with a median survival of 10 to 60 months with a local response rate of 63% to 97%. In another series of patients who underwent laser-induced interstitial thermotherapy for a variety of different types of hepatic metastases, among 127 patients with BCLM local tumor control was achieved in 98.2% at 6 months with a mean survival of 51 months.[21] Reports of microwave ablation of BCLM have noted similar findings with high rates of tumor control, but a modest 5-year survival of 29%.[22]

Abbas and colleagues[23] reported their institutional experience of 61 patients with BCLM who underwent liver resection (n = 23), RFA (n = 11), or chemotherapy alone (n = 27). Although median OS among patients who underwent hepatic resection (49 months) was better than patients who received chemotherapy alone (20 months; P<.001), the difference comparing resection with RAF (37 months; P = .854) was not statistically different. Of note, patients who underwent hepatic resection had a lower burden of disease (median of 1.6 ± 1 metastasis) compared with patients who had RFA (2.6 ± 2.7) or chemotherapy along (5.5 ± 2.9).[23] Moreover, median disease-free survival (surgery: 25 months; range, 0–72 months; RFA: 28 months; range 15–91 months) did not differ among patients treated with resection versus ablation, yet outcomes in both these cohorts were superior to patients who received chemotherapy alone. In turn, the authors concluded that ablation might be equally appropriate as resection in select patients.[23] Xiao and colleagues[24] performed a metanalysis of 14 studies to compare the therapeutic efficacy of resection versus ablation among patients with BCLM. Despite a lower incidence of postoperative complications and a shorter hospital stay among patients who underwent RFA, hepatic resection was associated with improved 5-year OS (odds ratio, 0.38; 95% CI, 0.32–0.46; P<.001) and 5-year disease-free survival (odds ratio, 0.51; 95% CI, 0.40–0.66; P<.001).

SUMMARY

Metastatic breast cancer is common and generally carries a poor prognosis. Given that BCLM represents systemic disease in most women, systemic therapy is the cornerstone of therapy. In a rare and highly select subset of patients, hepatic resection or other locoregional therapies should be considered. The data supporting prolonged survival after hepatic resection or ablation for BCLM are limited and poor. The data are retrospective, derive from small case series, and are highly susceptible to the effects of selection bias. Even larger series that used propensity matching were still subject to selection bias and confounding. As such, the use of hepatic resection for BCLM needs to be judicious and performed only in the multidisciplinary setting. Based on the limited data available, the best candidates for resection of BCLM are women who have a limited tumor burden in the liver, a longer disease-free interval between the primary breast and BCLM diagnoses, and individuals with the HER2-enriched and triple-negative subtypes who have responded to systemic therapy. Surgery should involve complete resection with no particular emphasis on the extent of resection needed to achieve this goal. In the era of modern effective systemic chemotherapy for BCLM, local regional therapies, such as resection or ablation, are warranted, yet only in well-selected patients following discussion in a multidisciplinary setting.

The Medical Oncology Perspective

Chasing a cure for metastatic breast cancer: can surgery be part of the catch?
Each year more than 40,000 individuals die from breast cancer. The sobering reality of this fact is that most of these deaths are caused by progressive stage IV disease. Patients, clinicians, and researchers have worked for decades to find better targeted treatments that prolong life while preserving quality of life. Although progress has been made, the drive to discover a cure for metastatic breast cancer remains as relevant and pressing as it was decades ago. The question remains, whether this is wishful thinking or is a cure for metastatic cancer a reality in select individuals?

In this article, the authors conduct a thorough and balanced appraisal of the published literature regarding outcomes of patients with BCLM with and without liver resection. They conclude that the best candidates for resection of BCLM are individuals who are carefully selected and managed by a multidisciplinary team and who have (1) limited tumor burden, (2) longer disease-free interval, and (3) certain subtypes of breast cancer with sustained response to systemic therapy.

Limited tumor burden was identified as one potential criterion for selecting candidates for resection of BCLM. This finding highlights the clinical significance of oligometastatic disease, which is characterized by a distinct group of patients who have one or limited detectable metastatic lesions confined to a single organ. This unique group consists of less than 10% of newly diagnosed patients with metastatic breast cancer and they tend to have superior clinical outcomes. Many observational studies have demonstrated that some patients with oligometastatic disease may achieve a complete remission or a prolonged disease-free interval. As such, these are the patients that could benefit the most from a multidisciplinary approach including "curative" surgery or ablative radiation, for the primary tumor when present and for distant disease.

In clinical practice, there is currently tremendous variability in oligometastatic disease management, which is driven by the predilection of the clinician and personal wishes of the patient. Well-designed, randomized trials are needed to critically evaluate the most evidence-based approach for the management of this unique patient population. A prospective randomized study (NRG-BR002) is currently ongoing and aims to evaluate standard of care therapy with or without stereotactic body radiotherapy for oligometastatic breast cancer (NCT02364557, https://clinicaltrials.gov/ct2/show/NCT02364557).[2] The study is designed to evaluate if stereotactic body radiotherapy and/or resection of all oligometastatic sites improves PFS compared with standard of care in patients who have received up to 12 months of first-line systemic therapy without progression. The study completed accrual for the phase II portion of the trial and will precede to the phase III study if interim analysis findings are favorable.

Subtype differences in breast cancer and response to systemic therapy are also important considerations when selecting candidates for surgical management of BCLM. Appraisal of the completed studies to date demonstrate that patients with HER2 neu overexpressing and triple-negative breast cancer who are also responding to systemic therapy may be better candidates for such an approach. Importantly, these tumor subtypes are historically labeled as the most aggressive breast cancer subtypes. However, in recent years, there have been several important advances in targeting the unique biology of these subtypes, including multiple Food and Drug Administration–approved HER2 neu targeted therapies, and the first approved immunotherapy drug for metastatic triple-negative breast cancer. It is not surprising that these subtypes tend to benefit the most from resection of BCLM. Many of these tumor subtypes, but not all, tend to respond quickly to targeted systemic therapies. By allowing additional time for the intrinsic biology of the disease to manifest itself, more judicial multidisciplinary decisions may be made regarding the relative benefit of surgery.

Ultimately, metastatic breast cancer is a systemic process and the importance of targeted chemotherapy and immunotherapies is a critical consideration before any surgical decision making. However, systemic therapy alone is not the sole answer if we are chasing a cure for metastatic disease because resistance to systemic therapy is likely over time. More importantly, the cumulative toxicity burden of ongoing systemic therapy can have debilitating consequences. In the appropriate candidate, surgical management of BCLM may allow for potential de-escalation of toxic systemic therapies and/or prolong the time before more aggressive systemic therapy needs to be initiated.

As the authors articulate, observational studies can suffer from biases and limitations that can only be delineated in the context of a prospective randomized study. Given the small numbers of patient with oligometastatic disease of the liver who are surgical candidates, such a potential study would be a tremendous undertaking and may not be feasible. If the results of NRG-BR002 favor targeting oligometastatic disease, perhaps there will be a renewed interest in a study that focuses on surgical management of BCLM. In the interim, we are left with making the best interpretation of the current limited data, using shared multidisciplinary decision making.

When we think about the intricacies of precision medicine and how to deliver the most personalized therapy options for our patients living with metastatic breast cancer, such care is not solely about genomic markers and disease genetics, but about a more comprehensive, holistic, individualized way of caring for those living with cancer. These considerations include selecting the most precise systemic therapies, evaluating individual response/tolerability, patient preferences, and considering locoregional therapies, such as resection or ablation, in the patients most likely to benefit. Ultimately, if we can chase and catch a cure in a few individuals with metastatic breast cancer, this is critical progress and is life changing.

CLINICS CARE POINTS

- The best candidates for resection of BCLM are individuals who have limited tumor burden, longer disease-free interval, and certain subtypes of breast cancer with sustained response to systemic therapy.
- In clinical practice, there is currently tremendous variability in oligometastatic disease management, which is driven by the predilection of the clinician and personal wishes of the patient.
- Well-designed, randomized trials are needed to critically evaluate the most evidence-based approach for the management of this unique patient population.

DISCLOSURE

The authors have nothing to disclose.

REFERENCES

1. DeSantis CE, Ma J, Gaudet MM, et al. Breast cancer statistics, 2019. CA Cancer J Clin 2019;69(6):438–51.
2. American Cancer Society. Cancer facts & figures, 2020. 2020. Available at: https://www.cancer.org/content/dam/cancer-org/research/cancer-facts-and-statistics/annual-cancer-facts-and-figures/2020/cancer-facts-and-figures-2020.pdf. Accessed March 1, 2020.
3. Mariotto AB, Etzioni R, Hurlbert M, et al. Estimation of the number of women living with metastatic breast cancer in the United States. Cancer Epidemiol Biomarkers Prev 2017;26(6):809–15.
4. Insa A, Lluch A, Prosper F, et al. Prognostic factors predicting survival from first recurrence in patients with metastatic breast cancer: analysis of 439 patients. Breast Cancer Res Treat 1999;56(1):67–78.
5. Hoe AL, Royle GT, Taylor I. Breast liver metastases: incidence, diagnosis and outcome. J R Soc Med 1991;84(12):714–6.
6. Jardines L, Callans LS, Torosian MH. Recurrent breast cancer: presentation, diagnosis, and treatment. Semin Oncol 1993;20(5):538–47.
7. Eichbaum MH, Kaltwasser M, Bruckner T, et al. Prognostic factors for patients with liver metastases from breast cancer. Breast Cancer Res Treat 2006;96(1):53–62.
8. Zinser JW, Hortobagyi GN, Buzdar AU, et al. Clinical course of breast cancer patients with liver metastases. J Clin Oncol 1987;5(5):773–82.
9. Pocard M, Pouillart P, Asselain B, et al. Hepatic resection in metastatic breast cancer: results and prognostic factors. Eur J Surg Oncol 2000;26(2):155–9.
10. Pocard M, Salmon RJ. [Hepatic resection for breast cancer metastasis. The concept of adjuvant surgery]. Bull Cancer 1997;84(1):47–50.
11. Sadot E, Lee SY, Sofocleous CT, et al. Hepatic resection or ablation for isolated breast cancer liver metastasis: a case-control study with comparison to medically treated patients. Ann Surg 2016;264(1):147–54.
12. Margonis GA, Buettner S, Sasaki K, et al. The role of liver-directed surgery in patients with hepatic metastasis from primary breast cancer: a multi-institutional analysis. HPB (Oxford) 2016;18(8):700–5.
13. He X, Zhang Q, Feng Y, et al. Resection of liver metastases from breast cancer: a multicentre analysis. Clin Transl Oncol 2020;22(4):512–21.
14. Ercolani G, Zanello M, Serenari M, et al. Ten-year survival after liver resection for breast metastases: a single-center experience. Dig Surg 2018;35(4):372–80.

15. Labgaa I, Slankamenac K, Schadde E, et al. Liver resection for metastases not of colorectal, neuroendocrine, sarcomatous, or ovarian (NCNSO) origin: a multicentric study. Am J Surg 2018;215(1):125–30.
16. Bergenfeldt M, Jensen BV, Skjoldbye B, et al. Liver resection and local ablation of breast cancer liver metastases: a systematic review. Eur J Surg Oncol 2011; 37(7):549–57.
17. Feng Y, He XG, Zhou CM, et al. Comparison of hepatic resection and systemic treatment of breast cancer liver metastases: a propensity score matching study. Am J Surg 2020 Oct;220(4):945–51.
18. Chun YS, Mizuno T, Cloyd JM, et al. Hepatic resection for breast cancer liver metastases: impact of intrinsic subtypes. Eur J Surg Oncol 2020;46(9):1588–95.
19. Spolverato G, Vitale A, Bagante F, et al. Liver resection for breast cancer liver metastases: a cost-utility Analysis. Ann Surg 2017;265(4):792–9.
20. Vogl TJ, Farshid P, Naguib NN, et al. Thermal ablation therapies in patients with breast cancer liver metastases: a review. Eur Radiol 2013;23(3):797–804.
21. Mack MG, Straub R, Eichler K, et al. Percutaneous MR imaging-guided laser-induced thermotherapy of hepatic metastases. Abdom Imaging 2001;26(4): 369–74.
22. Liang P, Dong B, Yu X, et al. Prognostic factors for percutaneous microwave coagulation therapy of hepatic metastases. AJR Am J Roentgenol 2003;181(5): 1319–25.
23. Abbas H, Erridge S, Sodergren MH, et al. Breast cancer liver metastases in a UK tertiary centre: outcomes following referral to tumour board meeting. Int J Surg 2017;44:152–9.
24. Xiao YB, Zhang B, Wu YL. Radiofrequency ablation versus hepatic resection for breast cancer liver metastasis: a systematic review and meta-analysis. J Zhejiang Univ Sci B 2018;19(11):829–43.

Surgical Management of Neuroendocrine Tumor Liver Metastases

Catherine G. Tran, MD[a], Scott K. Sherman, MD[b],
Chandrikha Chandrasekharan, MBBS[c], James R. Howe, MD[b],*

KEYWORDS

- Neuroendocrine tumor • Liver • Metastasis • Surgery

KEY POINTS

- Cytoreduction of neuroendocrine tumor liver metastases can relieve symptoms and is associated with improved survival.
- Data suggest the target for cytoreduction threshold should be lowered from 90% to 70% because cytoreduction of at least 70% of neuroendocrine liver tumor burden is associated with improved outcomes.
- Parenchymal-sparing procedures (eg, enucleation, ablation, and wedge resections) should be used when possible for cytoreduction.
- For patients who are not surgical candidates, liver-directed and systemic therapies can palliate symptoms and can prolong survival.

INTRODUCTION

Neuroendocrine tumors (NETs) are a group of heterogeneous neoplasms arising from cells of the neuroendocrine system. The term neuroendocrine neoplasia encompasses both well-differentiated NETs and poorly differentiated neuroendocrine carcinomas. NETs produce neurosecretory granules, express characteristic neuroendocrine differentiation markers, and secrete vasoactive substances responsible for carcinoid syndrome. More than one-third of patients with NETs present with distant disease, and the liver is the most common site of distant metastasis.[1,2] Patients

[a] Department of Surgery, University of Iowa Hospitals & Clinics, 200 Hawkins Drive, Iowa City, IA 52242, USA; [b] Department of Surgery, Division of Surgical Oncology and Endocrine Surgery, University of Iowa Carver College of Medicine, 200 Hawkins Drive, Iowa City, IA 52242, USA; [c] Department of Internal Medicine, Division of Hematology, Oncology and Blood and Marrow Transplantation, University of Iowa Carver College of Medicine, 200 Hawkins Drive, Iowa City, IA 52242, USA
* Corresponding author.
E-mail address: james-howe@uiowa.edu

Surg Oncol Clin N Am 30 (2021) 39–55
https://doi.org/10.1016/j.soc.2020.08.001
surgonc.theclinics.com
1055-3207/21/© 2020 Elsevier Inc. All rights reserved.

with NET liver metastases (NETLMs) can have significant hormonal symptoms and worse outcomes compared with patients with isolated locoregional disease.

Treatment of NETs therefore should include effective management of NETLMs, and multiple treatment modalities are available depending on primary site, disease extent, and tumor characteristics. There are 3 categories of treatment options: hepatic resection and cytoreduction, nonsurgical liver-directed therapies, and systemic therapies. This article reviews the epidemiology, presentation, diagnosis, and management of NETLMs.

EPIDEMIOLOGY

The incidence of NETs has increased from 1.09 per 100,000 persons in 1973 to 6.98 per 100,000 persons in 2012,[2] in part because of increased imaging, as well as increased screening and surveillance endoscopy. NET prevalence increased from a 20-year limited-duration prevalence of 0.006% in 1993 to 0.048% in 2012 as a result of increased incidence, the relatively indolent course of these tumors, and improvements in treatment.[2] Approximately 12% to 27% of all patients with NETs present with distant metastasis,[2–4] and the liver is the most frequent site for NET metastasis regardless of primary site.[1] The proportions of patients with pancreatic, cecal, colonic, and small bowel NETs presenting with distant disease are 64%, 44%, 32%, and 30%, respectively.[3] Metastatic disease negatively affects survival, and patients presenting with distant metastases have a 4-fold increased risk of death compared with those with localized disease.[2]

CLINICAL PRESENTATION

Clinical presentation of NETs depends on their primary site, tumor functionality, and patterns of metastasis. Functional small bowel NETs (SBNETs) can secrete bioactive amines such as serotonin, histamine, kallikrein, and tachykinins, causing carcinoid syndrome.[5] Carcinoid syndrome involves a classic triad of diarrhea, flushing, and wheezing. Less common symptoms include valvular heart disease and telangiectasias.[6] Serotonin is thought to cause fibrotic endocardial thickening that distorts the tricuspid and pulmonic valves, leading to valvular regurgitation or stenosis. When severe, carcinoid heart disease causes right-sided heart failure.[5] The liver often inactivates bioactive products released by functional NETs, so patients with carcinoid symptoms have a large tumor burden or liver metastases whose secretory products bypass hepatic inactivation.[5] Pancreatic NETs (PNETs) are nonfunctional in more than 70% of cases, but may also make several hormones, including gastrin, which results in Zollinger-Ellison syndrome and severe ulcer diathesis; insulin, which causes recurrent hypoglycemia; vasoactive intestinal peptide (VIP), which causes hypokalemia, achlorhydria, and watery diarrhea (Verner-Morrison syndrome); glucagon, which leads to hyperglycemia, stomatitis, weight loss, and a migratory necrolytic rash; somatostatin, associated with diabetes, steatorrhea, diarrhea, and cholelithiasis; adrenocorticotrophic hormone (ACTH), producing Cushing syndrome; and parathyroid hormone–related peptide (PTHrP), leading to severe hypercalcemia.[7]

DIAGNOSIS

Diagnosis of NETLMs involves multiple modalities, including biochemical testing, imaging, and pathologic examination. In patients with classic carcinoid symptoms, biochemical testing can confirm a diagnosis of carcinoid syndrome. A 24-hour urinary collection for 5-hydroxyindoleacetic acid (5-HIAA), a product of serotonin metabolism, is the preferred method for carcinoid syndrome diagnosis,[8] although the test is cumbersome and difficult to collect. Blood tumor markers are preferred for monitoring disease progression, recurrence, and response to treatment. Tumor biomarkers used for monitoring NETs include chromogranin A, pancreastatin, neurokinin A, pancreatic polypeptide, substance P, and neuron-specific enolase.[9] Chromogranin A is the most commonly monitored biomarker, although recent data suggest pancreastatin is more sensitive, specific, and accurate for detecting disease progression.[10,11] Hormones can also serve as biomarkers in functional tumors, such as gastrin, insulin, and C peptide, VIP, glucagon, somatostatin, ACTH, or PTHrP.[7]

In patients without classic hormonal symptoms, imaging for abdominal pain or unrelated indications may reveal hepatic lesions that, on biopsy, reveal the diagnosis of NETLM. Work-up and staging of NETs may use anatomic and/or functional imaging. Anatomic imaging includes computed tomography (CT), MRI, and ultrasonography. Functional imaging uses radiolabeled somatostatin analogues, such as [111]indium pentetreotide scintigraphy (Octreoscan) and [68]gallium PET-CT (DOTATATE, DOTATOC, or DOTANOC). NETs with somatostatin receptors take up these radiolabeled somatostatin analogues, facilitating tumor localization and staging (**Fig. 1**A).

CT is often the initial imaging tool used and helps identify the primary tumor and characterize nodal metastases. However, MRI is more sensitive for detecting hepatic

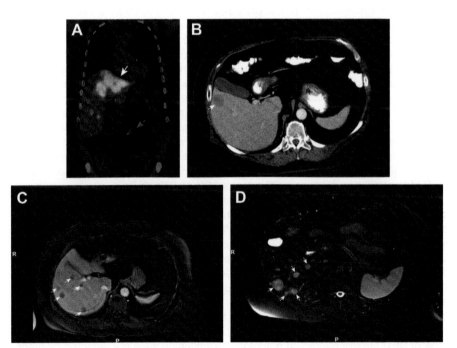

Fig. 1. (A) Coronal ^{68}Ga-DOTATOC PET/CT image of numerous neuroendocrine liver metastases (*white arrow*) from a primary small bowel NET (*red arrow*). (B) Axial CT image of a hypodense neuroendocrine liver metastasis (*white arrow*). (C) Axial T1-weighted MRI of multifocal neuroendocrine liver metastases (*white arrows*). Neuroendocrine liver metastases appear hypointense on T1-weighted MRI. (D) Axial T2-weighted MRI of multifocal neuroendocrine liver metastases (*white arrows*). Neuroendocrine liver metastases appear hyperintense on T2-weighted MRI.

metastasis because of its high contrast resolution.[12,13] Sensitivities for MRI, CT, somatostatin scintigraphy using indium octreotide, and ^{68}Ga-DOTATATE PET-CT for detecting well-differentiated gastroenteropancreatic NETLMs are 95%, 79%, 49%, and 81%, respectively.[12,14] NETs tend to be hypervascular and are best seen on arterial-phase imaging with intravenous contrast. These metastases typically show bright enhancement on arterial-phase CT (**Fig. 1**B), hypointensity on unenhanced T1-weighted MRI (**Fig. 1**C), and hyperintensity on T2-weighted MRI (**Fig. 1**D).[15]

In addition to imaging, pathologic examination of liver biopsy specimens confirms an NET diagnosis. Immunohistochemistry (IHC) staining for neuroendocrine markers, such as synaptophysin and chromogranin A, as well as staining for keratin and somatostatin receptors distinguishes NETLMs from other neoplasms.[16] Pathologic examination should include quantification of Ki-67 proliferative index, which determines the tumor's grade. When the primary site remains unknown despite imaging and endoscopy, extended IHC panels or gene expression classifiers can distinguish small bowel from pancreatic NETs.[17] Positive CDX2 staining suggests a midgut primary, whereas positive PAX6 or ISL1 staining suggests a pancreatic primary.[18]

HEPATIC RESECTION
Resection

Resection or cytoreduction is the preferred first-line treatment of NETLMs, when feasible. Resection or cytoreduction is associated with improved survival, offers relief from hormonal symptoms, and prevents sequelae of carcinoid syndrome, such as carcinoid heart disease. Randomized prospective data are lacking, but retrospective studies suggest that patients who undergo NETLM resection have better symptom relief and prolonged survival compared with patients not undergoing resection. In patients who can be optimally cytoreduced (>90% tumor burden), resection improves symptoms in up to 95% of patients,[19,20] whereas medical treatment alone improves symptoms in 25% to 80% of patients.[20,21] Although comparisons between nonrandomized surgical and medical studies are highly susceptible to the effects of selection bias and carry many caveats, resection of NETLMs is associated with reported 5-year overall survival (OS) rates of 61% to 74%,[19,20,22,23] whereas series of medical NETLM treatment report 5-year OS rates of 25% to 67%.[20,24,25]

Complete resection is the only treatment that offers a potential for cure, although cure is rare. In general, complete resection is only achievable in about 44% to 53% of patients and almost all patients recur after resection.[19,23] Mayo and colleagues[22] found a 5-year recurrence rate of 94% in their series of 339 patients that had resection of NETLMs. Sarmiento and colleagues[19] reported a similar 5-year recurrence rate of 84%, and, even after apparent R0 resections (n = 75), the 5-year recurrence rate was 76%. This finding is caused in part by underestimation of tumor burden by preoperative imaging. Elias and colleagues[26] compared the number of tumors present in 5-mm slices of hepatectomy specimens with those detected by preoperative imaging in patients undergoing hepatectomy for NETLMs (n = 37). The investigators found that 50% of NETLMs discovered on pathologic examination were not detected by preoperative imaging or intraoperative exploration, which used manual palpation and ultrasonography. Half of patients had hepatic metastases smaller than 2 mm, and the accuracy of somatostatin receptor scintigraphy, CT, and MRI in detecting NETLMs was only 24%, 38%, and 29%, respectively.[26] These data show that unrecognized small metastases are present in most patients, and a realistic goal for resection should be to control, rather than to eliminate, disease.

Resection Thresholds

The optimal thresholds for cytoreduction of NETLMs have not been established. With regard to resection margin, more complete resection is associated with improved progression-free survival (PFS) in some series.[19,23] Sarmiento and colleagues[19] found that complete (R0) resection was associated with longer PFS compared with incomplete resection (5-year recurrence rate 76% vs 91%, median PFS 30 vs 16 months, P<.001). In the series by Elias and colleagues,[23] the percentages of patients without progression at 5 years for R0, R1, and R2 resections were 66%, 46%, and 30%, respectively.

In other studies, margin status was not clearly associated with risk of death or progression.[22,27,28] For example, Mayo and colleagues[22] found that margin status was not associated with a statistically significant difference in recurrence, although R0/R1 resection was associated with improved OS compared with R2 resection. Glazer and colleagues[27] did not find a significant correlation with margin status and risk of death, and Graff-Baker and colleagues[28] found that R0 resection was not associated with disease-specific survival compared with R2 resection. The existence of unrecognized low-burden disease even in patients with apparently R0 resections likely explains such findings. Given these data, the North American Neuroendocrine Tumor Society (NANETS) recommends pursuing surgical cytoreduction even when complete resection cannot be obtained, because removal of most of the gross disease can improve symptoms and extend survival.[29]

The optimal threshold of expected cytoreduction to justify an attempt at R2 resection is controversial and continues to evolve. Historically, liver-directed surgery was pursued when at least 90% of liver metastases could be resected. This threshold is attributed to the study by McEntee and colleagues[30] in 1990, but as early as 1977 Foster and Berman[31] and Foster and Lundy[32] suggested that 95% cytoreduction of NETLMs was necessary to palliate symptoms in patients with NETLMs. The notion of a threshold for cytoreduction does not appear in the body of the McEntee and colleagues[30] article, but the discussion introduces it, where the investigators note that patients only experienced symptom relief when 90% of visible tumors were removed.[29] Que and colleagues[33] (n = 74) and Sarmiento and colleagues[19] (n = 170) used this 90% debulking threshold in their series, finding that resection of NETLMs improved symptoms and had favorable outcomes compared with previous studies of patients with unresected NETLMs.

However, recent data suggest that lower debulking thresholds still offer improvement in symptoms and are associated with prolonged survival. In a series by Chambers and colleagues,[34] a 70% or greater reduction of tumor burden effectively palliated carcinoid syndrome symptoms. Graff-Baker and colleagues[28] also used this 70% threshold and compared patients (n = 52) based on the percentage of gross NETLMs resected: 70% to 89%, 90% to 99%, and 100%. Importantly, percentage of disease resected did not correlate with rate of progression or Kaplan-Meier estimates of PFS or disease-free survival. Median liver PFS was 71.6 months and 5-year disease-specific survival was 90%. These outcomes were not significantly improved with increased resection percentage.

Maxwell and colleagues[35] also found associated oncologic value with this 70% threshold in a study of 108 patients with small bowel and pancreatic NETLMs. This series included patients who had a wide range of percentage of NETLMs debulked, from less than 50% to greater than 90%. Patients who had greater than or equal to 70% cytoreduction of NETLMs had improved PFS (median PFS 3.2 vs 1.3 years, P<.001) and OS (median OS not reached vs 6.5 years, P = .009) compared with patients who had less than 70% cytoreduction. Patients who had greater than or equal to 90% cytoreduction did have prolonged PFS compared with those who had less than 90% cytoreduction (median PFS 3.8 vs 1.5 years, $P<.001$), but no difference in OS (median OS not reached vs 6.5 years, $P = .12$). This series also showed that parenchymal-sparing procedures, such as ablation and enucleation, could achieve the 70% cytoreduction threshold, resulting in survival outcomes comparable with those from resection.

In an update and expansion of this series, Scott and colleagues[36] found that this 70% threshold could be reliably obtained in patients with 1 to 5, 6 to 10, or greater than 10 hepatic lesions treated (n = 188; 128 SBNETs, 41 PNETs, and 19 other primary sites). Furthermore, there was no significant difference in PFS in the 3 groups (median PFS 23.3 vs 21.6 vs 21.8 months, $P = .55$) or OS (median OS 80 vs 131.5 vs 89 months, $P = .55$). There were no differences in biochemical response in tumor markers (defined by reduction in hormone levels by >50%, which occurred in 69% of patients), and complication rates between these groups. Grade 3 tumors were associated with worse OS compared with grade 1 (hazard ratio [HR], 11.69; $P<.01$). Overall, greater than or equal to 70% cytoreduction was achieved in 79% of patients, which was determined through careful comparison of preoperative and postoperative anatomic imaging studies. This outcome could be achieved more often in patients with less than 45% liver replacement and when there were fewer than 30 lesions. The median OS was 37.6 months for the less than 70% cytoreduction group, 134.3 months for the 70% to 90% group, and was not reached in those with greater than 90% cytoreduction ($P<.01$ for <70% vs 70%–90% cytoreduction; $P = .6$ for 70%–90% vs >90% cytoreduction). Corresponding PFS was 10.8 months, 20.6 months, and 56.1 months, respectively, for these 3 categories of cytoreduction ($P<.01$ for each comparison). This study showed that cytoreduction was possible in most patients, even when many lesions were present, and that, although PFS improved with increasing levels of cytoreduction, OS was similar whether 70% to 90% or greater than 90% was achieved.

Morgan and colleagues[37] studied the potential value of the 70% threshold in a study of 44 patients with duodenal and pancreatic NETs, which found no significant differences in progression rates between patients who underwent greater than or equal to 70% debulking versus greater than or equal to 90% debulking. Median liver PFS was much lower in these tumors from this primary site (11 months) than their previous reports on SBNETs (71.6 months),[28] but 5-year OS was still high at 81%. Only size greater than 5 cm of the largest resected liver metastasis and formal hepatic resection correlated with rates of liver progression.

Guidelines now recommend considering resection when a 70% debulking threshold is possible.[29,38] Patients with numerous NETLMs, Ki-67 less than 20%, and extrahepatic disease may still be candidates for resection if at least 70% of their NETLMs can be cytoreduced based on careful preoperative imaging evaluation.[36] Guidelines also recommend parenchymal-sparing procedures when possible. Superficial metastases can be enucleated or resected with wedge resections, whereas radiofrequency or microwave ablation can reach deeper lesions, without sacrifice of large volumes of normal liver that anatomic resections might require.[35] Patients with poor performance status, significant comorbidities, severe hepatic dysfunction, or untreated carcinoid heart disease may not benefit from surgery. Patients with high-grade NETLMs or extensive liver replacement with tumor (tumor burden >50%–70%) are also unlikely to benefit from resection.[29,38]

Resection of Primary Tumors with Unresectable Metastases

Whether to resect the primary tumor in patients with unresectable metastases depends on the site, functional status, and symptoms from the primary. In patients with SBNETs, the primary tumor can cause obstruction, mesenteric ischemia, mesenteric fibrosis, and gastrointestinal bleeding. Resection of the small bowel primary can relieve or prevent these symptoms[34] and may improve survival even with unresectable NETLMs. A systematic review of 6 retrospective studies found that resection of the primary in midgut NETs was associated with a trend toward improved survival compared with nonsurgical management of the primary tumor (median OS, 75–139 vs 50–88 months).[39] In comparison, Daskalakis and colleagues[40] performed propensity matching in their retrospective series and concluded that prophylactic resection of asymptomatic primary tumors in patients with stage IV SBNETs was not associated with improved survival compared with no surgery or surgery delayed for greater than 6 months. However, the fact that 58% of patients in the delayed surgery group eventually underwent surgery makes it difficult to conclude that there was no benefit to surgery. Other retrospective series showing benefit are affected by selection bias, so this remains an unanswered question.

Resection of PNETs can improve hormonal symptoms and may extend survival. Franko and colleagues[41] found that patients with nonfunctional PNETs and distant metastases (n = 614) had an associated prolonged survival with resection of the primary tumor compared with no surgical treatment (median survival 8.4 vs 1.1 years, $P<.001$). A recent study evaluating the benefit of peptide receptor radionuclide therapy (PRRT) alone versus resection of the PNET followed by PRRT found longer survival of the latter group (median of 140 vs 58 months in 335 patients; HR, 2.91).[42] Because there are no randomized data regarding the removal of primary PNETs in the setting of unresectable NETLMs, and selection bias is present in retrospective series, these results are difficult to interpret. Guidelines recommend evaluating patients' symptoms, overall health, and tumor characteristics, such as grade and the location of the pancreatic tumor (distal pancreatectomy is less morbid than a Whipple procedure), and potential to improve response to PRRT.[38]

Other Surgical Options

Cytoreduction with heated intraperitoneal chemotherapy (HIPEC) is used in the treatment of appendiceal, colorectal, and mesothelial neoplasms with peritoneal metastases.[43–46] A retrospective French study compared patients with NET peritoneal metastases (n = 41) treated with cytoreduction and HIPEC versus those treated with cytoreduction alone; the 28 HIPEC plus cytoreduction patients were treated from 1994 to 2007, and the 13 cytoreduction-only patients from 2008 to 2012, after the authors had stopped doing HIPEC in these patients.[47] The 2 groups had similar 2-year OS of 81% and 73% (P = .73), and liver recurrence rates (2-year liver metastasis–free survival rates of 61% vs 38%, respectively; P = .12). The study had several significant limitations, including short follow-up time, heterogeneous treatment groups, and treatment of cohorts at different time periods. Current guidelines from neuroendocrine and peritoneal surface malignancy societies do not support HIPEC for treatment of NET peritoneal metastases.[29,48]

The impact of liver transplantation is unknown and its role in the management of NETLM remains controversial. In 1 retrospective European study of 213 patients undergoing liver transplant for NETLMs, median OS was 67 months and PFS was 24 months.[49] Postoperative mortality was 10%, and 11% of patients had to be retransplanted during the first 3 months.[49] A systematic review found that recurrence after liver transplant for NETLMs ranged from 31% to 57%.[50] Given the high rate of recurrence, patient selection is paramount with the understanding that disease-free survival is likely to be limited. Patients considered for transplant should have low-grade tumors, stable disease, their primary tumor removed before transplant, and absence of extrahepatic disease.[51]

Perioperative Considerations

Patients with carcinoid heart disease have increased operative complications, and significant valvular disease should be treated before surgery.[29,52] Even in the absence of hormonal symptoms of carcinoid syndrome, physicians should prepare for possible carcinoid crisis, which is hemodynamic instability thought to be caused by release of vasoactive substances resulting from anesthesia or tumor manipulation.[53] Features of carcinoid crisis include hypotension, flushing, chest pain, pruritus, and paresthesias. The incidence of carcinoid crisis is estimated between 3% and 35% in operations for SBNETs, and octreotide has been used to prevent carcinoid crisis.[54,55] The hormonal basis of carcinoid crisis has not been proved, and some investigators question the role of perioperative octreotide.[54,56] Nevertheless, octreotide may decrease the incidence of carcinoid crisis, the drug is inexpensive, and it does not seem to increase operative complications.[52,55] It is our practice to infuse octreotide at 100 μg/h throughout operations for NETLMs and additional fluids and vasopressors are provided if necessary. We wean the octreotide infusion postoperatively by 25 μg/h every 6 to 8 hours.[57]

LIVER-DIRECTED THERAPY
Ablation

Ablation can be performed during laparotomy for cytoreduction, laparoscopically, or percutaneously by interventional radiology. Ablative techniques include radiofrequency ablation, microwave ablation, cryotherapy, and irreversible electroporation. As an adjunct to resection, ablation can minimize the loss of normal liver tissue and allows improved cytoreduction by destroying tumors not amenable to resection. Intraoperative ultrasonography guides identification of lesions and ablation probe placement.[35,58] Smaller tumors (<3 cm in diameter) are more amenable to ablation and have decreased likelihood of local recurrence.[51] Ablation is not recommended for tumors near vital structures or tumors greater than 5 cm in diameter because of increased risk of complication and recurrence, based on studies of hepatocellular carcinoma and colorectal liver metastases.[59,60]

Prospective data are lacking, but ablation alone seems to be effective for palliation of symptoms and may provide some survival benefit. Akyildiz and colleagues[61] reported in a retrospective study of 89 patients that ablation of NETLM improved hormonal symptoms in 97% of patients for a median of 14 months. Disease-free survival in that study was 15 months, with 60% of patients developing new liver or extrahepatic metastases, and OS was 6 years.[61] The 5-year survival rate was 57%, which is lower than the 5-year survival rate of 74% reported in the study by Mayo and colleagues[22] of patients undergoing surgical resection and ablation.[61] Ablation seems relatively safe, with a morbidity rate around 6%.[61] Most of the patients reported by Scott and colleagues[36] had ablations performed with or without resection, with median OS of 134 months when greater than 70% cytoreduction could be achieved, with no mortality and a complication rate of 52% (15% Clavien-Dindo grade III–IV). Complications include hemorrhage, hematoma, pneumothorax, and neuritis where the probe enters the skin.[61,62]

Intra-arterial Therapies

Hepatic arterial embolization is another useful option for improving hormonal symptoms and slowing tumor growth in patients with NETLMs. Hypervascular NETLMs derive most of their blood supply from the hepatic artery, whereas the hepatic parenchyma has a dual blood supply but receives most from the portal vein.[62] Occlusion of arterial branches to NETLMs therefore induces tumor ischemia and necrosis with relative sparing of hepatic parenchyma. Types of embolization include bland transarterial embolization (TAE); transarterial chemoembolization (TACE), which administers doxorubicin or other chemotherapeutic agents to the tumor; and radioembolization with radionuclide ^{90}yttrium, which uses smaller bead sizes to enhance distribution of particles in more distal tumor vessels.

Intra-arterial therapies are generally used for palliation in patients whose hepatic tumor burden precludes surgical cytoreduction, and for less invasive treatment of symptoms. Bland embolization and chemoembolization can induce symptomatic improvements in 53% to 100% of patients for a duration of 10 to 55 months.[62] Five-year OS rates range from 40% to 83%.[62] Mayo and colleagues[63] compared 753 patients with NETLMs who underwent resection with those who underwent intra-arterial therapy (TAE, TACE, placement of drug-eluting beads, or selective internal radiation therapy with ^{90}yttrium). Propensity score matching was used to determine a subset of patients who underwent intra-arterial therapy with similar baseline characteristics to the surgical cohort. The study found that surgery and intra-arterial therapy had no difference in survival for patients with greater than 25% liver tumor burden and no symptoms, suggesting intra-arterial therapy may be an appropriate strategy in this cohort of patients. In comparison, surgery was associated with better survival in patients with less than 25% liver tumor burden (survival 84 vs 39 months for embolization, $P = .045$).

Morbidity with intra-arterial therapies occurs in approximately 25% of patients. A common complication is postembolization syndrome, which manifests as fever, leukocytosis, and abdominal pain and can be particularly sever in patients with high tumor burdens.[62,64] Absolute and relative contraindications to TAE and TACE include portal vein thrombosis, hepatic insufficiency, and history of a Whipple procedure (because of increased risk of hepatic abscess formation).[51]

SYSTEMIC THERAPIES
Somatostatin Analogues

In addition to treating hormonal symptoms, somatostatin analogues (SSAs) can stabilize tumor size and delay progression. The antitumor effect of SSAs was established by the phase III Placebo-Controlled, Double-Blind, Prospective, Randomized Study on the Effect of Octreotide LAR in the Control of Tumor Growth in Patients with Metastatic Neuroendocrine Midgut Tumors (PROMID) trial.[65] This study found that long-acting octreotide (30 mg intramuscularly every 4 weeks) stabilized tumor growth and decreased the risk of progression (HR, 0.33; $P<.001$) in patients with advanced (unresectable or metastatic) well-differentiated midgut NETs (n = 85).[65] Longer-term follow-up did not reveal a statistically significant difference in OS between placebo-treated and octreotide-treated groups, but the high rate of crossover to the treatment group on progression limited the ability to interpret the OS outcomes.[24] The Controlled Study of Lanreotide Antiproliferative Response in Neuroendocrine Tumors (CLARINET) trial confirmed the antitumor effects of SSAs in metastatic gastroenteropancreatic NETs (n = 204), finding that lanreotide (120 mg subcutaneously every 4 weeks) improved PFS compared with placebo (median PFS not reached vs 18 months,

$P<.002$).[66] As in the PROMID study, there were no significant differences in quality of life or OS, and the CLARINET study was also complicated by crossover from the placebo to the treatment group after progression. Taken together, these studies show that SSAs are an effective first-line treatment of hormonal symptoms and stabilization of disease in metastatic gastroenteropancreatic NETs.

Molecularly Targeted Therapies

Everolimus, a mammalian target of rapamycin (mTOR) inhibitor, is a treatment option for patients who progress on SSAs. The RAD001 in Advanced Neuroendocrine Tumors (RADIANT)-3 trial studied the efficacy of everolimus (10 mg/d orally) in patients with advanced low-grade or intermediate-grade PNETs (n = 410).[67] This study found that PFS was longer in patients treated with everolimus compared with placebo (median PFS, 11 vs 4.6 months; $P<.001$). Treated patients were also less likely to progress or die (HR, 0.35; $P<.001$). In the RADIANT-4 trial, the efficacy of everolimus was confirmed for advanced, well-differentiated, grade 1 or 2 NETs of the lung and gastrointestinal tract. In this phase III trial (n = 302), patients treated with everolimus had longer median PFS compared with those treated with placebo (median PFS, 11.0 vs 3.9 months; $P<.001$) and decreased risk of progression or death (HR, 0.48; $P<.001$).[68]

Another molecularly targeted therapy for advanced NETs is sunitinib, a vascular endothelial growth factor inhibitor. Sunitinib was studied in a randomized controlled study of 171 patients with progressive, advanced, well-differentiated pancreatic NETs. Patients treated with sunitinib (37.5 mg/d orally) had improved PFS compared with those in the placebo group (median PFS, 11.4 vs 5.5 months; HR for progression or death, 0.42; $P<.001$).[69] Sunitinib also stabilized disease and improved OS (HR of death, 0.41; $P = .02$). The study was terminated early because of the risk of adverse events, progression, and death in the placebo group. Based on this trial, sunitinib was US Food and Drug Administration approved for use in progressive, unresectable, and advanced pancreatic NETs.

Peptide Receptor Radionuclide Therapy

PRRT is a treatment option for patients who progress on SSAs, and involves the administration of a radionuclide, primarily [90]yttrium or [177]lutetium, conjugated to an SSA to selectively deliver radiation to NET cells.[70] The phase III Neuroendocrine Tumors Therapy (NETTER)-1 trial randomized patients to ^{177}Lu-DOTATATE and low-dose octreotide or high-dose long-acting octreotide (60 mg every 4 weeks) in 299 patients. The ^{177}Lu-DOTATATE treatment group had improved 20-month PFS rate compared with the control group (65% vs 11%), with HR for progression or death of 0.21 ($P<.001$). Median PFS was improved in the ^{177}Lu-DOTATATE group (median PFS not reached vs 8.4 months), and the HR for death in the ^{177}Lu-DOTATATE group compared with control was 0.4 ($P = .004$). There was also improved tumor response with PRRT compared with octreotide (objective response rate 18% vs 3%, $P<.001$). Therefore, PRRT is an effective treatment of metastatic well-differentiated NETs that express somatostatin receptors and have progressed despite SSA therapy.

Chemotherapy

Chemotherapy is generally indicated for higher-grade NETs such as neuroendocrine carcinomas, and advanced PNETs.[51,71] Neuroendocrine carcinomas (poorly differentiated, Ki-67>20%) are generally treated with platinum-based regimens, such as cisplatin or carboplatin in combination with etoposide.[72,73] Response rates to this regimen are only about 30% and prognosis remains poor, with median PFS of 4 months and median OS of 11 months.[74] In PNETs, streptozocin-based regimens with 5-fluorouracil or doxorubicin have been used with response rates of around 40% in older series, but are not commonly used currently.[75] The regimen of capecitabine and temozolamide (CAPTEM) has promising results in preliminary studies of advanced PNETs, with response rates greater than 50%.[76,77] The Eastern Cooperative Oncology Group (ECOG) 2211 trial resulted in preliminary data that CAPTEM (capecitabine 750 mg/m^2 by mouth twice day on days 1–14, temozolomide 200 mg/m^2 by mouth days 10–14) improved PFS compared with temozolamide alone (median PFS, 22.7 vs 14.4 months; $P = .023$).[78] CAPTEM shows lower efficacy in gastrointestinal NETs, with overall response rates of around 15%.[79] It remains an option for patients with progressive intestinal NETs who have failed other treatments.[51]

SUMMARY

A significant number of patients with NETs develop hepatic metastases, which can cause hormonal symptoms and negatively affect survival. Although prospective data comparing resection with other treatment modalities are lacking, resection and cytoreduction seem to improve symptoms and are associated with better survival outcomes. Cytoreduction should be considered when at least 70% of a patient's NETLMs can be resected, with treatment decisions depending on patient factors, tumor characteristics, and tumor burden. Instead of major formal hepatic resections, parenchymal-sparing procedures, such as wedge resections, enucleations, and ablations, should be used when possible. Liver-directed and systemic therapies can palliate symptoms and improve survival in patients who are not surgical candidates. Treatment of NETLMs requires a multidisciplinary approach, and patients with NETLMs should be referred to centers with experience caring for such patients to optimize patient quality of life and outcomes.

The medical oncologist's perspective

Surgical management of liver metastases is considered in select gastrointestinal cancers, including colon cancer, gastrointestinal stromal tumors, and NETs. In addition to resectability, many other factors, such as the primary site of origin, grade and differentiation of the tumor, hormone hypersecretion, and patient symptoms, have to be taken into account before considering surgical resection of NETLMs. Although a randomized controlled clinical trial will best answer the question of whether surgery for NETLMs improves OS in advanced gastroenteropancreatic (GEP) NETs, conducting such a trial is impractical because of the indolent nature of the tumor and inherent selection bias, among other factors. Thus, the authors rely largely on the retrospective single-institutional and multi-institutional series discussed in detail in this article. While reviewing these data, remember that some series predate widespread availability of newer therapeutic options such as everolimus, sunitinib, or PRRT that have shown improvement in PFS and a trend toward improved OS in rigorous randomized clinical trials. Furthermore, with the increasing use of the sensitive [68]gallium-DOTATATE PET/CT imaging for initial staging, surgical plans may be altered to include more invasive or less invasive approaches based on detection of additional sites of disease.[80,81]

In a recent meta-analysis of 11 cohort studies that included 1108 patients, 5 studies (n = 506) reported outcomes on liver metastases resection versus no liver metastases resection.[82] Although the meta-analysis showed that 5-year OS was in favor of liver metastases resection (OR, 0.15; 95% confidence interval, 0.05–0.42; $P = .0003$), the authors noted a high risk of selection bias and significant heterogeneity. The European working group on neuroendocrine liver metastases recommended liver resection as the first choice for patients with completely resectable grade 1 and grade 2 liver metastases and no resectable extrahepatic disease. However, the group also noted that the role of cytoreductive surgery when alternative nonsurgical options are available is unknown.[83] The recently published NANETS guidelines on surgical management of pancreatic NETs addressed the question of liver cytoreduction in detail.[38] Although more than half the panel thought that symptom control and survival could be improved with more than 70% cytoreduction, this was noted to be a controversial area with level III evidence. There is perhaps even more controversy about whether resection of the primary tumor is warranted in patients with unresectable liver metastases because of the lack of prospective data. Although removal of the primary tumor may have a role in preventing symptoms caused by the location of the tumor, especially in SBNETs, the premise that this may prevent further liver metastases, or seeding, has very weak evidence in the literature.

Because most patients undergoing surgery for NETLM have recurrent disease and surgery is not curative, the morbidity of the surgery has to be weighed against other available therapeutic options in individual patients. When surgery is offered, it is also important to discuss with the patient the goal of this intervention: whether the primary objective of surgical cytoreduction is symptom control or for a potential survival advantage. A one-size-fits-all approach based on an algorithm is clearly not suitable for this disease. All patients with NET deserve a multidisciplinary approach to help them make an informed choice regarding their care. Despite the lack of prospective trial data, surgery at high-volume centers with expertise remains an important part of the treatment paradigm in advanced gastroenteropancreatic NETs.

CLINICS CARE POINTS

- Cytoreduction of neuroendocrine tumor liver metastases can improve symptoms and survival.
- Systemic therapies are associated with improved survival outcomes in patients with metastatic neuroendocrine tumors.
- Patients with neuroendocrine tumors often benefit from multidisciplinary care at specialized centers.

ACKNOWLEDGMENTS

This work was supported by NIH grants no. T32CA148062 (C.G. Tran), T32CA078586 (S.K. Sherman), and Specialized Programs of Research Excellence grant no. P50 CA174521-01 (J.R. Howe).

DISCLOSURE

Dr C. Chandrasekharan serves on the advisory board of Lexicon Pharmaceuticals. The other authors have nothing to disclose.

REFERENCES

1. Riihimäki M, Hemminki A, Sundquist K, et al. The epidemiology of metastases in neuroendocrine tumors. Int J Cancer 2016;139(12):2679–86.
2. Dasari A, Shen C, Halperin D, et al. Trends in the Incidence, Prevalence, and Survival Outcomes in Patients With Neuroendocrine Tumors in the United States. JAMA Oncol 2017;3(10):1335–42.
3. Yao JC, Hassan M, Phan A, et al. One hundred years after "carcinoid": epidemiology of and prognostic factors for neuroendocrine tumors in 35,825 cases in the United States. J Clin Oncol 2008;26(18):3063–72.
4. Modlin IM, Lye KD, Kidd M. A 5-decade analysis of 13,715 carcinoid tumors. Cancer 2003;97(4):934–59.
5. Vinik AI, Chaya C. Clinical Presentation and Diagnosis of Neuroendocrine Tumors. Hematol Oncol Clin North Am 2016;30(1):21–48.
6. Modlin IM, Kidd M, Latich I, et al. Current status of gastrointestinal carcinoids. Gastroenterology 2005;128(6):1717–51.

7. Scott AT, Howe JR. Evaluation and Management of Neuroendocrine Tumors of the Pancreas. Surg Clin North Am 2019;99(4):793–814.

8. Shah MH, Goldner WS, Halfdanarson TR, et al. NCCN Guidelines Insights: Neuroendocrine and Adrenal Tumors, Version 2.2018. J Natl Compr Canc Netw 2018; 16(6):693–702.

9. Modlin IM, Bodei L, Kidd M. Neuroendocrine tumor biomarkers: From monoanalytes to transcripts and algorithms. Best Pract Res Clin Endocrinol Metab 2016; 30(1):59–77.

10. Sherman SK, Maxwell JE, O'Dorisio MS, et al. Pancreastatin predicts survival in neuroendocrine tumors. Ann Surg Oncol 2014;21(9):2971–80.

11. Tran CG, Sherman SK, Scott AT, et al. It Is Time to Rethink Biomarkers for Surveillance of Small Bowel Neuroendocrine Tumors. Ann Surg Oncol 2020. https://doi.org/10.1245/s10434-020-08784-0.

12. Dromain C, de Baere T, Lumbroso J, et al. Detection of liver metastases from endocrine tumors: a prospective comparison of somatostatin receptor scintigraphy, computed tomography, and magnetic resonance imaging. J Clin Oncol 2005;23(1):70–8.

13. Dromain C, de Baere T, Baudin E, et al. MR imaging of hepatic metastases caused by neuroendocrine tumors: comparing four techniques. AJR Am J Roentgenol 2003;180(1):121–8.

14. Haug AR, Cindea-Drimus R, Auernhammer CJ, et al. The role of 68Ga-DOTATATE PET/CT in suspected neuroendocrine tumors. J Nucl Med 2012;53(11):1686–92.

15. Horton KM, Kamel I, Hofmann L, et al. Carcinoid Tumors of the Small Bowel: A Multitechnique Imaging Approach. Am J Roentgenol 2004;182(3):559–67.

16. Klimstra DS, Modlin IR, Adsay NV, et al. Pathology reporting of neuroendocrine tumors: application of the Delphic consensus process to the development of a minimum pathology data set. Am J Surg Pathol 2010;34(3):300–13.

17. Sherman SK, Maxwell JE, Carr JC, et al. Gene expression accurately distinguishes liver metastases of small bowel and pancreas neuroendocrine tumors. Clin Exp Metastasis 2014;31(8):935–44.

18. Maxwell JE, Sherman SK, Stashek KM, et al. A practical method to determine the site of unknown primary in metastatic neuroendocrine tumors. Surgery 2014; 156(6):1359–65 [discussion: 1365–6].

19. Sarmiento JM, Heywood G, Rubin J, et al. Surgical treatment of neuroendocrine metastases to the liver: a plea for resection to increase survival. J Am Coll Surg 2003;197(1):29–37.

20. Touzios JG, Kiely JM, Pitt SC, et al. Neuroendocrine hepatic metastases: does aggressive management improve survival? Ann Surg 2005;241(5):776–83 [discussion: 783–5].

21. Strosberg JR, Benson AB, Huynh L, et al. Clinical benefits of above-standard dose of octreotide LAR in patients with neuroendocrine tumors for control of carcinoid syndrome symptoms: a multicenter retrospective chart review study. The oncologist 2014;19(9):930–6.

22. Mayo SC, de Jong MC, Pulitano C, et al. Surgical management of hepatic neuroendocrine tumor metastasis: results from an international multi-institutional analysis. Ann Surg Oncol 2010;17(12):3129–36.

23. Elias D, Lasser P, Ducreux M, et al. Liver resection (and associated extrahepatic resections) for metastatic well-differentiated endocrine tumors: a 15-year single center prospective study. Surgery 2003;133(4):375–82.

24. Rinke A, Wittenberg M, Schade-Brittinger C, et al. Placebo-Controlled, Double-Blind, Prospective, Randomized Study on the Effect of Octreotide LAR in the

Control of Tumor Growth in Patients with Metastatic Neuroendocrine Midgut Tumors (PROMID): Results of Long-Term Survival. Neuroendocrinology 2017; 104(1):26–32.

25. Yao JC, Pavel M, Lombard-Bohas C, et al. Everolimus for the Treatment of Advanced Pancreatic Neuroendocrine Tumors: Overall Survival and Circulating Biomarkers From the Randomized, Phase III RADIANT-3 Study. J Clin Oncol 2016;34(32):3906–13.

26. Elias D, Lefevre JH, Duvillard P, et al. Hepatic Metastases From Neuroendocrine Tumors With a "Thin Slice" Pathological Examination: They are Many More Than You Think. Ann Surg 2010;251(2):307–10.

27. Glazer ES, Tseng JF, Al-Refaie W, et al. Long-term survival after surgical management of neuroendocrine hepatic metastases. HPB (Oxford) 2010;12(6):427–33.

28. Graff-Baker AN, Sauer DA, Pommier SJ, et al. Expanded criteria for carcinoid liver debulking: Maintaining survival and increasing the number of eligible patients. Surgery 2014;156(6):1369–76 [discussion: 1376–7].

29. Howe JR, Cardona K, Fraker DL, et al. The Surgical Management of Small Bowel Neuroendocrine Tumors: Consensus Guidelines of the North American Neuroendocrine Tumor Society. Pancreas 2017;46(6):715–31.

30. McEntee GP, Nagorney DM, Kvols LK, et al. Cytoreductive hepatic surgery for neuroendocrine tumors. Surgery 1990;108(6):1091–6.

31. Foster JH, Berman MM. Solid liver tumors. Major Probl Clin Surg 1977;22:1–342.

32. Foster JH, Lundy J. Liver metastases. Curr Probl Surg 1981;18(3):157–202.

33. Que FG, Nagorney DM, Batts KP, et al. Hepatic resection for metastatic neuroendocrine carcinomas. Am J Surg 1995;169(1):36–42 [discussion: 42–3].

34. Chambers AJ, Pasieka JL, Dixon E, et al. The palliative benefit of aggressive surgical intervention for both hepatic and mesenteric metastases from neuroendocrine tumors. Surgery 2008;144(4):645–51 [discussion: 651–3].

35. Maxwell JE, Sherman SK, O'Dorisio TM, et al. Liver-directed surgery of neuroendocrine metastases: What is the optimal strategy? Surgery 2016;159(1):320–33.

36. Scott AT, Breheny PJ, Keck KJ, et al. Effective cytoreduction can be achieved in patients with numerous neuroendocrine tumor liver metastases (NETLMs). Surgery 2019;165(1):166–75.

37. Morgan RE, Pommier SJ, Pommier RF. Expanded criteria for debulking of liver metastasis also apply to pancreatic neuroendocrine tumors. Surgery 2018; 163(1):218–25.

38. Howe JR, Merchant NB, Conrad C, et al. The North American Neuroendocrine Tumor Society Consensus Paper on the Surgical Management of Pancreatic Neuroendocrine Tumors. Pancreas 2020;49(1):1–33.

39. Capurso G, Rinzivillo M, Bettini R, et al. Systematic review of resection of primary midgut carcinoid tumour in patients with unresectable liver metastases. Br J Surg 2012;99(11):1480–6.

40. Daskalakis K, Karakatsanis A, Hessman O, et al. Association of a Prophylactic Surgical Approach to Stage IV Small Intestinal Neuroendocrine Tumors With Survival. JAMA Oncol 2018;4(2):183–9.

41. Franko J, Feng W, Yip L, et al. Non-functional neuroendocrine carcinoma of the pancreas: incidence, tumor biology, and outcomes in 2,158 patients. J Gastrointest Surg 2010;14(3):541–8.

42. Kaemmerer D, Twrznik M, Kulkarni HR, et al. Prior Resection of the Primary Tumor Prolongs Survival After Peptide Receptor Radionuclide Therapy of Advanced Neuroendocrine Neoplasms. Ann Surg 2019. March 1, 2019 - Volume Publish Ahead of Print - Issue - https://doi.org/10.1097/SLA.0000000000003237.

43. Glehen O, Gilly FN, Boutitie F, et al. Toward curative treatment of peritoneal carcinomatosis from nonovarian origin by cytoreductive surgery combined with perioperative intraperitoneal chemotherapy: a multi-institutional study of 1,290 patients. Cancer 2010;116(24):5608–18.
44. Jacobson R, Sherman SK, Dahdaleh F, et al. Peritoneal Metastases in Colorectal Cancer. Ann Surg Oncol 2018;25(8):2145–51.
45. The Chicago Consensus on Peritoneal Surface Malignancies: Management of Appendiceal Neoplasms. Ann Surg Oncol 2020;27(6):1753–60.
46. The Chicago Consensus on peritoneal surface malignancies: Management of peritoneal mesothelioma. Cancer 2020;126(11):2547–52.
47. Elias D, David A, Sourrouille I, et al. Neuroendocrine carcinomas: optimal surgery of peritoneal metastases (and associated intra-abdominal metastases). Surgery 2014;155(1):5–12.
48. Chicago Consensus Working Group. The Chicago Consensus on Peritoneal Surface Malignancies: Management of Neuroendocrine Tumors. Ann Surg Oncol 2020;27(6):1788–92.
49. Le Treut YP, Gregoire E, Klempnauer J, et al. Liver transplantation for neuroendocrine tumors in Europe-results and trends in patient selection: a 213-case European liver transplant registry study. Ann Surg 2013;257(5):807–15.
50. Moris D, Tsilimigras DI, Ntanasis-Stathopoulos I, et al. Liver transplantation in patients with liver metastases from neuroendocrine tumors: A systematic review. Surgery 2017;162(3):525–36.
51. Pavel M, Baudin E, Couvelard A, et al. ENETS Consensus Guidelines for the management of patients with liver and other distant metastases from neuroendocrine neoplasms of foregut, midgut, hindgut, and unknown primary. Neuroendocrinology 2012;95(2):157–76.
52. Kinney MA, Warner ME, Nagorney DM, et al. Perianaesthetic risks and outcomes of abdominal surgery for metastatic carcinoid tumours. Br J Anaesth 2001;87(3): 447–52.
53. Kahil ME, Brown H, Fred HL. The Carcinoid Crisis. Arch Intern Med 1964; 114(1):26–8.
54. Condron ME, Jameson NE, Limbach KE, et al. A prospective study of the pathophysiology of carcinoid crisis. Surgery 2019;165(1):158–65.
55. Woltering EA, Wright AE, Stevens MA, et al. Development of effective prophylaxis against intraoperative carcinoid crisis. J Clin Anesth 2016;32:189–93.
56. Massimino K, Harrskog O, Pommier S, et al. Octreotide LAR and bolus octreotide are insufficient for preventing intraoperative complications in carcinoid patients. J Surg Oncol 2013;107(8):842–6.
57. Tran CG, Sherman SK, Howe JR. Small bowel neuroendocrine tumors. Curr Probl Surg, in press. 2020:100823. https://doi.org/10.1016/j.cpsurg.2020.100823
58. Gamblin TC, Christians K, Pappas SG. Radiofrequency ablation of neuroendocrine hepatic metastasis. Surg Oncol Clin N Am 2011;20(2):273–9, vii-viii.
59. Elias D, Baton O, Sideris L, et al. Hepatectomy plus intraoperative radiofrequency ablation and chemotherapy to treat technically unresectable multiple colorectal liver metastases. J Surg Oncol 2005;90(1):36–42.
60. N'Kontchou G, Mahamoudi A, Aout M, et al. Radiofrequency ablation of hepatocellular carcinoma: long-term results and prognostic factors in 235 Western patients with cirrhosis. Hepatology 2009;50(5):1475–83.
61. Akyildiz HY, Mitchell J, Milas M, et al. Laparoscopic radiofrequency thermal ablation of neuroendocrine hepatic metastases: long-term follow-up. Surgery 2010; 148(6):1288–93 [discussion: 1293].

62. Vogl TJ, Naguib NN, Zangos S, et al. Liver metastases of neuroendocrine carcinomas: interventional treatment via transarterial embolization, chemoembolization and thermal ablation. Eur J Radiol 2009;72(3):517–28.

63. Mayo SC, de Jong MC, Bloomston M, et al. Surgery versus intra-arterial therapy for neuroendocrine liver metastasis: a multicenter international analysis. Ann Surg Oncol 2011;18(13):3657–65.

64. Ruutiainen AT, Soulen MC, Tuite CM, et al. Chemoembolization and bland embolization of neuroendocrine tumor metastases to the liver. J Vasc Interv Radiol 2007;18(7):847–55.

65. Rinke A, Muller HH, Schade-Brittinger C, et al. Placebo-controlled, double-blind, prospective, randomized study on the effect of octreotide LAR in the control of tumor growth in patients with metastatic neuroendocrine midgut tumors: a report from the PROMID Study Group. J Clin Oncol 2009;27(28):4656–63.

66. Caplin ME, Pavel M, Cwikla JB, et al. Lanreotide in metastatic enteropancreatic neuroendocrine tumors. N Engl J Med 2014;371(3):224–33.

67. Yao JC, Shah MH, Ito T, et al. Everolimus for advanced pancreatic neuroendocrine tumors. N Engl J Med 2011;364(6):514–23.

68. Yao JC, Fazio N, Singh S, et al. Everolimus for the treatment of advanced, nonfunctional neuroendocrine tumours of the lung or gastrointestinal tract (RADIANT-4): a randomised, placebo-controlled, phase 3 study. Lancet 2016; 387(10022):968–77.

69. Raymond E, Dahan L, Raoul JL, et al. Sunitinib malate for the treatment of pancreatic neuroendocrine tumors. N Engl J Med 2011;364(6):501–13.

70. Sherman SK, Howe JR. Translational research in endocrine surgery. Surg Oncol Clin N Am 2013;22(4):857–84.

71. Kunz PL, Reidy-Lagunes D, Anthony LB, et al. Consensus guidelines for the management and treatment of neuroendocrine tumors. Pancreas 2013;42(4):557–77.

72. Garcia-Carbonero R, Rinke A, Valle JW, et al. ENETS Consensus Guidelines for the Standards of Care in Neuroendocrine Neoplasms: Systemic Therapy - Chemotherapy. Neuroendocrinology 2017;105(3):281–94.

73. Moertel CG, Kvols LK, O'Connell MJ, et al. Treatment of neuroendocrine carcinomas with combined etoposide and cisplatin. Evidence of major therapeutic activity in the anaplastic variants of these neoplasms. Cancer 1991;68(2):227–32.

74. Sorbye H, Welin S, Langer SW, et al. Predictive and prognostic factors for treatment and survival in 305 patients with advanced gastrointestinal neuroendocrine carcinoma (WHO G3): the NORDIC NEC study. Ann Oncol 2013;24(1):152–60.

75. Kouvaraki MA, Ajani JA, Hoff P, et al. Fluorouracil, doxorubicin, and streptozocin in the treatment of patients with locally advanced and metastatic pancreatic endocrine carcinomas. J Clin Oncol 2004;22(23):4762–71.

76. Cives M, Ghayouri M, Morse B, et al. Analysis of potential response predictors to capecitabine/temozolomide in metastatic pancreatic neuroendocrine tumors. Endocr Relat Cancer 2016;23(9):759–67.

77. Strosberg JR, Fine RL, Choi J, et al. First-line chemotherapy with capecitabine and temozolomide in patients with metastatic pancreatic endocrine carcinomas. Cancer 2011;117(2):268–75.

78. Kunz PL, Catalano PJ, Nimeiri HS, et al. A randomized study of temozolomide or temozolomide and capecitabine in patients with advanced pancreatic neuroendocrine tumors: A trial of the ECOG-ACRIN Cancer Research Group (E2211). J Clin Oncol 2015;33(15_suppl):TPS4145.

79. de Mestier L, Walter T, Brixi H, et al. Comparison of Temozolomide-Capecitabine to 5-Fluorouracile-Dacarbazine in 247 Patients with Advanced Digestive

Neuroendocrine Tumors Using Propensity Score Analyses. Neuroendocrinology 2019;108(4):343–53.

80. Ilhan H, Fendler WP, Cyran CC, et al. Impact of (68)Ga-DOTATATE PET/CT on the surgical management of primary neuroendocrine tumors of the pancreas or ileum. Ann Surg Oncol 2015;22(1):164–71.

81. Crown A, Rocha FG, Raghu P, et al. Impact of initial imaging with gallium-68 do-tatate PET/CT on diagnosis and management of patients with neuroendocrine tu-mors. Surg Oncol 2020;121(3):480–5.

82. Kaçmaz E, Heidsma CM, Besselink MGH, et al. Treatment of Liver Metastases from Midgut Neuroendocrine Tumours: A Systematic Review and Meta-Analysis. J Clin Med 2019;8(3):403.

83. Frilling A, Modlin IM, Kidd M, et al. Recommendations for management of pa-tients with neuroendocrine liver metastases. Lancet Oncol 2014;15(1):e8–21.

Surgical Management of Sarcoma Metastatic to Liver

Brett L. Ecker, MD[a],*, Robert G. Maki, MD, PhD[b], Michael J. Cavnar, MD[c],
Ronald P. DeMatteo, MD[a]

KEYWORDS

- Sarcoma • Metastasis • Gastrointestinal stromal tumor • GIST • Imatinib
- Hepatic tumor

KEY POINTS

- Sarcomas represent a diverse group of uncommon tumors.
- Systemic therapies are often of limited benefit in many sarcomas.
- Partial hepatectomy may improve long-term outcomes in certain histologies, of which GIST and leiomyosarcoma are the most frequently studied.
- Liver resection in highly selected patients with GIST can achieve prolonged disease control when combined with tyrosine kinase inhibitors.
- Further advances for many of the sarcoma subtypes will depend on the development of improved systemic therapies.

INTRODUCTION

Sarcomas are rare mesenchymal tumors that comprise more than 70 subtypes and have a propensity for hematogenous metastasis. Hepatic metastases are uncommon for soft tissue tumors of the extremities, but may be observed in approximately 16% of patients with retroperitoneal sarcomas and 62% of patients with visceral sarcomas.[1] Gastrointestinal stromal tumor (GIST) is the most common histologic subtype of sarcoma[2] and the most common source of hepatic metastases, both overall and in the subset of patients who undergo partial hepatectomy.[3] Current therapeutic modalities for sarcoma metastatic to the liver include targeted therapy and chemotherapy, tumor ablation, trans-arterial embolization, and resection.

SYSTEMIC THERAPIES

Chemotherapy alone for patients with advanced non-GIST soft tissue sarcoma with hepatic metastasis is associated with poor response rates. In pooled analyses of

[a] Department of Surgery, University of Pennsylvania, 3400 Spruce st, Philadelphia, PA 19104, USA; [b] Department of Medicine, University of Pennsylvania, 3400 Spruce st, Philadelphia, PA 19104, USA; [c] Department of Surgery, University of Kentucky, 800 Rose St First Floor, Lexington, KY 40536, USA
* Corresponding author.
E-mail address: Brett.Ecker@uphs.upenn.edu

Surg Oncol Clin N Am 30 (2021) 57–67
https://doi.org/10.1016/j.soc.2020.08.002
surgonc.theclinics.com

European Organization for Research and Treatment of Cancer (EORTC) trials of doxorubicin-containing or epirubicin-containing regimens, median overall survival (OS) was 10 months.[4] Likewise, analyses of EORTC trials for advanced soft tissue sarcoma using first-line ifosfamide-containing regimens demonstrated median OS of 12 months, and patients with unresectable hepatic metastases had worse response rates and inferior progression-free survival relative to those with metastases to other sites.[5] There are no completed randomized trials comparing surgery versus systemic therapy for hepatic metastasis of any sarcoma histology, underscoring the rarity of this clinical entity and the infrequent use of liver resection for non-GIST sarcomas.

Metastatic GIST is unresponsive to conventional cytotoxic agents, with response rates generally less than 5%.[6] GIST typically harbors a mutation in *KIT*, or less frequently in *PDGFRA*. Targeted therapy directed against the oncogenic KIT and PDGFR tyrosine kinases has been proven highly effective. The median OS in the landmark trial of imatinib, in which 95% of patients had hepatic involvement, was 57 months.[7,8] However, one-sixth of all GISTs demonstrate primary resistance to imatinib. Furthermore, in tumors that initially respond to imatinib, secondary resistance develops at a median of 2 years due to accumulation of drug-resistant, secondary mutations.[9,10] Thus, there is rationale to combine tyrosine kinase inhibition with other therapeutic modalities.

LOCOREGIONAL THERAPIES

Percutaneous thermal ablation (ie, radiofrequency ablation [RFA], cryotherapy, or microwave ablation) and intra-arterial therapies (ie, bland embolization, chemoembolization, and radioembolization) are therapeutic modalities used with palliative intent for unresectable liver metastases or in conjunction with resection. The choice to use these local strategies and which particular locoregional therapy to use is highly dependent on institutional preferences, as high-quality data are lacking.

There are several small series of percutaneous RFA for both GIST and non-GIST sarcoma liver metastasis. Hakime and colleagues[11] reported on 17 patients with GIST liver metastases. There were no technical failures of RFA and, after a mean follow-up of 49 months, there were no local recurrences. Jones and colleagues[12] reported the results of RFA for 13 patients with GIST, in whom the median time to local progression at the RFA site was 28 months. Given the small numbers in each series, direct comparison of these disparate outcomes is limited. Jones and colleagues[12] additionally treated 6 patients with non-GIST histologies (50% leiomyosarcoma), in whom a complete treatment was achieved in 5 and the median time to local progression at the RFA site was 9 months. Thus, the long-term outcomes for patients with non-GIST histologies are poor, paralleling the inferior responses also observed with systemic therapy. In a series from MD Anderson Cancer Center, intraoperative RFA was combined with resection in 66 patients with metastatic sarcoma (GIST 55%; leiomyosarcoma 27%).[13] The rates of recurrence were significantly higher for patients treated with RFA in combination with surgical resection (89%), as compared with resection alone (57%); yet, the rate of liver-only recurrence was similar between treatment strategies, suggesting that patient selection likely underlies the apparent differences in efficacy. There are no randomized data comparing RFA alone versus surgery alone. RFA is the most commonly reported ablation technique, but cryoablation and microwave ablation have also been combined with surgical resection[14] or used independently[15] with an acceptable safety profile. Evaluation of efficacy is prohibited by the small sample sizes and diverse histologies described. We now prefer to use microwave ablation instead of RFA, because the extent of the ablation is more predictable and can be monitored well with ultrasound. Microwave ablation can be used alone or in combination with resection.

Arterial therapies used for sarcoma metastases to the liver include bland embolization,[16,17] chemoembolization,[18–20] and radioembolization.[18] Each series demonstrates that arterial therapy is a safe salvage option. In a series from Memorial Sloan Kettering Cancer Center, bland embolization of the liver achieved a radiographic response in 8 of 16 patients with metastatic GIST, but only 1 of 6 patients with leiomyosarcoma; the latter cohort of patients had a median OS of 18 months.[16] Modern series of hepatic arterial therapy for metastatic GIST are composed of patients who are not candidates for resection and who progress on imatinib therapy, where OS ranges between 14.9 and 23.8 months.[17] The difference in outcome between liver metastases from GIST and leiomyosarcoma presumably relates to the fact that GIST is more vascular.

Hepatic artery infusion of chemotherapy is not used because of its lack of efficacy.[21]

SURGICAL RESECTION

Liver resection is an increasingly used therapy in the management of hepatic sarcoma metastasis. Over 2 decades (from 1983 to 2004), there was a 16-fold increase in the utilization of hepatic resections for patients with noncolorectal, nonendocrine liver metastases. A better appreciation of anatomy and surgical technique improved the safety of hepatectomy, which then broadened the indications for surgery.[22] Criteria to determine candidacy for hepatic resection follow those for liver metastasis from other primaries, namely a hepatic distribution of disease that can be removed while preserving adequate hepatic reserve. Extrahepatic disease is not necessarily a contraindication for surgical therapy as long as the overall treatment plan addresses all tumor sites.[23] Hepatic resection can be combined with resection of primary disease site in the setting of synchronous metastasis or has occasionally been performed in a staged fashion, depending on the magnitude of the required procedures.[24] In the case of GIST, where effective systemic therapies are available, the primary goal is to remove all macroscopic disease. In selected patients, resection is sometimes performed just to remove a progressing tumor (ie, resistant clones to tyrosine kinase inhibition), especially when the patient is symptomatic, while leaving macroscopic disease that is still responsive to therapy.

The favorable safety profile of hepatectomy for sarcoma metastasis is summarized in **Table 1**. Single-institution series from high-volume centers report successful hepatectomies with no mortality,[3] whereas some nationwide registries report perioperative mortality rates less than 3%.[25] The perioperative morbidity, which ranged from 15% to 20% in major series, is significantly higher than that observed with locoregional therapy, and thus the application of surgery must be justified by a potentially favorable impact on prognosis, beyond that achieved with nonsurgical therapy. There have been no major clinical trials comparing surgery with locoregional or systemic therapies. The strongest evidence for the oncologic value of resectional therapy derives from the longest observed survival for metastatic sarcoma in *surgical* series. Long-term (5-year) survival has been observed in 30% to 50% of patients with non-GIST histologies and 70% for those with metastatic GIST (see **Table 1**). However, the precise therapeutic value of surgery cannot be disentangled from the patient and disease factors that dictate management paradigms. These are the careful selection of patients for surgery after consideration of the patient's overall health, extent of disease, tumor histologic subtype, and duration between the primary tumor and the development of

Table 1
Summary of perioperative and long-term outcomes after hepatic resection of sarcoma metastasis

Author	Years	No. Patients (%)			90-d Morbidity, %	90-d Mortality, %	5-y Survival, %
		Total	GIST	Non-GIST			
DeMatteo et al,[3] 2001	1982–2000	56	34	22	NA	0	30[a]
Adam et al,[22] 2006	1983–2004	158	33	123	14.0 "local" 15.0 "general"	2.3	GIST: 70 Non-GIST: 31
Groeschl et al,[40] 2012	1990–2009	98	NA	NA	20.0	1.9	32[a]
Pawlik et al,[13] 2006	1996–2005	66	36	30	15.2	4.5	54[a]
Marudanayagam et al,[41] 2011	1997–2009	36	5	31	NA	8.3	31.8[a]
Brudvik et al,[27] 2015	1998–2013	146	49	97	NA	NA	GIST: 55.3 Non-GIST: 44.9–48.4
Grimme et al,[25] 2019	1998–2014	38	0	38	15.8	2.6	54.6

Abbreviation: GIST, gastrointestinal stromal tumor.
[a] Survival not stratified by tumor histology.
Data from Refs.[3,22,25,27,40,41]

metastases. Disease rarity has been a barrier to a clinical trial that would overcome the selection bias inherent in these nonrandomized comparisons.

An important surgical consideration is the importance of margins. R2 is defined by gross tumor on the hepatic margin or elsewhere in the liver, whereas R1 is defined by microscopic positivity or viable tumor within 1 mm of the hepatic transection surface. R2 resection is equivalent to palliative debulking and is usually associated with survival comparable to those patients not receiving resectional therapy. We presented a single-institution surgical series in which 8 patients who underwent an R2 resection had a median survival of only 8 months.[3] In contrast, the prognostic value of R1 margins is less clearly defined. In the same series, R1 resection (n = 5; 9%) was not associated with inferior survival. This is consistent with American College of Surgeons Oncology Group (ACOSOG) Z9001 data, in which patients with R0 versus R1 margins after resection of primary GIST had similar outcomes (regardless of imatinib therapy).[26] In contrast, in a series of 146 patients from Brudvik and colleagues[27] where 8 patients (5.5%) underwent R1 resection, margin was significantly associated with survival in a multivariable model for patients with certain non-GIST histologies. However, margin was not prognostic for patients with metastatic GIST. Because the margin analysis from the study by DeMatteo and colleagues[3] did not differentiate between GIST and non-GIST histologies, it is not possible to reconcile this disparate finding between the 2 major series. Last, R0 is defined by the absence of tumor within 1 mm of the hepatic transection margin. One study compared recurrence risk based on the width of the negative margin. Pawlik and colleagues[13] compared the outcomes of 22 patients (42%) in whom the margin was negative by <10 mm with 30 patients (57%) in whom the margin was at least 10 mm; the extent of the margin was not associated with recurrence or OS.

HEPATIC RESECTION FOR GASTROINTESTINAL STROMAL TUMOR IN THE IMATINIB ERA

Imatinib is a small molecule tyrosine kinase inhibitor of KIT and PDGFRA, among other receptor tyrosine kinases, and a highly effective targeted therapy for the management of localized and metastatic GIST. Maximal treatment response is often achieved within 6 to 9 months after imatinib initiation,[28] at which point surgery can be considered (**Fig. 1**). Surgery is associated with the longest survival when patients respond to preoperative imatinib, whereas the benefit of an aggressive surgical strategy is likely limited for patients with progressive disease.[24,29,30] In a series of metastatic disease to the liver, peritoneum, and/or other sites, patients with multifocal resistance (ie, more than 1 tumor enlarging on imatinib) had a median time to progression of as little as 3 months after surgery.[24,31] Yet patients with metastatic disease that was either stable or responsive to preoperative imatinib achieved a median progression-free survival of more than 10 years with extensive resection.[30] In a subset of patients with liver-only metastases adapted from the series published by Cavnar and colleagues,[23] there were 100 patients who underwent curative-intent resection: 27 in the pre-imatinib era (26% had synchronous primary resection) and 73 in the imatinib era (49% had synchronous primary resection) (**Fig. 2**). Median OS in the imatinib era was significantly longer (9.2 vs 2.9 years), with a greater proportion of 10-year actuarial survivors (40% vs 22%). Thus, the combination of imatinib with the judicious application of surgery can achieve prolonged disease control beyond that observed with other treatment modalities, although as proof, it is unlikely that the study of systemic therapy alone versus systemic therapy with surgery can ever be performed.

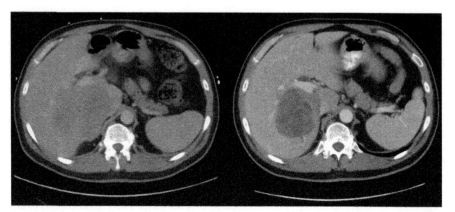

Fig. 1. Typical radiographic response of a liver metastasis from an intestinal GIST. At diagnosis (*left*), the tumor enhances homogeneously. After 4 months of imatinib (*right*), the tumor is much smaller in size and there are areas of reduced contrast uptake.

The precise benefit of surgery in patients with metastatic GIST whose disease responds to imatinib remains an unanswered question. Complete response rates are less than 10%. Moreover, given that secondary resistance to imatinib develops at a median of 2 years, there is a theoretic advantage to consider resection even in treatment-responsive patients to preempt the development of resistant clones. Prospective, randomized trials designed to compare metastasectomy plus imatinib to imatinib alone were attempted without success. We initially proposed a US-based trial for patients with responsive or stable disease after 6 months of imatinib, which was never approved by the National Cancer Institute, whereas multicenter trials in Europe (EORTC Trial NCT00956072) and China (ChiCTR-TRC-00000244) closed because of

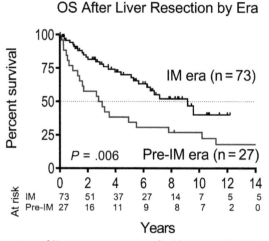

Fig. 2. OS after resection of liver metastasis, stratified by imatinib (IM) era. IM era defined by earliest date that any patient in group received IM. Median OS was significantly longer in the IM era (9.2 vs 2.9 years, P = .006). (*Data from* Cavnar MJ, Seier K, Curtin C, et al. Outcome of 1000 Patients With Gastrointestinal Stromal Tumor (GIST) Treated by Surgery in the Pre and Post-imatinib Eras. Ann Surg. 2019.)

poor accrual. In a small (n = 41), single-institution randomized controlled trial from China, resection of GIST liver metastasis combined with imatinib was superior to imatinib alone (3-year OS: 90% vs 60%).[32] Unfortunately, validation of these underpowered results is unlikely to occur. There are inherent limitations to a trial in which randomization to surgery is required, including disparate beliefs of clinicians of the risk and value of surgery. Moreover, because GIST metastasectomy may be associated with morbidity,[33] patients may not accept a randomization that involves surgery. For instance, the failed ChiCTR-TRC-00000244 trial did not include any patients with liver metastasis, because patients at these hospitals "are more likely to choose less invasive treatment such as transcatheter arterial chemoembolization, stereotactic radiation and radiofrequency ablation."[34]

Regardless of strategy chosen, tyrosine kinase inhibition is continued indefinitely for patients with metastatic GIST, irrespective of whether their disease is resected. In patients managed without resectional therapy, imatinib interruption resulted in rapid progression in most patients with advanced GIST in a multicenter trial from the French Sarcoma Group, leading to premature closing of the trial.[35] Likewise, following complete metastasectomy, tyrosine kinase inhibition is continued to treat the likely existence of residual, microscopic disease. In the landmark ACOSOG Z9001 trial of imatinib versus placebo for resected primary GIST, in which imatinib was prescribed for 1 year, the recurrence-free survival curves eventually converged. Thus, imatinib does not eradicate microscopic disease with this duration of treatment but rather is cytostatic.[36] The fact that very few patients with metastatic GIST to the liver were cured after partial hepatectomy in the pre-imatinib era indicates that essentially all patients have residual microscopic disease. On a practical note, imatinib does not appear to adversely impact wound healing, and can be restarted within 2 weeks after surgery.

Imatinib is one of several drugs approved by the Food and Drug Administration (FDA) for the treatment of metastatic GIST. Sunitinib, regorafenib, and avapritinib are multi-targeted tyrosine kinase inhibitors used in the second line or beyond. Avapritinib is a highly selective and KIT/PDGFRα inhibitor with superior activity for GIST harboring a *PDGFRA* exon 18 D842V mutation and is the first-line therapy for this genetic profile. Ripretinib is a unique KIT and PDGFRα kinase switch pocket inhibitor that is under priority review by the FDA for metastatic GIST. The interaction between resection and these more novel agents is poorly characterized, but comparable results are expected.

Last, it should be noted that the subset of patients with SDH-deficient GIST, or other types of KIT/PDGFRA wild-type GIST, generally have more indolent disease and because effective therapies are lacking for these patients, partial hepatectomy is sometimes indicated for progressive disease when all disease can be addressed.

LIVER TRANSPLANTATION

Total hepatectomy with liver transplantation is a surgical therapy rarely used for sarcoma metastases, but has been described for patients with extensive hepatic disease without any extrahepatic tumor burden. In one of the largest series of 13 patients (GIST and non-GIST histologies), 12 patients (92%) suffered disease recurrence at a median time of 11.7 months, leading the study investigators to strongly discourage the use of scarce organ resources for this indication.[37] In contrast, there are 2 case reports of liver transplantation for wild-type metastatic GIST and the patients have been recurrence-free with nearly 4 years of follow-up.[38,39]

THE MEDICAL ONCOLOGIST'S PERSPECTIVE

Although systemic therapy can be active in sarcomas other than GIST that are metastatic to liver, responses are generally not durable. Conversely, surgery for liver metastatic disease can rapidly decrease tumor burden. However, nearly all data for such studies are descriptive. The heterogeneity of tumor presentation even in a single organ provides ample clinical and research challenges alike. Because sarcomas represent less than 1% of cancers that arise in the United States and comprise more than 70 subtypes, it is unsurprising that there are not better outcome data on sarcomas metastatic to liver. Indeed, liver metastatic only or liver-predominant patterns are seen for only a few histologies. Nonetheless, it is becoming appreciated that despite their rarity, sarcomas should be treated on subtype-specific trials whenever possible. Although such studies are slow to accrue, subtype or molecularly defined trials will lead the way to better outcomes and reveal the activity of novel agents in a specific sarcoma. The principles that have been advanced by trials of metastatic GIST can be applied to even less common sarcomas.

SUMMARY

Sarcomas metastatic to the liver provide clinical challenges for surgeons, medical oncologists, radiation oncologists, and interventional radiologists alike. Impactful studies are difficult to perform owing to the heterogeneity of disease presentations, and the number of different histologies involved. Cooperation will be needed to advance the field. Combining resources from multiple centers, it is possible to propose treatment standards that can be tested and challenged in prospective trials.

DISCLOSURE

Drs B.L. Ecker, M.J. Cavnar, and R.P. DeMatteo do not have any relevant conflicts of interest to disclose. Dr R.G. Maki reports research support to the institution from SARC: Sarcoma Alliance for Research through Collaboration.

REFERENCES

1. Jaques DP, Coit DG, Casper ES, et al. Hepatic metastases from soft-tissue sarcoma. Ann Surg 1995;221(4):392–7.
2. Ducimetiere F, Lurkin A, Ranchere-Vince D, et al. Incidence of sarcoma histotypes and molecular subtypes in a prospective epidemiological study with central pathology review and molecular testing. PLoS One 2011;6(8):e20294.
3. DeMatteo RP, Shah A, Fong Y, et al. Results of hepatic resection for sarcoma metastatic to liver. Ann Surg 2001;234(4):540–7 [discussion: 547–8].
4. Van Glabbeke M, van Oosterom AT, Oosterhuis JW, et al. Prognostic factors for the outcome of chemotherapy in advanced soft tissue sarcoma: an analysis of 2,185 patients treated with anthracycline-containing first-line regimens–a European Organization for Research and Treatment of Cancer Soft Tissue and Bone Sarcoma Group Study. J Clin Oncol 1999;17(1):150–7.
5. Sleijfer S, Ouali M, van Glabbeke M, et al. Prognostic and predictive factors for outcome to first-line ifosfamide-containing chemotherapy for adult patients with advanced soft tissue sarcomas: an exploratory, retrospective analysis on large series from the European Organization for Research and Treatment of Cancer-Soft Tissue and Bone Sarcoma Group (EORTC-STBSG). Eur J Cancer 2010; 46(1):72–83.

6. Dematteo RP, Heinrich MC, El-Rifai WM, et al. Clinical management of gastrointestinal stromal tumors: before and after STI-571. Hum Pathol 2002;33(5):466–77.

7. Demetri GD, von Mehren M, Blanke CD, et al. Efficacy and safety of imatinib mesylate in advanced gastrointestinal stromal tumors. N Engl J Med 2002;347(7): 472–80.

8. Blanke CD, Demetri GD, von Mehren M, et al. Long-term results from a randomized phase II trial of standard- versus higher-dose imatinib mesylate for patients with unresectable or metastatic gastrointestinal stromal tumors expressing KIT. J Clin Oncol 2008;26(4):620–5.

9. Vadakara J, von Mehren M. Gastrointestinal stromal tumors: management of metastatic disease and emerging therapies. Hematol Oncol Clin North Am 2013; 27(5):905–20.

10. Antonescu CR, Besmer P, Guo T, et al. Acquired resistance to imatinib in gastrointestinal stromal tumor occurs through secondary gene mutation. Clin Cancer Res 2005;11(11):4182–90.

11. Hakime A, Le Cesne A, Deschamps F, et al. A role for adjuvant RFA in managing hepatic metastases from gastrointestinal stromal tumors (GIST) after treatment with targeted systemic therapy using kinase inhibitors. Cardiovasc Intervent Radiol 2014;37(1):132–9.

12. Jones RL, McCall J, Adam A, et al. Radiofrequency ablation is a feasible therapeutic option in the multi modality management of sarcoma. Eur J Surg Oncol 2010;36(5):477–82.

13. Pawlik TM, Vauthey JN, Abdalla EK, et al. Results of a single-center experience with resection and ablation for sarcoma metastatic to the liver. Arch Surg 2006; 141(6):537–43 [discussion: 543–4].

14. Chua TC, Chu F, Morris DL. Outcomes of single-centre experience of hepatic resection and cryoablation of sarcoma liver metastases. Am J Clin Oncol 2011; 34(3):317–20.

15. Perrodin S, Lachenmayer A, Maurer M, et al. Percutaneous stereotactic image-guided microwave ablation for malignant liver lesions. Sci Rep 2019;9(1):13836.

16. Maluccio MA, Covey AM, Schubert J, et al. Treatment of metastatic sarcoma to the liver with bland embolization. Cancer 2006;107(7):1617–23.

17. Takaki H, Litchman T, Covey A, et al. Hepatic artery embolization for liver metastasis of gastrointestinal stromal tumor following imatinib and sunitinib therapy. J Gastrointest Cancer 2014;45(4):494–9.

18. Chapiro J, Duran R, Lin M, et al. Transarterial chemoembolization in soft-tissue sarcoma metastases to the liver - the use of imaging biomarkers as predictors of patient survival. Eur J Radiol 2015;84(3):424–30.

19. Rajan DK, Soulen MC, Clark TW, et al. Sarcomas metastatic to the liver: response and survival after cisplatin, doxorubicin, mitomycin-C, Ethiodol, and polyvinyl alcohol chemoembolization. J Vasc Interv Radiol 2001;12(2):187–93.

20. Kobayashi K, Gupta S, Trent JC, et al. Hepatic artery chemoembolization for 110 gastrointestinal stromal tumors: response, survival, and prognostic factors. Cancer 2006;107(12):2833–41.

21. Melichar B, Voboril Z, Nozicka J, et al. Hepatic arterial infusion chemotherapy in sarcoma liver metastases: a report of 6 cases. Tumori 2005;91(1):19–23.

22. Adam R, Chiche L, Aloia T, et al. Hepatic resection for noncolorectal nonendocrine liver metastases: analysis of 1,452 patients and development of a prognostic model. Ann Surg 2006;244(4):524–35.

23. Cavnar MJ, Seier K, Curtin C, et al. Outcome of 1000 patients with gastrointestinal stromal tumor (GIST) treated by surgery in the pre and post-imatinib eras. Ann Surg 2019.

24. DeMatteo RP, Maki RG, Singer S, et al. Results of tyrosine kinase inhibitor therapy followed by surgical resection for metastatic gastrointestinal stromal tumor. Ann Surg 2007;245(3):347–52.

25. Grimme FAB, Seesing MFJ, van Hillegersberg R, et al. Liver resection for hepatic metastases from soft tissue sarcoma: a nationwide study. Dig Surg 2019;36(6): 479–86.

26. McCarter MD, Antonescu CR, Ballman KV, et al. Microscopically positive margins for primary gastrointestinal stromal tumors: analysis of risk factors and tumor recurrence. J Am Coll Surg 2012;215(1):53–9 [discussion: 59–60].

27. Brudvik KW, Patel SH, Roland CL, et al. Survival after resection of gastrointestinal stromal tumor and sarcoma liver metastases in 146 patients. J Gastrointest Surg 2015;19(8):1476–83.

28. Verweij J, Casali PG, Zalcberg J, et al. Progression-free survival in gastrointestinal stromal tumours with high-dose imatinib: randomised trial. Lancet 2004; 364(9440):1127–34.

29. Gronchi A, Fiore M, Miselli F, et al. Surgery of residual disease following molecular-targeted therapy with imatinib mesylate in advanced/metastatic GIST. Ann Surg 2007;245(3):341–6.

30. Bauer S, Rutkowski P, Hohenberger P, et al. Long-term follow-up of patients with GIST undergoing metastasectomy in the era of imatinib – analysis of prognostic factors (EORTC-STBSG collaborative study). Eur J Surg Oncol 2014;40(4):412–9.

31. Fairweather M, Balachandran VP, Li GZ, et al. Cytoreductive surgery for metastatic gastrointestinal stromal tumors treated with tyrosine kinase inhibitors: a 2-institutional analysis. Ann Surg 2018;268(2):296–302.

32. Xia L, Zhang MM, Ji L, et al. Resection combined with imatinib therapy for liver metastases of gastrointestinal stromal tumors. Surg Today 2010;40(10):936–42.

33. Fairweather M, Cavnar MJ, Li GZ, et al. Prediction of morbidity following cytoreductive surgery for metastatic gastrointestinal stromal tumour in patients on tyrosine kinase inhibitor therapy. Br J Surg 2018;105(6):743–50.

34. Du CY, Zhou Y, Song C, et al. Is there a role of surgery in patients with recurrent or metastatic gastrointestinal stromal tumours responding to imatinib: a prospective randomised trial in China. Eur J Cancer 2014;50(10):1772–8.

35. Blay JY, Le Cesne A, Ray-Coquard I, et al. Prospective multicentric randomized phase III study of imatinib in patients with advanced gastrointestinal stromal tumors comparing interruption versus continuation of treatment beyond 1 year: the French Sarcoma Group. J Clin Oncol 2007;25(9):1107–13.

36. Dematteo RP, Ballman KV, Antonescu CR, et al. Adjuvant imatinib mesylate after resection of localised, primary gastrointestinal stromal tumour: a randomised, double-blind, placebo-controlled trial. Lancet 2009;373(9669):1097–104.

37. Husted TL, Neff G, Thomas MJ, et al. Liver transplantation for primary or metastatic sarcoma to the liver. Am J Transplant 2006;6(2):392–7.

38. Iesari S, Mocchegiani F, Nicolini D, et al. Liver transplantation for metastatic wild-type gastrointestinal stromal tumor in the era of molecular targeted therapies: Report of a first case. Am J Transplant 2019;19(10):2939–43.

39. Benitez C, Inzunza M, Riveros S, et al. First report of living donor liver transplantation for imatinib-resistant GIST liver metastases. A new therapeutic option in transplant oncology. Liver Transpl 2020.

40. Groeschl RT, Nachmany I, Steel JL, et al. Hepatectomy for noncolorectal non-neuroendocrine metastatic cancer: a multi-institutional analysis. J Am Coll Surg 2012;214(5):769–77.
41. Marudanayagam R, Sandhu B, Perera MT, et al. Liver resection for metastatic soft tissue sarcoma: an analysis of prognostic factors. Eur J Surg Oncol 2011;37(1): 87–92.

Surgical Management of Gynecologic Cancers

Kiran H. Clair, MD[a],*, Juliet Wolford, MD[a], Jason A. Zell, DO[b], Robert E. Bristow, MD[c]

KEYWORDS

- Metastatic gynecologic cancer • Stage IV uterine • Ovarian
- Cervical cancer with liver metastases

KEY POINTS

- Randomized data on the role of liver resection in gynecologic cancers are limited, and the role of aggressive surgery remains controversial.
- Residual disease remains an important predictive for survival in ovarian cancer.
- Gynecologic cancers that metastasize to the liver usually do so in the setting of disseminated disease; hepatic resection should be considered when disease can be completely resected to achieve optimal surgical cytoreduction.

INTRODUCTION

An estimated 113,520 women will be diagnosed with a gynecologic cancer in the United States in 2020, and 33,620 deaths will be attributed to the disease.[1] Worldwide, 1.3 million women were diagnosed in 2018 with an estimated 609,000 disease-related deaths.[1,2] Despite improved screening programs and the implementation of the human papillomavirus vaccine, cervical cancer remains the most common gynecologic cancer worldwide. In the United States, uterine cancer is the most commonly diagnosed; however, ovarian cancer remains the most fatal largely because of the proportion of patients with advanced disease at the time of diagnosis, because they are relatively asymptomatic until the cancer has progressed to an advanced stage. Surgical management with platinum-based chemotherapy remains the cornerstone of ovarian cancer treatment; however, this paradigm is rapidly evolving with the use of novel genetic/molecular targeted therapies. There remains continued debate over the role of radical surgery in the management of hepatic metastasis in primary and recurrent disease.

As with most cancers, stage IV gynecologic cancers confer poorer survival outcomes.[2] In ovarian cancer, the liver is the most common site of metastasis followed

[a] Division of Gynecologic Oncology, University of California, 333 City Boulevard West, Suite 1400, Orange, CA 92868, USA; [b] Division of Hematology/Oncology, Department of Medicine, University of California, 333 City Boulevard West, Suite 1400, Orange, CA 92868, USA; [c] Department of Obstetrics and Gynecology, University of California, 333 City Boulevard West, Suite 1400, Orange, CA 92868, USA
* Corresponding author.
E-mail address: jclair@hs.uci.edu

Surg Oncol Clin N Am 30 (2021) 69–88
https://doi.org/10.1016/j.soc.2020.09.004
1055-3207/21/© 2020 Elsevier Inc. All rights reserved.

by the lung, bone, and brain.[3–5] In uterine and cervical cancers, disease is more likely to metastasize to the lung, followed by the liver, brain, and bone.[4] Patients with ovarian cancer with liver metastases have relatively better survival compared with those whereby the disease has spread to the brain, lung, or bone.[3] Contrary to this, patients with uterine cancer with bone metastasis have relatively better survival compared with those with lesions in the liver, lung, or brain. Recently, a retrospective analysis using SEER data evaluated stage IV uterine and ovarian cancers and found that liver metastasis had the highest survival compared with bone and brain metastasis.[4]

The International Federation of Gynecology and Oncology staging for ovarian cancer distinguishes perihepatic surface lesions as stage III and liver parenchymal disease as stage IV.[6] Ovarian cancer cells circulate in peritoneal fluid within the abdominal cavity in a clockwise direction, a result of intestinal peristalsis and diaphragmatic movement. Because of this pattern, the liver capsule and right hemidiaphragm have a higher propensity for metastatic disease.[7] The first hepatic resection for metastatic gynecologic cancer was described by Brunschwig[8] at the Memorial Hospital in 1963. Nearly 45 years later, the Memorial group published a series of 12 patients with gynecologic cancer with isolated metastasis to the liver who underwent resection.[9] Since then, several studies have demonstrated that the amount of residual disease after cytoreductive surgery for advanced ovarian cancer is a significant prognostic factor for survival.[10–13] Additional studies have explored the survival benefit of hepatic resection at the time of primary and secondary surgery to achieve no gross residual disease.[13–16]

In this article, the authors review indications for the surgical resection of liver metastasis from gynecologic cancers in the treatment of both primary and recurrent disease. They highlight relevant clinical trials regarding short-term complications and long-term oncologic outcomes of liver resection. Data supporting the use of nonsurgical options are also discussed. Finally, the authors highlight several ongoing trials evaluating the role of liver resection and the challenges faced in study design and data interpretation.

OVARIAN CANCER

In the United States, there are 21,750 patients who will be diagnosed with ovarian cancer in 2020 and 13,940 who will die from the disease.[2] In 1975, Griffiths[17] presented the landmark study describing the correlation between the amount of residual disease after surgical cytoreduction and overall survival in advanced ovarian cancer. Since that time, surgical cytoreduction in combination with taxane- and platinum-based chemotherapy has become the basis for the management of advanced ovarian cancer. No gross residual disease at the completion of surgery continues to be an important predictor of survival.[18] The debate surrounding whether tumor biology or the quality of cytoreductive surgery (with minimal residual disease) is most influential in the prognosis of ovarian cancer largely persists because of the lack of consensus over the quality of studies available for interpretation. A Cochrane review in 2011 evaluated studies with ultraradical (extensive) surgery compared with standard surgery for primary cytoreduction and suggested that the available evidence pointed to radical surgery leading to improved survival; however, it cited low-quality evidence comparing the 2 arms.[19]

Primary Cytoreductive Surgery

Several case series have reported the outcome of patients who have undergone resection for liver metastasis from ovarian cancer (**Table 1**). One of the earliest studies, by Chi and colleagues,[9] reported a series of 12 patients who underwent surgical resection with a median survival of 27 months and no associated perioperative

Table 1
Studies reporting surgical management of hepatic metastases from ovarian and endometrial cancers

Author, Year	Study Type	Patients	Primary	Median Overall Survival (mo)	Factors Associated with Survival
Neumann et al,[80] 2012	Retrospective	41	Ovary	42 (R0), 4 (R1), 6 (R2)	Postoperative residual tumor
Kamel et al,[81] 2011	Retrospective	52	Ovary	53; 5-y survival 41%	Not reported
Lim et al,[82] 2009	Retrospective	14	Ovary	5-y overall survival (OS) stage IIIC 55%, stage IV 51%	Not reported
Bristow et al,[33] 2009	Retrospective	56	Endometrial	34 mo	Residual disease ($P = .0001$), performance status ($P = .043$), age ($P = .023$)
Winter et al,[11] 2008	Retrospective	64	Ovary	20.7 mo	Microscopic residual disease
Aletti et al,[22] 2007	Retrospective	49	Ovary	38 mo	Residual disease and radical surgical procedures ($P<.001$), extent of peritoneal disease, parenchymal liver metastases, and ASA associated with suboptimal cytoreduction
Van Wijk et al,[83] 2009	Retrospective	67	Endometrial	5-y survival 65.6%	Optimal cytoreduction (5-y survival 65.6% vs 40.6%)
Loizzi et al,[84] 2005	Retrospective	8	Ovary	19 mo	Number of hepatic lesions, presence of extrahepatic metastasis, performance status, histology
Lambrou et al,[85] 2004	Retrospective	85	Endometrial	17.8 mo	Optimal cytoreduction (17.8 vs 6.7 mo, $P = .001$)
Ayhan et al,[86] 2002	Retrospective	37	Endometrial	25 mo	Extraabdominal metastases, suboptimal cytoreduction, cervical invasion associated with worse survival

(continued on next page)

Table 1
(continued)

Author, Year	Study Type	Patients	Primary	Median Overall Survival (mo)	Factors Associated with Survival
Fan et al,[87] 2001	Retrospective	18	Ovary (immature teratoma)	5-y survival 55.6%	Not reported
Naik et al,[88] 2000	Retrospective	37	Ovary	11 mo; 5-y survival 9%	Optimal cytoreduction with residual <2 cm ($P = .0029$) or <1 cm ($P = .0086$)
Bristow et al,[10] 1999	Retrospective	37	Ovary	50.1 mo (optimal extrahepatic and hepatic); 27 mo (optimal extrahepatic with residual hepatic tumor)	Optimal extrahepatic resection ($P = .0001$)
Elias et al,[89] 1998	Retrospective	6	Gynecologic	5-y survival 45%	Not reported

mortality. Similarly, the Mayo Clinic reported 26 patients with hepatic resection for metastatic ovarian cancer with a median survival of 26.3 months, morbidity of 23%, and no perioperative mortality.[15]

Bristow and colleagues[10] retrospectively reviewed patients with stage IV ovarian cancer who underwent hepatic cytoreduction for liver metastasis ($\leq$1 cm residual disease) and observed a median survival of 50.1 months. Optimal hepatic cytoreduction was only achieved in 16% of patients, and nearly 30% of patients achieved optimal extrahepatic disease but suboptimal hepatic disease, resulting in a median survival of 27 months. When stratified by both optimal hepatic and extrahepatic cytoreduction (6 patients), median survival was 50.1 months compared with 27 months for suboptimal hepatic and optimal extrahepatic residual disease (11 patients). Patients who had both suboptimal hepatic and extrahepatic disease had a median survival of 7.6 months (20 patients). Further analysis also demonstrated that the number of parenchymal liver lesions correlated with survival; median survival for 1 to 2 lesions was 20.9 months compared with 6.4 months when 3+ lesions were present ($P = .0012$). Although the study has significant limitations given the small sample size, it demonstrates the difficulty in achieving optimal hepatic cytoreduction. Even when hepatic cytoreduction was not achieved, there remained a survival advantage when extrahepatic residual disease was minimal.

Chi and colleagues[20] evaluated the incorporation of radical procedures into the surgical management of advanced ovarian cancer on cytoreduction rates and overall survival. With an institutional practice change to incorporate extensive upper-abdominal surgery, 378 patients were randomized to undergo standard surgery or surgery with extensive upper-abdominal procedures. Patients who underwent aggressive upper-abdominal surgery had an improved median overall survival compared with those who underwent standard surgery (54 months vs 43 months, $P = .03$). The proportion of patients who achieved no gross residual disease also increased to 27% from 11% without an increase in postoperative complications.

A metaanalysis from Chang and colleagues[18] evaluated survival differences associated with the amount of residual disease after cytoreductive surgery and found an inverse correlation with survival. With every 10% increase in cytoreduction to no visible disease, a survival benefit of 2.3 months was observed. Although the interpretation of how best to achieve no gross residual disease remains a debate between the underlying tumor biology versus surgical aggressiveness, the survival benefit of achieving complete cytoreduction is predictive of improved survival.

Aletti and colleagues[21] highlighted the significant variation that exists among surgeons by examining their propensity to perform aggressive radical surgeries. Patients with stage IIIC ovarian cancer were retrospectively reviewed and found that the only predictor of survival was the performance of radical surgery ($P = .047$). After adjusting for other variables, the 5-year overall survival was significantly higher for surgeons who performed aggressive radical procedures, 44%, compared with 17% for surgeons who operated with standard surgery ($P<.001$). Aletti and colleagues[22] also reviewed 30-day morbidity and 3-month mortality across 3 centers, which were 18.4% and 4.5%, respectively. Endogenous patient factors, albumin ($P = .001$) and American Society of Anesthesiolgists Classification (ASA Class) ($P = .008$), and complexity of surgery were the strongest predictors of morbidity, whereas age ($P = .002$) and ASA ($P = .001$) most strongly correlated with mortality.

Neoadjuvant Chemotherapy

The role of neoadjuvant chemotherapy (NACT) in the primary management of advanced ovarian cancer remains a debated topic. Previously, as many as 45.5% of surgeons in the Society of Gynecologic Oncology (SGO) reported that the primary rationale against aggressive surgical resection was largely due to the lack of evidence.[23] Since then, recommendations regarding the decision-making process of primary cytoreduction versus NACT have been based on the results of 4 randomized clinical trials.[24–27] The SGO and the American Society of Clinical Oncology provided clinical practice guidelines for the use of NACT for newly diagnosed, advanced ovarian cancer.

In a Cochrane review, 3 of the 4 randomized trials were included in analysis. There were 1713 patients who were randomly assigned to NACT or primary cytoreductive surgery (CRS). Pooled results from these studies showed no difference in regard to overall survival (hazard ratio [HR] 1.06; 95% confidence interval [CI] 0.94–1.19) or progression-free survival (HR 1.02; 95% CI 0.92–1.13). When considering adverse events, NACT was favored, including the need for blood transfusion, infection, and venous thromboembolism. NACT also reduced the need for bowel resection, stoma formation, and perioperative mortality.[28] In EORTC 55971 (ClinicalTrials.gov, NCT00003636), 42% of patients randomized to primary CRS achieved residual tumor of 1 cm or less compared with 81% of the NACT arm. Perioperative mortality and morbidity were similar between the 2 groups. In subgroup analysis, stage IIIC patients with less extensive metastatic disease had improved survival with primary CRS, whereas patients with stage IV disease and larger metastatic disease burden had improved survival with NACT. In the CHORUS trial (ClinicalTrial.gov, NCT00075712), patients who underwent primary cytoreduction achieved ≤1 cm of gross residual disease in 41% of cases compared with 73% in the NACT arm (P = .0001).[25] The SCORPION trial (ClinicalTrials.gov, NCT01461850) found that the median operative time was shorter in the NACT arm in addition to fewer major postoperative complications and length of hospital stay.[26] NACT followed by interval CRS is a safe alternative in patients with advanced, large-volume disease, or poor performance status. However, even at the time of interval debulking, residual disease remains the strongest predictor of overall survival. There remain limited data regarding the extent and frequency of radical liver resection in these trials.

Future Studies

The limitations of the existing 4 randomized trials evaluating primary surgery versus chemotherapy include lower than expected median overall survival, mean operative time, and rates of optimal cytoreduction. Given these concerns, the TRUST trial (ClinicalTrials.gov, NCT02826818), a multicenter, international, randomized control trial (RCT) evaluating primary surgery versus NACT in advanced stage ovarian cancer, is underway.[29] To ensure high surgical quality, participating centers are required to fulfill specific criteria (ie, ≥50% complete resection rate in upfront surgery, ≥36 debulking surgeries per year). The intention of the study is complete tumor resection according to guidelines. Ancillary studies with molecular subtype analysis of which patients may be best treated with aggressive resection of hepatic lesions are also needed.

Secondary Cytoreductive Surgery

Most (80%) patients with ovarian cancer will experience disease recurrence. With 10-year disease-free survival rates of less than 15% in the recurrent setting, it becomes imperative to understand which patients may benefit from secondary surgery.[30] Current National Comprehensive Cancer Network guidelines recommend secondary cytoreduction as a treatment option for patients with ovarian cancer with at least 6 months of a treatment-free interval after completion of chemotherapy.[31]

Clinical factors, including a longer platinum-free interval (>6 months), in addition to isolated or small-volume disease (<0.5 cm) at the time of recurrence have been associated with improved benefit with secondary surgical resection.[32–35] Historically, studies evaluating the role of hepatic resection during secondary cytoreduction were limited to single-institution, retrospective data, and metaanalyses. There are a limited number of studies that have focused specifically on the role of hepatic resection during secondary cytoreduction (**Table 2**).[14,15,33,36]

The evaluation of single- versus multi-segmental liver resection in ovarian cancer has largely remained unaddressed, because of the small number of eligible patients. Historically, liver resection was performed in patients with single liver metastasis; however, both Kolev and colleagues[36] and Merideth and colleagues[15] present case series that found no difference in survival when solitary versus multilesion liver resections were performed ($P = .97$). Thus, despite the lack of randomized data, the resection of multiple liver masses with a multidisciplinary team at the time of secondary cytoreduction is considered safe and feasible.

More recently, Gynecologic Oncology Group (GOG)-0213 (Clinicaltrials.gov, NCT00565851) was an open-label, phase 3, multicenter randomized trial that evaluated secondary cytoreduction followed by chemotherapy with chemotherapy alone in platinum-sensitive recurrent ovarian cancer.[37] The trial enrolled 485 patients with recurrent ovarian cancer who were candidates for secondary cytoreduction based on historic criteria (1 prior therapy, platinum-free interval of at least 6 months, small-volume disease). Patients were determined to have disease amenable to resection by the investigator, and more 67% of patients in the surgery arm underwent complete gross resection. All patients received platinum-based chemotherapy, and 84% of patients also received bevacizumab with chemotherapy.

The median overall survival was statistically similar between the 2 groups (50.6 months surgery group vs 64.7 months chemotherapy only, $P = .08$). Consistent with other studies, patients who underwent complete cytoreduction benefited in overall and progression-free survival compared with patients with residual disease (56.0 months complete gross resection vs 37.8 months incomplete resection; HR 0.61, 95% CI 0.40–0.93). Although the study was not powered for the specific evaluation of hepatic metastasis, sub-group analysis for patients with liver metastasis did not show a survival benefit when surgical resection was performed (HR 0.89; 95% CI 0.39–2.01). Although statistical significance was not achieved, there was an advantage to surgery with respect to progression-free survival (18.9 months surgery vs 16.2 months chemotherapy only; HR 0.82, 95% CI 0.66–1.01). Secondary surgical cytoreduction remains a safe and feasible option in platinum-sensitive recurrent ovarian cancer; however, the benefit in overall survival was not observed in the surgical group, suggesting a case-by-case evaluation for select patients.

Future Studies

The lack of benefit observed in GOG-0213 when secondary cytoreduction was performed prompts the question of which specific patient population may gain a survival advantage from surgical intervention. There are currently 3 ongoing phase 3 trials to evaluate the role of surgery and chemotherapy versus chemotherapy alone. Desktop III (ClinicalTrials.gov, NCT01166737) uses a similar selection criterion as GOG-0213; however, it only includes patients with complete gross resection at the completion of primary surgery and limits the proportion of patients receiving bevacizumab to 20%.[38] A second trial, SOC 1 (Clinicaltrials.gov, NCT01611766), is being conducted in China with primary endpoints including overall and progression-free survival, and the secondary endpoint, including the validation of iMODEL, a patient selection risk model. The third trial, SOCceR (Netherlands Trial Register number NL3137), is also evaluating the role of secondary cytoreduction.

Table 2
Studies reporting surgical management of hepatic metastases from recurrent ovarian of endometrial cancer

Author, Year	Study Type	Patients	Primary	Median Overall Survival	Outcomes/Significance
Kolev et al,[36] 2014	Retrospective	27	Ovary	12 mo (2–190)	Secondary cytoreduction to <1 cm ($P = .014$); interval >24 mo from primary surgery ($P = .044$)
Roh et al,[90] 2011	Retrospective	18	Ovary	38 mo (3–78)	Optimal cytoreduction (40 vs 9 mo, $P = .0004$), negative margin status of hepatic resection (40 vs 9 mo, $P = .02$), less abdominal than pelvic disease (38 vs 11 mo, $P = .032$)
Pekmezci et al,[91] 2010	Retrospective	8	Ovary	Disease-free survival 39 mo	Not reported
Knowles et al,[60] 2010	Retrospective	5	Endometrioid (ovary or uterine)	OS not reported; disease-free survival 8–66 mo	Not reported
Loizzi et al,[84] 2005	Retrospective	29	Ovary	OS 24 mo (1st recurrence), 10 mo (2nd recurrence)	Not reported
Weitz et al,[92] 2005	Retrospective	19	(Ovary/fallopian 68.4%, endometrium 21.1%)	3-y disease free 58%	Time interval disease free from primary diagnosis
Meredith et al,[93] 2003	Retrospective	26	Ovary	26.3 mo	Interval >12 mo from original diagnosis (27.3 vs 5.7 mo, $P = .004$); ≤1 cm residual disease
Yoon et al,[14] 2003	Retrospective	24	Ovary	62 mo (6–94)	No significant factors identified
Chi et al,[9] 1997	Retrospective	12	Gynecologic (ovary/fallopian 70%, endometrium 17%)	27 mo, (8–94)	Not reported

CHALLENGES OF SURGICAL TRIAL DESIGN

The design of randomized surgical trials to improve decision-making capacity as to which patients may benefit from hepatic resection is challenging in the primary and recurrent disease setting. Not only are the surgical interventions difficult to standardize but also the inherent bias in patient selection and interpretation of prior studies are hard to overcome. This bias is further complicated with the limited number of prospective, randomized trials and a lack of prognostic factors to inform clinical decision making.

Selection bias is an important consideration in the design of a trial evaluating the role of liver resection. For example, patients who are enrolled in a primary or secondary cytoreductive surgery trial may be those individuals that an investigator thinks is an ideal candidate to achieve microscopic or no gross residual disease, thus narrowing the inclusion of patients who could potentially benefit. Even in GOG-0213, the investigators noted that patient selection bias was still present despite randomization, as patients had relatively limited tumor volume with fewer sites of recurrent disease and significantly longer periods of platinum-free interval.[37] Baseline tumor volume in GOG-0213 enrollees was also low with most patients having 2 or fewer sites of recurrent disease, which could reflect the investigator's desire to achieve complete gross section.

In addition, most studies that have evaluated radical surgery for advanced ovarian cancer have used residual disease as the primary outcome instead of overall survival. Several studies evaluating radical surgery did not use patients who underwent standard surgery as a reference group, whereas other studies have had a heterogenous patient population with the inclusion of those with recurrent disease.[19] Given the challenge of recruiting a significant number of patients, studies may not be statistically powered to adequately analyze subgroups with hepatic resection, making any favorable findings less persuasive.

Surgical trials also have the inherent difficulty of adequate standardization of complex procedures and access to hepatobiliary specialists, which may also limit a center's ability to participate in a trial. Selection criteria of surgeons, including baseline outcomes, volume, and standardization of technique, are needed to ensure study uniformity. When RCTs are not feasible, high-quality prospective studies could be implemented across multiple centers in addition to the indirect evidence obtained from retrospective comparisons.

Successful clinical trials should be convincing enough to resolve disagreement among clinicians. The ideal study design preserves the patient-physician relationship while also providing results that are clinically relevant and consistent with modern technologies. Although RCTs are considered the gold standard of statistical validity, they are not the only way to demonstrate efficacy or safety of an experimental therapy. RCTs are often not feasible or definitive and should not be considered the only valid approach to medical progress. Alternatives to RCTs should be considered when ethical obligations from the traditional patient-physician relationship are significant enough to outweigh the need to perform the most statistically rigorous study. RCTs often demand uniformity and consistency within the interventional technique (hepatic surgical resection arm), and quality of the intervention at the end of a trial may be significantly different from the beginning of the trial because of practical aspects, such as low study accrual, surgical learning curves, changes in clinical practice, and surgeon volume.

PREOPERATIVE CONSIDERATIONS

The amount of residual disease after cytoreductive surgery for ovarian cancer is an important prognostic factor for patients; therefore, the preoperative assessment of the extent of gross tumor involving the liver parenchyma is critical. The distribution of metastatic liver disease and whether the disease appears close to major vascular or biliary structures on preoperative imaging may compromise the ability to achieve complete cytoreduction and is considered a contraindication to aggressive surgery. Intraoperative ultrasound can be considered to assess the depth and relation of tumor to intraparenchymal vessels. In addition, the anticipated liver volume is also taken into consideration by using the ratio of future liver remnant volume to total liver volume, which has an inverse correlation with the risk of death.

Other considerations include the patient's medical comorbidities, including nutritional status and cardiac, pulmonary, and renal disease that can be optimized before surgery. Any underlying liver disease should be thoroughly evaluated, as the severity and underlying pathogenesis may dictate if the surgery is contraindicated.

The availability of an intradisciplinary surgical team for complex hepato-pancreatobiliary (HPB) procedures and higher-volume centers and surgeons is associated with improved perioperative outcomes.[39,40] The collaboration with a specialized HPB team before surgery should be confirmed.

SURGICAL TECHNIQUES

Optimizing exposure is an important key step for any surgical procedure. When extrahepatic disease is anticipated, a midline vertical incision is usually performed allowing for a comprehensive assessment of metastatic disease. If isolated disease recurrence occurs within the liver parenchyma, a subcostal incision can also be considered. In order to access the relevant liver segment or segments that contain metastatic disease, the liver must be adequately mobilized with detachment of its ligaments and ligation of appropriate vascular pedicles. Throughout the procedure, hemostasis should be pursued with sufficient blood products available if needed. In the case of massive hemorrhage, a plan should be in place for timely management. Depending on the extent of disease, nonanatomic procedures, such as wedge resection, can be performed by an experienced gynecologic oncologist, whereas anatomic resections should be performed by a hepatobiliary surgeon.

Superficial Hepatic Lesions

With the transcoelomic spread of ovarian cancer cells, superficial implants involving the liver are often present in advanced disease. Ablation or cauterization of these implants may be sufficient for treating nonbulky lesions, and the liver surface surrounding the lesion can also be cauterized to allow for an adequate margin. Bleeding from the resection site can be controlled using an argon beam coagulator or with hemostatic agents. Superficial implants along the posterior liver are more difficult to reach and require adequate mobilization.

Nonanatomic Resection of Parenchymal Disease

Nonanatomic resections of parenchymal disease generally do not clearly distinguish the segmental anatomy and are often limited to wedge resections. Lesions generally less than 4 cm in dimension are considered for these types of resections, allowing for preservation of parenchymal volume. A combination of cautery and coagulation is generally sufficient for dissection and hemostasis. Wedge resections may be associated with a higher rate of intraoperative bleeding owing to limited vascular occlusion.

Nonmajor Anatomic Resection of Parenchymal Disease

For small-volume disease requiring the removal of a single liver segment, nonmajor anatomic resection will limit the vascular flow and control blood loss, allowing for the safe excision of tumor. In ovarian cancer, unisegmentectomy of 5 or 6 is more commonly required. With the conservation of hepatic volume, patients with underlying liver disease or function may benefit from this more limited approach.

Major (Anatomic) Resection of Parenchymal Disease

Commonly described major resections are generally described by their anatomic locations. Right hepatectomy involves segments 5, 6, 7, and 8, whereas left is the removal of segments 2, 3, and 4. Left lobectomy includes the removal of segments 2 and 3. Extended right hepatectomy removes segments 5, 6, 7, 8, and 4, whereas extended left includes segments 2, 3, 4, 5, and 8. If these larger resections are required for complete cytoreduction, a hepatobiliary surgeon is recommended to assist in the resection.

POSTOPERATIVE CONSIDERATIONS

Because of the pattern of tumor spread in ovarian cancer, the en bloc removal of liver metastasis often extends into the diaphragm peritoneum, musculature, and tendons. The acute care of these patients postoperatively in an intensive unit allows for precise monitoring and early recognition of complications. Because ovarian cancer surgery can predispose patients to develop ascites and have increased interstitial retention, strict fluid and electrolyte management in addition to early mobilization is recommended. Early nutrition (oral or enteral feeding) is an important component to support liver regeneration. Prophylactic anticoagulation is typically recommended in patients with gynecologic cancer undergoing abdominal surgery postoperatively. In the setting of liver resection, coagulation laboratory test parameters generally are self-limited and resolve without intervention. Therefore, in addition to early mobilization, thromboprophylaxis should be started pending no additional risk factors for bleeding.[41]

With the right diaphragm commonly being included in the radical dissection for liver metastasis, patients are at increased risk of pleural effusions and pneumothorax. A catheter is often placed within the thoracic cavity while closing the defect to allow the pneumothorax to be evacuated and the lung to expand. Prophylactic chest tubes have also been considered to decrease the risk of complications attributed to pleural effusions. Additional considerations inherent to liver resection include the risk of bile, which may present with peritonitis, or obstructive jaundice and posthepatectomy liver failure, which can be associated with an increased international normalized ratio (INR) or bilirubin after postoperative day 5.[41]

Nasser and colleagues[42] retrospectively reviewed postoperative complications in patients who underwent right upper-quadrant radical surgery as part of cytoreduction for primary or relapsed ovarian cancer. Of 132 patients who underwent some combination of diaphragmatic peritoneal stripping, full-thickness resection, portahepatis tumor resection, and partial hepatectomy, 74% (98/132) had an increase in their liver function tests postoperative with a peak at 24 hours. They reported 1 case fatality on postoperative day 3, and although there were no major complications intraoperatively, there was greater than expected blood loss of 2 L with eventual clinical decompensation.

NONSURGICAL TECHNIQUES

Currently, there are no randomized trial data regarding the nonsurgical management of liver metastasis from gynecologic cancer. Data are limited to case series and reports that have reviewed the role of hepatic artery chemotherapy, radiofrequency ablation (RFA), microwave ablation, and computed tomographic (CT)–guided high-dose brachytherapy.[43,44] Although the technological details of these therapies are reviewed in later articles, the authors evaluate the data to support the use of these interventions in gynecologic cancer.

Local therapies, such as radiofrequency and microwave ablation, can be performed via minimally invasive techniques and should be considered in patients with contraindications to anesthesia or surgery. RFA delivers high-frequency alternating current using an electrode to the tissue surrounding the tumor leading to cell death.[45] Tumors that are generally larger than 5 cm should not be treated with RFA because of concern of incomplete necrosis leading to higher recurrence rates.[46] There are very limited data for the use of RFA in metastatic gynecologic cancer.[47,48]

RFA is generally limited to patients who are not ideal candidates for surgical resection, but have disease limited to the liver. Consideration for this treatment could also be made intraoperatively when the surgical treatment plan includes optimal extrahepatic cytoreduction; however, the patient may not be deemed amenable to liver resection. For patients who are not ideal candidates for resection, the minimally invasive approach of RFA may allow for treatment of metastatic liver lesions, intraoperatively avoiding the morbidity of liver resection and allowing for the prompt initiation of systemic chemotherapy.[43] Given the lack of randomized trials, the application of RFA should be limited to a case-by-case basis.

CT-guided high-dose-rate brachytherapy for targeted cytoreduction of metachronous ovarian cancer metastases to the liver has been reported in a case series.[44] Intralesional injections for hepatic lesions and intraarterial therapy have also been described in the literature.[49–51] These studies have shown that such therapies are feasible in metastatic gynecologic cancers; however, no randomized trials have been conducted to assess the long-term efficacy.

GENETIC AND MOLECULAR PROGNOSTIC MARKERS

As the paradigm for frontline chemotherapy shifts to incorporate molecular and genetic signatures in treatment decisions, the role of these prognostic markers in surgical decision making should also be evaluated. There are limited data evaluating the benefit of surgical resection of hepatic lesions in patients with BRCA mutations. Gallotta and colleagues[52] published a series of 34 patients with recurrent ovarian cancer that underwent hepatic resection with a 3-year progression-free survival of 49.1% and overall survival of 72.9%. On univariate analysis, BRCA mutational status played a statistically favorable role with 3-year progression-free survival of 81.0% compared with 15.2% in wild-type patients ($P = .001$). More recently, Moore and colleagues[53] published the results of the phase 3 randomized trial, SOLO1 (ClinicalTrials.gov, NCT01844986), which showed a substantial benefit in the progression-free survival of patients with advanced stage BRCA 1/2 ovarian cancer who received maintenance therapy with the polyadenosine diphosphate-ribose polymerase inhibitor, olaparib. Patients who received olaparib had a 70% lower risk of disease recurrence compared with the placebo group, and final survival analysis is still pending. This practice-changing study highlights the significant role tumor biology and biomarkers will have in assessing which patients may benefit from aggressive surgical intervention. Other investigators have evaluated the predictive model of specific gene expression data; however, there remains a need for additional studies to validate potential molecular prognostic markers that correlate with surgical outcomes.[54]

UTERINE CANCER

Uterine cancer is the most common gynecologic cancer in the United States.[2] Most patients generally present with symptoms, such as postmenopausal bleeding, and as a result are diagnosed at earlier stages. Patients with advanced staged disease only comprise 10% to 15% of new cases, but more than half of uterine cancer deaths. The optimal treatment of advanced uterine cancer is still not clearly defined; however, several retrospective studies have evaluated the role of surgical cytoreduction in the management of advanced and recurrent endometrial cancer. There remain limited data regarding the management of stage IV disease and the potential benefit of aggressive hepatic resection.

Similar to the paradigm of optimal cytoreduction for ovarian cancer, complete cytoreduction of visible disease is associated with improved overall and progression-free survival in advanced endometrial cancer.[55–58] A metaanalysis performed by Barlin and colleagues[59] reviewed retrospective studies investigating the role of cytoreductive surgery in advanced or recurrent endometrial cancer. In this pooled analysis, complete cytoreduction and adjuvant radiation were both positively associated with survival, whereas adjuvant chemotherapy was associated with decreased survival. With each 10% increase in the proportion of patients undergoing complete cytoreduction, survival improved by 9.3 months.

A case series from Knowles and colleagues[60] reviewed patients with recurrent endometrial cancer who underwent hepatic resection with a disease-free survival ranging from 8 to 66 months following resection. More recently, the use of NACT has been investigated in the treatment of stage IV endometrial cancer; however, patients with liver metastasis were excluded from surgical management.[61] Currently, there are no RCTs evaluating the role of aggressive surgical management or NACT for advanced uterine cancer.

CERVICAL CANCER

Metastatic cervical cancer overall has a poor prognosis. There are conflicting data regarding whether the organ-specific location of metastatic disease in cervical cancer affects survival.[4,62] Compared with lung and bone metastasis, liver metastasis is less likely to be isolated to a single organ.[63,64] There remains a lack of clear understanding of the hematogenous spread of cervical cancer to the liver. Data regarding the role of hepatic resection are limited to case reports and series that have reported the safety and feasibility of hepatic resection for metastatic cervical cancer when isolated metastasis is suspected.[65–67]

RARE TUMORS

Uterine sarcomas are uncommon and typically metastasize via hematogenous spread. The peritoneal cavity/omentum is the most frequently involved site of metastasis followed by the lung and pelvic lymph nodes.[68] Given this pattern, surgery has largely been limited to early-stage disease with curative intent or for palliation. Uterine leiomyosarcoma (LMS) is a rare uterine cancer that is highly aggressive with an increased risk of disease recurrence regardless of stage. Studies evaluating the role of surgical management of metastatic and recurrent disease are primarily retrospective studies. Much like the ovarian cancer studies, complete cytoreduction is associated with improved progression-free interval.[69] Given the limited number of therapeutic options, surgical resection of metastatic LMS should be carefully balanced with the potential morbidity given the small sample sizes and retrospective nature of the studies showing benefit in progression-free survival.[70–72] Patients with isolated hepatic recurrence with long disease-free intervals should be considered for secondary resection on a case by case basis.

Gestational trophoblastic neoplasia is considered a highly chemosensitive disease; however, patients with liver metastasis still have worse survival.[73] Barber and colleagues[74] recently reviewed the outcomes of patients with gestational trophoblastic neoplasia with hepatic metastasis and reported an improved survival after the introduction of systemic chemotherapy with EMA-CO (etoposide, methotrexate, actinomycin D, cyclophosphamide, vincristine). The risk of hemorrhage from liver metastases typically occurs after the initiation of chemotherapy leading to necrosis and bleeding as a result of vascular malformations from the tumor. The use of transcatheter angiographic embolization of the hepatic artery has been reported in case series as an effective form of treatment for acute hemorrhage.[73]

Of particular interest is the role of aggressive liver resection in the management of tumors that are not highly chemosensitive. Mizuno and colleagues[75] investigated whether stage IV nonserous, nonendometrioid ovarian cancers, such as mucinous and clear cell histology, were associated with similar benefits from complete cytoreductive surgery. In this retrospective study, non-S/E (serous/endometrioid) groups had worse median overall survival compared with S/E tumors (0.9 years vs 3.1 years; P<.001). For patients with non-S/E cancers, improved prognosis was associated with single-organ metastasis (except for liver and distant lymph nodes), no residual tumor, and resection of metastasis. Granulosa cell tumors of the ovary are rare and associated with delayed recurrences that can be highly chemoresistant. Madhuri and colleagues[76] report a case series of 3 patients who underwent secondary CRS with liver resection without significant complications. Additional investigators have also evaluated the role of RFA in granulosa cell tumors metastatic to the liver.[77] Given the tendency of chemoresistance, aggressive surgical resection may be beneficial in cases with isolated liver metastasis; however, further studies are needed.

MEDICAL ONCOLOGIST PERSPECTIVE

While systemic chemotherapy and biologic therapy may be curative in the setting of advanced hematologic malignancy, rarely does this hold true for solid tumors (testicular cancer being a notable exception). As such, among the vast majority of advanced solid tumors: surgery is a *sine qua non* for curative-intent treatment. During the 1980s and 1990s, advances in liver surgery (e.g., intraoperative ultrasound, portal vein embolization), followed by laparoscopic techniques in the 2000s led to major advances in resection of primary and metastatic liver tumors.[78] Perhaps the greatest evidence in support of resecting hepatic metastases emanates from the literature on colorectal liver metastasis (CLM). In the era of modern chemotherapeutics and biologic agents, advanced CRC rarely is curable without surgery (5-year relative survival rate is 14%)[2], and yet clinical trials have demonstrated impressive 47-60% 5-year OS rates in select CRC patients undergoing hepatic tumor resection.[79] Of course, success after hepatic resection in metastatic CRC does not necessarily translate to other solid tumor sites. In this context the present article provides a current appraisal of the literature on surgical management of liver metastases in patients with gynecologic cancers.

Consensus is lacking for treatment of hepatic metastases in the major gynecologic malignancies. The major problem we see from the extant literature is simply the lack of randomized controlled clinical-trial-based evidence. Beyond case series and anecdotal reports, there is a lack of clear evidence supporting hepatic tumor resection in uterine cancer, and cervical cancer. There are defined roles for surgery of metastatic disease (regardless of metastatic site) for specific, less common gynecologic cancers such as uterine leiomyosarcomas. The bulk of evidence supporting hepatic resection in gynecologic malignancies comes from studies on ovarian cancer. In the setting of primary cytoreductive surgery, a number of retrospective studies are discussed, reporting impressive survival outcomes (exceeding 50 months OS) among ovarian cancer patients treated with hepatic resection.[10,36] These studies are limited in sample size and of course one must strongly consider selection bias given their retrospective nature. In the setting of secondary cytoreductive surgery, GOG-0213 (Clinicaltrials.gov NCT 00565851) stands out as a landmark randomized controlled clinical trial of secondary cytoreductive surgery followed by chemotherapy or chemotherapy alone.[37] No statistical difference in OS was observed between the groups. However, a borderline significant 18% decreased risk of progression was noted in the surgery group, accompanied by a non-significant 11% decreased risk of death. Given that the trial was not powered to examine progression-free survival (PFS) or OS differences by presence of liver metastasis – these results are interesting, if not compelling, and would appear to warrant further study. Lack of randomized controlled clinical trial-based evidence does not necessarily indicate a lack of benefit. Through this review of the literature, it is clear that hepatic resection of ovarian liver metastases can be safe (especially in select patients having oligome tastic disease) and associated with excellent outcomes. A multidisciplinary approach (together with hepatobiliary surgery in case of tumors requiring segmental resections) is often warranted, and further considerations regarding the timing of neoadjuvant and/or adjuvant chemotherapy must be refined. Unique characteristics of ovarian cancer are highlighted, including direct spread in ovarian cancer with en bloc hepatic resections often dictating additional extended diaphragmatic resections. Such disease characteristics complicate treatment and make it difficult to extrapolate directly from the literature on surgical approaches to non-ovarian cancers.

   While data for surgical resection of liver metastases in ovarian cancer are promising, the present review highlights both challenges unique to the field and the need for additional clinical trial-based evidence. What might the optimal clinical trial study design look like? Perhaps a randomized controlled trial of primary (or secondary) cytoreduction and chemotherapy vs. chemotherapy alone, restricted to patients having hepatic (with or without extrahepatic) metastases. Such a trial would be narrow in scope, requiring a large group effort (as could be done in through the U.S. National Clinical Trials Network). This trial would need sufficient power to convincingly address the role of hepatic resection in select ovarian cancer patients, with OS and PFS primary and secondary endpoints, respectively. However, smaller, phase I/II trials could also be considered- perhaps restricted to a genetic cohort (e.g., BRCA1/2 mutation), with surrogate endpoint markers or safety/feasibility endpoints, and containing robust translational correlative science (ie, circulating tumor DNA and/or plasma exome analyses). Such smaller trials would substantially improve our understanding of the disease process while providing valuable information on how best to approach ovarian cancer-associated liver metastases.

SUMMARY

With the rapid approval of biomarker-driven novel therapeutics, the role of aggressive surgery, including the resection of liver metastasis, remains controversial. Although the data supporting aggressive resection of liver metastasis are largely retrospective and case based, the randomized control data to address neoadjuvant versus chemotherapy have been widely criticized. Residual disease remains an important predictor for survival. If a patient cannot achieve near optimal cytoreduction, radical cytoreductive procedures, such as hepatic resection, should be considered for palliation only. When hepatic resection is considered to achieve complete surgical cytoreduction, a collaborative approach with hepatobiliary surgeons should be emphasized to allow for individualized treatment plans with consideration given to the patient's performance status and the extent of liver disease.

DISCLOSURE

Research reported in this publication was supported by the National Cancer Institute of the National Institutes of Health under Award Number T32CA060396.

REFERENCES

1. Bray F, Ferlay J, Soerjomataram I, et al. Global cancer statistics 2018: GLOBO-CAN estimates of incidence and mortality worldwide for 36 cancers in 185 countries. CA Cancer J Clin 2018;68(6):394–424.
2. Siegel RL, Miller KD, Jemal A. Cancer statistics, 2020. CA Cancer J Clin 2020; 70(1):7–30.
3. Deng K, Yang C, Tan Q, et al. Sites of distant metastases and overall survival in ovarian cancer: a study of 1481 patients. Gynecol Oncol 2018;150(3):460–5.
4. Gardner AB, Charo LM, Mann AK, et al. Ovarian, uterine, and cervical cancer patients with distant metastases at diagnosis: most common locations and outcomes. Clin Exp Metastasis 2020;37(1):107–13.
5. Rose PG, Piver MS, Tsukada Y, et al. Metastatic patterns in histologic variants of ovarian cancer. An autopsy study. Cancer 1989;64(7):1508–13.
6. Berek JS, Kehoe ST, Kumar L, et al. Cancer of the ovary, fallopian tube, and peritoneum. Int J Gynecol Obstet 2018;143(S2):59–78.
7. Nakayama K, Nakayama N, Katagiri H, et al. Mechanisms of ovarian cancer metastasis: biochemical pathways. Int J Mol Sci 2012;13(9):11705–17.
8. Brunschwig A. Hepatic lobectomy for metastatic cancer. Cancer 1963;16: 277–82.
9. Chi DS, Fong Y, Venkatraman ES, et al. Hepatic resection for metastatic gynecologic carcinomas. Gynecol Oncol 1997;66(1):45–51.
10. Bristow RE, Montz FJ, Lagasse LD, et al. Survival impact of surgical cytoreduction in stage IV epithelial ovarian cancer. Gynecol Oncol 1999;72(3):278–87.
11. Winter WE 3rd, Maxwell GL, Tian C, et al. Tumor residual after surgical cytoreduction in prediction of clinical outcome in stage IV epithelial ovarian cancer: a Gynecologic Oncology Group Study. J Clin Oncol 2008;26(1):83–9.
12. Curtin JP, Malik R, Venkatraman ES, et al. Stage IV ovarian cancer: impact of surgical debulking. Gynecol Oncol 1997;64(1):9–12.
13. Bristow RE, Tomacruz RS, Armstrong DK, et al. Survival effect of maximal cytoreductive surgery for advanced ovarian carcinoma during the platinum era: a meta-analysis. J Clin Oncol 2002;20(5):1248–59.
14. Yoon SS, Jarnagin WR, Fong Y, et al. Resection of recurrent ovarian or fallopian tube carcinoma involving the liver. Gynecol Oncol 2003;91(2):383–8.
15. Merideth MA, Cliby WA, Keeney GL, et al. Hepatic resection for metachronous metastases from ovarian carcinoma. Gynecol Oncol 2003;89(1):16–21.
16. Eisenhauer EL, Abu-Rustum NR, Sonoda Y, et al. The addition of extensive upper abdominal surgery to achieve optimal cytoreduction improves survival in patients with stages IIIC-IV epithelial ovarian cancer. Gynecol Oncol 2006;103(3):1083–90.
17. Griffiths CT. Surgical resection of tumor bulk in the primary treatment of ovarian carcinoma. Natl Cancer Inst Monogr 1975;42:101–4.
18. Chang SJ, Hodeib M, Chang J, et al. Survival impact of complete cytoreduction to no gross residual disease for advanced-stage ovarian cancer: a meta-analysis. Gynecol Oncol 2013;130(3):493–8.
19. Ang C, Chan KK, Bryant A, et al. Ultra-radical (extensive) surgery versus standard surgery for the primary cytoreduction of advanced epithelial ovarian cancer. Cochrane Database Syst Rev 2011;(4):CD007697.
20. Chi DS, Eisenhauer EL, Zivanovic O, et al. Improved progression-free and overall survival in advanced ovarian cancer as a result of a change in surgical paradigm. Gynecol Oncol 2009;114(1):26–31.

21. Aletti GD, Dowdy SC, Gostout BS, et al. Aggressive surgical effort and improved survival in advanced-stage ovarian cancer. Obstet Gynecol 2006;107(1):77–85.
22. Aletti GD, Santillan A, Eisenhauer EL, et al. A new frontier for quality of care in gynecologic oncology surgery: multi-institutional assessment of short-term outcomes for ovarian cancer using a risk-adjusted model. Gynecol Oncol 2007;107(1):99–106.
23. Eisenkop SM, Spirtos NM. What are the current surgical objectives, strategies, and technical capabilities of gynecologic oncologists treating advanced epithelial ovarian cancer? Gynecol Oncol 2001;82(3):489–97.
24. Wright AA, Bohlke K, Armstrong DK, et al. Neoadjuvant chemotherapy for newly diagnosed, advanced ovarian cancer: Society of Gynecologic Oncology and American Society of Clinical Oncology Clinical Practice Guideline. J Clin Oncol 2016;34(28):3460–73.
25. Kehoe S, Hook J, Nankivell M, et al. Primary chemotherapy versus primary surgery for newly diagnosed advanced ovarian cancer (CHORUS): an open-label, randomised, controlled, non-inferiority trial. Lancet 2015;386(9990):249–57.
26. Fagotti A, Ferrandina G, Vizzielli G, et al. Phase III randomised clinical trial comparing primary surgery versus neoadjuvant chemotherapy in advanced epithelial ovarian cancer with high tumour load (SCORPION trial): final analysis of peri-operative outcome. Eur J Cancer 2016;59:22–33.
27. Onda T, Satoh T, Saito T, et al. Comparison of treatment invasiveness between upfront debulking surgery versus interval debulking surgery following neoadjuvant chemotherapy for stage III/IV ovarian, tubal, and peritoneal cancers in a phase III randomised trial: Japan Clinical Oncology Group Study JCOG0602. Eur J Cancer 2016;64:22–31.
28. Coleridge SL, Bryant A, Lyons TJ, et al. Chemotherapy versus surgery for initial treatment in advanced ovarian epithelial cancer. Cochrane Database Syst Rev 2019;2019(10).
29. Reuss A, du Bois A, Harter P, et al. TRUST: Trial of Radical Upfront Surgical Therapy in advanced ovarian cancer (ENGOT ov33/AGO-OVAR OP7). Int J Gynecol Cancer 2019;29(8):1327–31.
30. Dood RL, Zhao Y, Armbruster SD, et al. Defining survivorship trajectories across patients with solid tumors: an evidence-based approach. JAMA Oncol 2018; 4(11):1519–26.
31. Morgan RJ Jr, Armstrong DK, Alvarez RD, et al. Ovarian cancer, version 1.2016, NCCN Clinical Practice Guidelines in Oncology. J Natl Compr Cancer Netw 2016; 14(9):1134–63.
32. Al Rawahi T, Lopes AD, Bristow RE, et al. Surgical cytoreduction for recurrent epithelial ovarian cancer. Cochrane Database Syst Rev 2013;(2):CD008765.
33. Bristow RE, Puri I, Chi DS. Cytoreductive surgery for recurrent ovarian cancer: a meta-analysis. Gynecol Oncol 2009;112(1):265–74.
34. Zang RY, Harter P, Chi DS, et al. Predictors of survival in patients with recurrent ovarian cancer undergoing secondary cytoreductive surgery based on the pooled analysis of an international collaborative cohort. Br J Cancer 2011; 105(7):890–6.
35. Chi DS, McCaughty K, Diaz JP, et al. Guidelines and selection criteria for secondary cytoreductive surgery in patients with recurrent, platinum-sensitive epithelial ovarian carcinoma. Cancer 2006;106(9):1933–9.
36. Kolev V, Pereira EB, Schwartz M, et al. The role of liver resection at the time of secondary cytoreduction in patients with recurrent ovarian cancer. Int J Gynecol Cancer 2014;24(1):70–4.
37. Coleman RL, Spirtos NM, Enserro D, et al. Secondary surgical cytoreduction for recurrent ovarian cancer. N Engl J Med 2019;381(20):1929–39.

38. Bois AD, Vergote I, Ferron G, et al. Randomized controlled phase III study evaluating the impact of secondary cytoreductive surgery in recurrent ovarian cancer: AGO DESKTOP III/ENGOT ov20. J Clin Oncol 2017;35(15_suppl):5501.

39. Nathan H, Cameron JL, Choti MA, et al. The volume-outcomes effect in hepato-pancreato-biliary surgery: hospital versus surgeon contributions and specificity of the relationship. J Am Coll Surg 2009;208(4):528–38.

40. Learn PA, Bach PB. A decade of mortality reductions in major oncologic surgery: the impact of centralization and quality improvement. Med Care 2010;48(12): 1041–9.

41. Longoria TC, Bristow RE. Technique of Liver Resection in Cytoreductive Surgery for Advanced Ovarian Cancer. In: Ayhan A, Reed N, Gultekin M, Dursun P. Textbook of Gynaecological Oncology. Vol 1. 3rd ed. Ankara, Turkey: Gunes Publishing; 2016: 801-808.

42. Nasser S, Lathouras K, Nixon K, et al. Impact of right upper quadrant cytoreductive techniques with extensive liver mobilization on postoperative hepatic function and risk of liver failure in patients with advanced ovarian cancer. Gynecol Oncol 2018;151(3):466–70.

43. Mateo R, Singh G, Jabbour N, et al. Optimal cytoreduction after combined resection and radiofrequency ablation of hepatic metastases from recurrent malignant ovarian tumors. Gynecol Oncol 2005;97(1):266–70.

44. Collettini F, Poellinger A, Schnapauff D, et al. CT-guided high-dose-rate brachytherapy of metachronous ovarian cancer metastasis to the liver: initial experience. Anticancer Res 2011;31(8):2597–602.

45. Chong WK. Radiofrequency ablation of liver tumors. J Clin Gastroenterol 2001; 32(5):372–4.

46. Kuvshinoff BW, Ota DM. Radiofrequency ablation of liver tumors: influence of technique and tumor size. Surgery 2002;132(4):605–11 [discussion: 11-2].

47. Bleicher RJ, Allegra DP, Nora DT, et al. Radiofrequency ablation in 447 complex unresectable liver tumors: lessons learned. Ann Surg Oncol 2003;10(1):52–8.

48. Bojalian MO, Machado GR, Swensen R, et al. Radiofrequency ablation of liver metastasis from ovarian adenocarcinoma: case report and literature review. Gynecol Oncol 2004;93(2):557–60.

49. Chao A, Lai CH, Hsueh S, et al. Intralesional injection for hepatic metastasis from cervical carcinoma. A report of two cases. J Reprod Med 2001;46(11):1008–12.

50. Seki A, Hori S, Sueyoshi S, et al. Local control and prognostic significance of transarterial treatment for limited recurrence of ovarian cancer as third-line and beyond therapy. Int J Clin Oncol 2014;19(6):1065–73.

51. Mambrini A, Caudana R, Zamagni D, et al. Intra-arterial hepatic chemotherapy in heavily pretreated patients with epithelial ovarian cancer. Ann Oncol 2005;16(2): 334–5.

52. Gallotta V, Conte C, D'Indinosante M, et al. Prognostic factors value of germline and somatic BRCA in patients undergoing surgery for recurrent ovarian cancer with liver metastases. Eur J Surg Oncol 2019;45(11):2096–102.

53. Moore K, Colombo N, Scambia G, et al. Maintenance olaparib in patients with newly diagnosed advanced ovarian cancer. N Engl J Med 2018;379(26): 2495–505.

54. Borley J, Wilhelm-Benartzi C, Brown R, et al. Does tumour biology determine surgical success in the treatment of epithelial ovarian cancer? A systematic literature review. Br J Cancer 2012;107(7):1069–74.

55. Goff BA, Goodman A, Muntz HG, et al. Surgical stage IV endometrial carcinoma: a study of 47 cases. Gynecol Oncol 1994;52(2):237–40.

56. Chi DS, Welshinger M, Venkatraman ES, et al. The role of surgical cytoreduction in stage IV endometrial carcinoma. Gynecol Oncol 1997;67(1):56–60.
57. Bristow RE, Duska LR, Montz FJ. The role of cytoreductive surgery in the management of stage IV uterine papillary serous carcinoma. Gynecol Oncol 2001; 81(1):92–9.
58. Memarzadeh S, Holschneider CH, Bristow RE, et al. FIGO stage III and IV uterine papillary serous carcinoma: impact of residual disease on survival. Int J Gynecol Cancer 2002;12(5):454–8.
59. Barlin JN, Ueda SM, Bristow RE. Cytoreductive surgery for advanced and recurrent endometrial cancer: a review of the literature. Womens Health (Lond) 2009; 5(4):403–11.
60. Knowles B, Bellamy CO, Oniscu A, et al. Hepatic resection for metastatic endometrioid carcinoma. HPB (Oxford) 2010;12(6):412–7.
61. Vandenput I, Van Calster B, Capoen A, et al. Neoadjuvant chemotherapy followed by interval debulking surgery in patients with serous endometrial cancer with transperitoneal spread (stage IV): a new preferred treatment? Br J Cancer 2009;101(2):244–9.
62. Gardner AB, Charo LM, Mann AK, et al. Ovarian, uterine, and cervical cancer patients with distant metastases at diagnosis: most common locations and outcomes. Clin Exp Metastasis 2020;37(1):107–13.
63. Kim GE, Lee SW, Suh CO, et al. Hepatic metastases from carcinoma of the uterine cervix. Gynecol Oncol 1998;70(1):56–60.
64. Yin Z, Tang H, Li L, et al. Impact of sites versus number of metastases on survival of patients with organ metastasis from newly diagnosed cervical cancer. Cancer Manag Res 2019;11:7759–66.
65. Kaseki H, Yasui K, Niwa K, et al. Hepatic resection for metastatic squamous cell carcinoma from the uterine cervix. Gynecol Oncol 1992;44(3):284–7.
66. Filipescu A, Balescu I, Bacalbasa N. Upper abdominal resection for isolated metastatic lesions in recurrent cervical cancer. Anticancer Res 2018;38(3):1659–63.
67. Bacalbasa N, Balescu I, Dima S, et al. Hepatic resection for liver metastases from cervical cancer is safe and may have survival benefit. Anticancer Res 2016;36(6): 3023–7.
68. Rose PG, Piver MS, Tsukada Y, et al. Patterns of metastasis in uterine sarcoma. An autopsy study. Cancer 1989;63(5):935–8.
69. Park JY, Kim DY, Suh DS, et al. Prognostic factors and treatment outcomes of patients with uterine sarcoma: analysis of 127 patients at a single institution, 1989-2007. J Cancer Res Clin Oncol 2008;134(12):1277–87.
70. Leitao MM Jr, Zivanovic O, Chi DS, et al. Surgical cytoreduction in patients with metastatic uterine leiomyosarcoma at the time of initial diagnosis. Gynecol Oncol 2012;125(2):409–13.
71. Giuntoli RL, Garrett-Mayer E, Bristow RE, et al. Secondary cytoreduction in the management of recurrent uterine leiomyosarcoma. Gynecol Oncol 2007; 106(1):82–8.
72. Leitao MM, Brennan MF, Hensley M, et al. Surgical resection of pulmonary and extrapulmonary recurrences of uterine leiomyosarcoma. Gynecol Oncol 2002; 87(3):287–94.
73. Lok CA, Reekers JA, Westermann AM, et al. Embolization for hemorrhage of liver metastases from choriocarcinoma. Gynecol Oncol 2005;98(3):506–9.
74. Barber EL, Schink JC, Lurain JR. Hepatic metastasis in gestational trophoblastic neoplasia: patient characteristics, prognostic factors, and outcomes. J Reprod Med 2014;59(5–6):199–203.

75. Mizuno M, Kajiyama H, Shibata K, et al. Prognostic value of histological type in stage IV ovarian carcinoma: a retrospective analysis of 223 patients. Br J Cancer 2015;112(8):1376–83.

76. Madhuri TK, Butler-Manuel S, Karanjia N, et al. Liver resection for metastases arising from recurrent granulosa cell tumour of the ovary–a case series. Eur J Gynaecol Oncol 2010;31(3):342–4.

77. Jacobs IA, Chang CK, Salti G. Hepatic radiofrequency ablation of metastatic ovarian granulosa cell tumors. Am Surg 2003;69(5):416–8.

78. Kokudo N, Takemura N, Ito K, Mihara F. The history of liver surgery: achievements over the past 50 years. Ann Gastroenterol Surg 2020;4:109–17.

79. Kow AWC. Hepatic metastasis from colorectal cancer. J Gastrointest Oncol 2019; 10:1274–98.

80. Neumann UP, Fotopoulou C, Schmeding M, et al. Clinical outcome of patients with advanced ovarian cancer after resection of liver metastases. Anticancer Res 2012;32(10):4517–21. PMID: 23060580.

81. Kamel SI, de Jong MC, Schulick RD, et al. The role of liver-directed surgery in patients with hepatic metastasis from a gynecologic primary carcinoma. World J Surg 2011;35(6):1345–54.

82. Lim MC, Kang S, Lee KS, et al. The clinical significance of hepatic parenchymal metastasis in patients with primary epithelial ovarian cancer. Gynecol Oncol 2009;112(1):28–34.

83. van Wijk FH, van der Burg ME, Burger CW, et al. Management of recurrent endometrioid endometrial carcinoma: an overview. Int J Gynecol Cancer 2009;19(3):314–20.

84. Loizzi V, Rossi C, Cormio G, et al. Clinical features of hepatic metastasis in patients with ovarian cancer. International Journal of Gynecological Cancer 2005; 15:26–31.

85. Lambrou NC, Gómez-Marín O, Mirhashemi R, et al. Optimal surgical cytoreduction in patients with Stage III and Stage IV endometrial carcinoma: a study of morbidity and survival. Gynecol Oncol 2004;93(3):653–8.

86. Ayhan A, Taskiran C, Celik C, et al. Surgical stage III endometrial cancer: analysis of treatment outcomes, prognostic factors and failure patterns. Eur J Gynaecol Oncol 2002;23(6):553–6.

87. Fan Q, Huang H, Lian L, et al. Characteristics, diagnosis and treatment of hepatic metastasis of pure immature ovarian teratoma. Chin Med J (Engl) 2001;114(5):506–9.

88. Naik R, Nordin A, Cross PA, et al. Optimal cytoreductive surgery is an independent prognostic indicator in stage IV epithelial ovarian cancer with hepatic metastases. Gynecol Oncol 2000;78(2):171–5.

89. Elias D, Cavalcanti de Albuquerque A, Eggenspieler P, et al. Resection of liver metastases from a noncolorectal primary: indications and results based on 147 monocentric patients. J Am Coll Surg 1998;187(5):487–93.

90. Roh HJ, Kim DY, Joo WD, et al. Hepatic resection as part of secondary cytoreductive surgery for recurrent ovarian cancer involving the liver. Arch Gynecol Obstet 2011;284(5):1223–9.

91. Pekmezci S, Saribeyoglu K, Aytac E, et al. Surgery for isolated liver metastasis of ovarian cancer. Asian J Surg 2010;33(2):83–8.

92. Weitz J, Blumgart LH, Fong Y, et al. Partial hepatectomy for metastases from noncolorectal, nonneuroendocrine carcinoma. Ann Surg 2005;241(2):269–76.

93. Merideth MA, Cliby WA, Keeney GL, et al. Hepatic resection for metachronous metastases from ovarian carcinoma. Gynecol Oncol 2003;89(1):16–21.

Surgical Management of Genitourinary Cancer Liver Metastases

Guillaume Martel, MD, MSc, FRCSC, FACS[a],*,
Kimberly A. Bertens, MD, MPH, FRCSC, FACS[a,b],
Christina Canil, MD, FRCPC[b]

KEYWORDS

- Renal cell carcinoma • Germ cell tumor • Prostate cancer • Bladder cancer
- Urothelial carcinoma • Liver metastasis • Hepatectomy

KEY POINTS

- Liver resection in select patients with metastatic renal cell cancer can lead to prolonged survival. Patients with metachronous and low-burden disease are most likely to benefit.
- Chemotherapy is first-line treatment for metastatic germ cell tumors. The role of liver resection is dependent on germ cell lineage and the initial response to chemotherapy.
- The prognosis of patients with liver metastases from prostate cancer is poor and liver-only lesions are rare. Liver resection is generally not indicated.
- The cumulative experience with liver resection for metastatic bladder cancer is extremely limited. Liver metastases are a poor prognostic indicator for surgical metastasectomy.
- Any consideration of liver metastasectomy for genitourinary cancers should be thoroughly discussed within a multidisciplinary group of experts.

INTRODUCTION

Genitourinary malignancies, including, but not limited to, renal cell carcinoma, germ cell tumors (GCTs), prostate cancer, and bladder cancer, are common and account for 20% of new cancer cases in the United States.[1] Yet, for liver surgeons, these malignancies remain an infrequent indication for hepatectomy. Although most liver surgeons have an excellent understanding of the behavior of gastrointestinal cancers, their knowledge base pertaining to urologic oncology may be more limited. Thus,

[a] Liver and Pancreas Unit, Department of Surgery, The Ottawa Hospital, University of Ottawa, 501 Smyth Road, Ottawa, Ontario K1H 8L6, Canada; [b] Division of Medical Oncology, Department of Medicine, The Ottawa Hospital, University of Ottawa, 501 Smyth Road, Ottawa, Ontario K1H 8L6, Canada
* Corresponding author.
E-mail address: gumartel@toh.ca
Twitter: @ChamoGui (G.M.); @BertensK (K.A.B.)

Surg Oncol Clin N Am 30 (2021) 89–102
https://doi.org/10.1016/j.soc.2020.08.003
1055-3207/21/© 2020 Elsevier Inc. All rights reserved.

this review provides a synopsis of the 4 most common genitourinary cancers, in addition to summarizing the data supporting or refuting the role of liver resection for metastases.

RENAL CELL CARCINOMA

Renal cell carcinoma (RCC) accounts for approximately 3% of all malignancies, and its incidence is increasing. Surgery remains the only curative approach for RCC. Traditional chemotherapy and radiation have limited efficacy, although molecularly targeted therapy and immunotherapy have improved overall survival (OS) in the metastatic setting in multicenter trials.[2,3] Despite these advancements, the prognosis for metastatic RCC remains poor, with a 5-year OS of 5% to 10%.[4] Synchronous metastases are present in 25% to 30% of patients with RCC and another 30% present with distant metastases after nephrectomy.[5,6] Although both bone and lung metastases are common, liver metastases are seen in only 20% of patients with distant disease.[7,8] Among the patients with hepatic metastases, only 5% have disease confined to the liver, with multiorgan metastases more prevalent.[8] Furthermore, hepatic metastases from RCC commonly are multiple, with solitary liver metastases occurring in less than 25% of cases.[9]

Metastasectomy may be considered with (1) synchronous metastases, performed concurrently with nephrectomy; (2) metachronous metastases after nephrectomy; or (3) minimal residual disease after response to initial systemic therapy. The role of surgical metastasectomy is most well established for pulmonary metastases, and patients with lung-only metastases have been shown to have a favorable prognosis.[10] Conversely, hepatic metastases are considered a poor prognostic factor and typically are a predictor of widespread disease.[11,12] Only approximately 1% of patients with liver metastases from RCC will undergo surgical management.[13]

The existing literature on hepatic resection for RCC metastases is scant and consists mostly of small, single-institution retrospective studies (**Table 1**). Much of the data are reported as pooled series of hepatic resections for noncolorectal and nonneuroendocrine (NCNNE) metastases, which limits the conclusions that can be drawn. Moreover, few studies include significant numbers of patients from the era of targeted therapy and immunotherapy.

Survival

The median survival post–liver resection for RCC ranges from 16 months to 142 months, when considering series of 10 or more patients.[11–21] OS at 3 years and 5 years ranged from 26% to 68% and from 26% to 62%, respectively. Likewise, 5-year disease-free survival in these selected patients was favorable, ranging from 11% to 25%.[11,12,16] The second largest series by Staehler and colleagues[17] compared 68 patients undergoing liver resection for RCC metastases to 20 patients with liver metastases who refused surgery. Their reported median survival and 5-year OS of 142 months and 62%, respectively, for the resected patients are outliers within the literature, although this cohort excluded patients with extrahepatic disease.[17] This is the only study to use a comparable group of patients that did not undergo surgery. The investigators reported that patients who did not undergo hepatic resection had significantly higher risk of death (hazard ratio [HR] 2.23; $P = .04$).[17] Importantly, the patients who underwent liver resection in these series represent a highly selected group of patients with favorable oncologic features. Greater than two-thirds of the patients had liver resection for metachronous metastases and 35% to 58% had a solitary liver lesion.[11,14,17,19,22]

Table 1
Outcomes of liver metastasectomy for renal cell carcinoma

Authors, Publication Year	Number of Patients	Solitary Lesion (%)	Synchronous (%)	Median Overall Survival (mo)	3-Year Overall Survival	5-Year Overall Survival	5-Year Disease-Free Survival
Stief et al,[13] 1997	13	—	—	16	—	—	—
Alves et al,[14] 2003	14	35.7	—	26	26	—	—
Aloia et al,[12] 2006	19	—	26	36	52	26	25
Adam et al,[15] 2006	85	—	—	36	—	38	—
Thelen et al,[16] 2007	31	—	19.4	48	54.3	38.9	26.1
Staehler et al,[17] 2010	68	38.2	—	142	—	62.2	—
Marudanayagam et al,[18] 2011	24	—	—	22.5	—	—	—
Ruys et al,[11] 2011	33[a]	57.6	30.3	33	47	43	11
Hatzaras et al,[22] 2012	43	55.8	—	—	62.1	—	—
Langan et al,[19] 2012	10	38.9	27.7	24	45	34	—
Schiergens et al,[20] 2016	28	—	—	50	68	—	—
Beetz et al,[21] 2020	40	—	7.5	37.8	52.6	38.0	—

[a] 4 patients had radiofrequency ablation.
Data from Refs.[11–21]

Prognostic Factors

Various prognostic factors for improved survival after liver resection for RCC have been published. Several studies have demonstrated improved survival with prolonged disease-free intervals between primary resection and metastasectomy. Alves and colleagues[14] reported that patients with more than 2 years between nephrectomy and liver resection had improved 2-year OS (71% vs 25%, $P = .05$). Similarly, metachronous metastases were found to be a favorable prognostic factor in multiple other cohorts.[11,19,21,22] Negative resection margins also have been found to be predictive of improved OS post–liver resection for RCC.[11,14,16] Hatzaras and colleagues[22] included patients with extrahepatic disease in their analysis and found that having liver-only metastases was associated with improved survival. Conversely, Langan and colleagues[19] did not find the presence of extrahepatic disease to have an impact on long-term outcomes. The number of liver metastases was not predictive of survival in multiple studies.[11,14,19,22] Most recently, Beetz and colleagues[21] specifically set out to examine the role of hepatectomy in the era of targeted therapy. They concluded that after the introduction of the tyrosine kinase inhibitor sunitinib in Europe (July 2006), there was a significantly improved median OS in patients undergoing hepatic resection for RCC (45.2 vs 27.5 months, $P = .04$).

GERM CELL CANCERS

Testicular cancer is the most common malignancy in young men between the ages of 15 years to 35 years.[23] Although overall oncological outcomes are excellent, careful staging at diagnosis, adequate chemotherapeutic treatment, and meticulous follow-up are paramount to effectively manage this cancer.[24] GCTs account for approximately 95% of testicular malignancies and are divided into seminomas and nonseminomas. Nonseminoma GCTs (NSGCTs) are less common but have more aggressive biology. They typically are made up of 1 or more of 4 cell types: embryonal carcinoma, choriocarcinoma, yolk sac tumor, and teratoma.[25] The serum tumor markers α-fetoprotein (AFP) and β-human chorionic gonadotropin (β-hCG) are critical in informing prognosis and detecting relapse. Pure seminomas do not exhibit elevations in AFP.

Chemotherapy is paramount in the treatment of GCT regardless of stage. Multimodal treatment with surgery and chemotherapy leads to long-term progression-free survival of greater than 90%, inclusive of those with metastatic disease.[26] The most common sites of metastases for GCTs include lung, liver, brain, and bone.[27] The International Germ Cell Cancer Collaborative Group (IGCCCG) classifies GCT into good-risk, intermediate-risk, and poor-risk groups. Nonpulmonary visceral metastases portend an intermediate-risk designation and poor-risk designation for seminomas and NSGCTs, respectively.[28] Although well-established guidelines exist on the surgical management of advanced testicular cancer in the form of retroperitoneal lymph node (LN) dissection, there are limited data on the role of surgery in patients with no-pulmonary metastases.[28] The indications for surgery vary depending on germ cell lineage.

Seminoma

After treatment with chemotherapy, patients with advanced stage seminoma should undergo computerized tomography (CT) imaging of the chest, abdomen, and pelvis as well as measurement of serum AFP and β-hCG. Patients with normal serum tumor markers and a residual mass of 3 cm or less should undergo surveillance alone because these patients have a negligible risk of harboring viable seminoma.[29,30] In patients with a residual mass larger than 3 cm, and normal serum tumor markers, viable tumor is present in up to 30% of cases.[31] Fluorodeoxyglucose (FDG)-PET can be utilized to distinguish between viable seminoma and necrotic or fibrotic tissue but should be reserved until at least 6 weeks postchemotherapy.[32] If the FDG-PET is positive, percutaneous biopsy or resection should be considered.[29]

Nonseminomatous Germ Cell Tumors

Patients with advanced metastatic NSGCTs to nonpulmonary visceral sites are considered to have poor-risk tumors, and 4 cycles of chemotherapy is recommended.[29] Fewer than half of patients treated in this have a durable complete response and 30% die of their disease.[28,33] After chemotherapy, CT of the chest, abdomen, and pelvis, as well as serum tumor markers are required to assess response. If there is complete radiological response and normal serum tumor markers, surveillance is warranted.[29] In those with partial response (with residual masses) and normal or near-normal (but stable) tumor markers, resection of all residual masses is recommended.[34] Patients with rising tumor markers should be assessed for further systemic therapy.

Liver Metastases

The published literature pertaining to surgical management of liver metastases from testicular GCT consists of only 4 retrospective single-institution reviews.[27,35–37] A majority of patients with liver metastases also have extrahepatic involvement.[35] Hahn and colleagues[35] published the largest series consisting of 57 patients, all of whom had testicular NSGCT. In this series, 16% of the lesions resected represented benign lesions, including necrotic tumor, 51% teratoma, and 33% active tumor. A majority of those with active tumor (14/19) had normal serum tumor markers, and the 2-year OS rate for these patients was 43%. The investigators recommended liver resection in all patients with residual liver masses postchemotherapy, except those with elevated serum tumor markers.[35] In Rivoire and colleagues'[36] report on 37 patients with GCT, 27 of these patients had primary testicular lesions. A significant number of patients (18/27) had necrosis only on final pathology, and this was more common when liver lesions were 1 cm or less. The 5-year OS for this population was 62%.[36] The investigators recommended surveillance of lesions of 1 cm or less, and resection for lesions measuring between 1 cm and 3 cm. Furthermore, they recommended against resection of hepatic tumors greater than 3 cm in men due to a poor outcomes.[36] Conversely, Copson and colleagues[27] advocate for conservative management in patients with residual liver disease after initial treatment. They identified 27 patients with GCT and liver metastases treated at a single center. Of these, 8 had a complete biochemical and radiologic response to chemotherapy, and 7 had residual radiologic abnormalities in the liver with normal tumor markers.[27] None of the 7 patients underwent resection and the median OS was 49 months, which was comparable to the survival reported in the surgical series.[27] These investigators recommend surgical resection of liver metastases only in cases of a marker-negative relapse.

PROSTATE CANCER

Prostate cancer is the most common cancer and second highest cause of cancer-related death in men in the United States.[1] Importantly, approximately 4% of patients have metastatic disease at presentation.[38] Androgen-deprivation therapy is the standard-of-care backbone in the setting of metastatic disease.[39] Recent data show that treatment intensification with docetaxel or androgen receptor axis-targeted (ARAT) agents, such as apalutamide, enzalutamide, and abiraterone, can improve OS for patients with metastatic hormone-sensitive disease. With progression to castration-resistant disease, additional treatment options include cabazitaxel and radium-223.[40]

Metastatic Disease Sites

LNs and bone are the most prevalent sites of metastases in prostate cancer. Visceral metastases are less common but can occur in the lungs, liver, and brain. Across the literature, the incidence of liver metastases varies between 4.3% and 25%, based on data source and castration-resistance status.[41–44] An autopsy study of 1589 men with prostate cancer identified hematogenous metastases in 35%, of which 90% had bony lesions, 46% lung lesions, and 25% liver lesions.[42] A meta-analysis of 9 phase 3 randomized trials of patient-level data with metastatic castration-resistant prostate cancer reported that 20.8% had visceral lesions, among whom 44% had liver metastases (8.6% of whole cohort).[41] Finally, a population-based study of 12,180 patients with metastatic prostate cancer identified liver lesions in 4.3% of patients and only 105 of 12,180 (0.9%) patients had liver-only disease.[43]

Among patients with metastatic disease, survival is associated significantly with the site of disease. More specifically, the presence of liver metastases usually portends a poor prognosis, irrespective of other sites of involvement.[41,43] In their meta-analysis of 8820 patients, Halabi and colleagues[41] noted that the presence of liver metastases carried the worst OS (median 13.5 months) compared with LN (31.6 months), bone (21.3 months), or lung (19.4 months). Similarly, Budnik and colleagues[43] noted that the presence of liver metastases, whether alone (HR 1.63 [1.24–2.13]) or together with bony lesions (HR 1.99 [1.70–2.34]) or with bone and lung lesions (HR 2.25 [1.82–2.80]), was associated with the worse risk-adjusted OS compared with bony metastases alone.

Metastatic Disease Burden

Multiple studies have shown that metastatic burden is an important prognostic factor in prostate cancer. Specifically, increasing metastatic disease volume is associated with worse OS and shorter time to progression to castration-resistant prostate cancer.[40,45] Francini and colleagues[45] have reported that hormone-sensitive patients with high-volume metastatic disease had a significantly worse risk-adjusted prognosis than those with low-volume disease, whether or not they presented de novo (median OS 43.2 months) or after prior local therapy (median OS 55.2 months).

In this context, the concept of oligometastatic prostate cancer is important. Oligometastatic disease increasingly is identified given the growing availability of improved imaging modalities, such as whole-body magnetic resonance imaging and prostate-specific membrane antigen (PSMA) PET/CT.[46] An evolving body of literature suggests that in select patients, early detection and targeted local therapy of limited metastatic lesions may delay the use of systemic therapies.[46–48] Although no definition is agreed on, oligometastatic disease generally can be considered biologically distinct from high-volume metastatic disease.[46] Existing studies have defined it on the basis of having a low disease burden (from ≤1 to ≤5 lesions, most commonly ≤3) and occasionally on the basis of having more favorable metastatic locations, such as bone or LN.[46] A vast majority of patients who have received metastasis-directed therapy have been those with bone or LN lesions.[46–48] Metastasis-directed therapy for liver, lung, or brain lesions has been exceedingly rare, likely in large part owing to the rarity of low-burden visceral metastases.

Role of Liver Resection

Liver-directed therapy for oligometastatic prostate cancer is so uncommon that it has been published primarily in individual case reports. An examination of the literature describing cases of liver resection for metastatic prostate cancer has identified only a handful of publications pertaining to 7 patients.[48–53] Among these, all except 1 had a metachronous presentation,[48] in some cases with several years of disease-free interval.[50–52] All except 1 patient had a single liver lesion.[48] All reported patients were disease-free at least 1 year post–liver resection. This review highlights the rarity of the set of conditions under which liver surgery ever could be contemplated for this disease. Liver resection generally is not indicated for metastatic prostate cancer. Although a few of the published patients have had excellent outcomes, liver resection for this disease remains a once-in-a-career statistical anomaly that should be vetted thoroughly by a multidisciplinary group of experts and weighted against other ablative modalities, such as stereotactic body radiation therapy.[54]

BLADDER CANCER

Bladder cancer is the sixth most prevalent cancer in the United States and the most common cancer of the urinary system.[1] Approximately three-quarters of cases occur in male patients, with a median age at presentation of 73 years. Urothelial carcinoma, also known as transitional cell carcinoma, accounts for 90% of bladder cancers in North America and Europe.[55] Three main phases of bladder cancer can be described: (1) nonmuscle invasive, (2) muscle-invasive, and (3) metastatic disease. Approximately 5% to 15% of patients have metastatic or unresectable disease at presentation.[56] In addition, approximately half of patients with muscle-invasive cancer relapse with LN or distant metastatic disease after initial intensive therapy.[56] With locally advanced inoperable or metastatic disease, the mainstay of treatment is platinum-based systematic chemotherapy, with which the initial response rate is high (40%–70%).[55,56] Despite this high response rate with modern chemotherapeutic agents, median survival is 15 months and 5-year survival is 15%.[55]

Metastatic Disease Sites

Metastatic urothelial carcinoma of the bladder can be separated into distant LNs (M1a) and visceral lesions (M1b). Bianchi and colleagues[57] have reported on 7543 patients with metastatic bladder cancer from the National Inpatient Sample, noting that the most common sites were LN (25%), bone (24%), urinary (23%), lung (19%), liver (18%), and brain (3%). The rate of multisite metastases was 29%. Another group examined 1862 patients from the Surveillance, Epidemiology, and End Results database, reporting that bone lesions were most frequent (43%), followed by lung (39%), distant LN (34%), and liver (26%) metastases.[58] Liver-only metastases were found in 9.2% of patients.

Not unexpectedly, OS and cancer-specific survival have been demonstrated to be significantly worse with visceral (M1b) metastases than with distant LNs (M1a).[56,58–60] As well, patients with a single site of metastatic disease fared significantly better than those with multiple sites.[56,58] Among patients with single-site metastasis, those with liver lesions had the worst overall outcomes.[58] Finally, poor performance status also has been identified as an important predictor of worsening survival.[59,60] This finding is important in the bladder cancer population, given the high median age at presentation and the associated high prevalence of renal insufficiency.

Surgical Metastasectomy

Despite the high response rate to chemotherapy in the setting of locoregional recurrence or distant metastases after cystectomy, most patients experience disease progression rapidly within a median of 7 months.[61] Some investigators have noted that progression occurs principally at the original metastatic site, which has provided a clinical rationale for considering surgical metastasectomy to improve oncologic outcomes.[62] This clinical rationale has been emboldened further by the reporting of favorable prognostic factors in published nomograms.[59,60]

Several publications have examined the role of metastasectomy after systemic chemotherapy for locally advanced disease and/or lymph-positive bladder cancer as well as for visceral metastases. A recent systematic review by Patel and colleagues[63] pooled data from 17 studies (1990–2015; n = 412) and reported that metastasectomy was associated with improved OS (HR 0.63 [0.49–0.81]) compared with nonoperative management. The 2 dominant metastasis groups in this review were distant LN and lung. The mean time to recurrence after metastasectomy was 14.3 months, whereas OS from metastasectomy ranged from 2 months to 60 months in included studies.

Abufaraj and colleagues[56] recently published a second systematic review, including 27 studies published between 1999 and 2016, reaching slightly different conclusions. The principal finding was that metastasectomy remains largely unproved. Moreover, the investigators commented that "anecdotal reports" have suggested a possible survival benefit with lung resection for metastatic bladder cancer in the context of a multimodal treatment plan in well-selected patients. The narrative evidence synthesis specifically identified metastasectomy in the absence of liver lesions as more favorable and more likely to lead to improved outcomes.

Role of Liver Resection

Liver resection for metastatic urothelial carcinoma rarely is reported in the literature. In total, 27 individual cases of liver resection for metastatic bladder/urothelial cancer have been identified in the liver surgery literature[48,64–66] (n = 6) and in the metastatic urology literature[63,67,68] (n = 21). No published series of hepatectomy has solely examined outcomes with metastatic bladder cancer. Similarly, some of the largest published multi-institutional series of liver resections for NCNNE metastases (n = 2037) were reviewed and were noted not to have included any case of metastatic bladder/urothelial cancer.[15,69,70] A systematic review of 3596 resections for NCNNE metastases published up to 2013 also did not include any relevant cases.[71]

The cumulative experience with liver resection for metastatic bladder cancer remains extremely limited. The conditions under which this operation might be considered are rare and include liver-only disease, minimal disease burden, or ideally single-lesion, good performance status, and objective response to systemic chemotherapy. The decision to perform a liver resection for metastatic bladder cancer should include input from experts in urologic oncology.

MEDICAL ONCOLOGY PERSPECTIVE

Many published series assessing the role of liver resection for NCNNE metastases report outcomes for genitourinary cancers as 1 entity, primarily because the number of cases was limited.[20,69,71,72] On review of individual cases, the genitourinary category often consisted of a heterogeneous group of cancers of renal, germ cell, adrenal, urothelial, and even ovarian origin. These cancers are very different in terms of tumor biology, patient population, prognosis, and systemic therapy options, making it difficult to determine the applicability of reported conclusions. In addition, due to better understanding of tumor biology and advancements in drug therapy, the management and outcomes of different genitourinary cancers has changed tremendously since these patients were reported and, therefore, would not accurately reflect current treatment paradigms.

Table 2
Prognostic factors with metastatic renal cell carcinoma treated with vascular endothelial growth factor receptor agents

Prognostic Factors	Score	Prognosis	Median Survival
Anemia Elevated calcium	0	Favorable	43.2 mo
Elevated neutrophils Elevated platelets	1–2	Intermediate	22.5 mo
Karnofsky performance status <80% Time from diagnosis to treatment <1 y	≥3	Poor	7.8 mo

Data from Heng DY, Xie W, Regan MM, Warren MA, Golshayan AR, Sahi C, et al. Prognostic factors for overall survival in patients with metastatic renal cell carcinoma treated with vascular endothelial growth factor-targeted agents: results from a large, multicenter study. J Clin Oncol 2009;27:5794–5799.

When considering resection of liver metastases, patient selection is imperative. For metastatic RCC, in the era of tyrosine kinase inhibitors and immunotherapy, the International Metastatic Renal Cell Carcinoma Database Consortium has identified 6 factors that can categorize patients into prognostic groups and be used to guide management (**Table 2**).[73] Patients with favorable disease can have prolonged, disease-free intervals with resection of oligometastases. Because liver metastases are associated with worse prognosis and often extrahepatic disease, however, patients may be best served with systemic therapy as initial management.[74]

Similarly, with metastatic GCT, by definition from the IGCCCG, the presence of liver metastases places patients in a poor prognostic category for nonseminomas.[28] Primary management of metastatic GCT is platinum-based triplet chemotherapy. In cases of nonseminoma, patients with radiological response and normalization of tumor markers undergo resection of residual disease, including liver metastases. It is essential that patients with metastatic GCT be managed at a center with high-volume expertise because data show improved outcomes for patients with poor prognostic disease.[75]

Primary management of metastatic urothelial cancers (bladder and upper tract disease) also consists of systemic therapy (chemotherapy and immunotherapy). Isolated liver metastases are rare and on multivariable analysis are considered a negative prognostic factor.[63,76] Therefore, resection of liver metastases does not play a prominent role in patient care. Initial management of metastatic prostate cancer is androgen deprivation therapy, often in combination with ARAT therapies or chemotherapy for treatment intensification.[77] With development of more accurate imaging modalities, such as PSMA-PET scans to identify metastatic sites, the management of oligometastatic disease is evolving rapidly and often involves focused radiation therapy techniques as opposed to surgical options, particularly because bone and LNs are by far the more common sites of metastases.

SUMMARY

In summary, it is of upmost importance that patients with genitourinary malignancies undergoing consideration of resection of liver metastases be discussed in a multidisciplinary setting, including expertise with knowledge of the natural history and systemic therapy options for the patients' specific cancer. This approach ensures appropriate selection of patients who are most likely to benefit from surgical intervention.

DISCLOSURE

The authors declare that they have no conflicts of interest.

REFERENCES

1. Siegel RL, Miller KD, Jemal A. Cancer statistics, 2020. CA Cancer J Clin 2020; 70:7–30.
2. Motzer RJ, Hutson TE, Tomczak P, et al. Overall survival and updated results for sunitinib compared with interferon alfa in patients with metastatic renal cell carcinoma. J Clin Oncol 2009;27:3584–90.
3. Motzer RJ, Tannir NM, McDermott DF, et al. Nivolumab plus ipilimumab versus sunitinib in advanced renal-cell carcinoma. N Engl J Med 2018;378:1277–90.
4. Gupta K, Miller JD, Li JZ, et al. Epidemiologic and socioeconomic burden of metastatic renal cell carcinoma (mRCC): a literature review. Cancer Treat Rev 2008; 34:193–205.
5. Mickisch GH, Garin A, van Poppel H, et al. Radical nephrectomy plus interferon-alfa-based immunotherapy compared with interferon alfa alone in metastatic renal-cell carcinoma: a randomised trial. Lancet 2001;358:966–70.
6. Hamada S, Ito K, Kuroda K, et al. Clinical characteristics and prognosis of patients with renal cell carcinoma and liver metastasis. Mol Clin Oncol 2015;3:63–8.
7. Bianchi M, Sun M, Jeldres C, et al. Distribution of metastatic sites in renal cell carcinoma: a population-based analysis. Ann Oncol 2012;23:973–80.
8. Weiss L, Harlos JP, Torhorst J, et al. Metastatic patterns of renal carcinoma: an analysis of 687 necropsies. J Cancer Res Clin Oncol 1988;114:605–12.
9. Janzen NK, Kim HL, Figlin RA, et al. Surveillance after radical or partial nephrectomy for localized renal cell carcinoma and management of recurrent disease. Urol Clin North Am 2003;30:843–52.
10. Kim DY, Karam JA, Wood CG. Role of metastasectomy for metastatic renal cell carcinoma in the era of targeted therapy. World J Urol 2014;32:631–42.
11. Ruys AT, Tanis PJ, Nagtegaal ID, et al. Surgical treatment of renal cell cancer liver metastases: a population-based study. Ann Surg Oncol 2011;18:1932–8.
12. Aloia TA, Adam R, Azoulay D, et al. Outcome following hepatic resection of metastatic renal tumors: the Paul Brousse Hospital experience. HPB (Oxford) 2006;8: 100–5.
13. Stief CG, Jáhne J, Hagemann JH, et al. Surgery for metachronous solitary liver metastases of renal cell carcinoma. J Urol 1997;158:375–7.
14. Alves A, Adam R, Majno P, et al. Hepatic resection for metastatic renal tumors: is it worthwhile? Ann Surg Oncol 2003;10:705–10.
15. Adam R, Chiche L, Aloia T, et al. Hepatic resection for noncolorectal nonendocrine liver metastases. Ann Surg 2006;244:524–35.
16. Thelen A, Jonas S, Benckert C, et al. Liver resection for metastases from renal cell carcinoma. World J Surg 2007;31:802–7.
17. Staehler MD, Kruse J, Haseke N, et al. Liver resection for metastatic disease prolongs survival in renal cell carcinoma: 12-year results from a retrospective comparative analysis. World J Urol 2010;28:543–7.
18. Marudanayagam R, Sandhu B, Perera MT, et al. Hepatic resection for noncolorectal, non-neuroendocrine, non-sarcoma metastasis: a single-centre experience. HPB (Oxford) 2011;13:286–92.
19. Langan RC, Ripley RT, Davis JL, et al. Liver directed therapy for renal cell carcinoma. J Cancer 2012;3:184–90.

20. Schiergens TS, Lüning J, Renz BW, et al. Liver resection for non-colorectal non-neuroendocrine metastases: where do we stand today compared to colorectal cancer? J Gastrointest Surg 2016;20:1163–72.
21. Beetz O, Söffker R, Cammann S, et al. Extended hepatic metastasectomy for renal cell carcinoma-new aspects in times of targeted therapy: a single-center experience over three decades. Langenbecks Arch Surg 2020;405:97–106.
22. Hatzaras I, Gleisner AL, Pulitano C, et al. A multi-institution analysis of outcomes of liver-directed surgery for metastatic renal cell cancer. HPB (Oxford) 2012;14: 532–8.
23. Tonyali S, Yazici S. Does solitary- and organ-confined metastasectomy really improve survival in advanced urologic malignancies? Int Urol Nephrol 2016;48: 671–80.
24. Albers P, Albrecht W, Algaba F, et al. EAU guidelines on testicular cancer: 2011 update. Eur Urol 2011;60:304–19.
25. Vasdev N, Moon A, Thorpe AC. Classification, epidemiology and therapies for testicular germ cell tumours. Int J Dev Biol 2013;57:133–9.
26. Oldenburg J, Fosså SD, Nuver J, et al. Testicular seminoma and non-seminoma: ESMO Clinical Practice Guidelines for diagnosis, treatment and follow-up. Ann Oncol 2013;24(Suppl 6):vi125–32.
27. Copson E, McKendrick J, Hennessey N, et al. Liver metastases in germ cell cancer: defining a role for surgery after chemotherapy. BJU Int 2004;94:552–8.
28. International Germ Cell Cancer Collaborative Group. International Germ Cell Consensus classification: a prognostic factor-based staging system for metastatic germ cell cancers. J Clin Oncol 1997;15:594–603.
29. National Comprehensive Cancer Network. NCCN Clinical Practice Guidelines in Oncology: Testicular Cancer. 2019. Available at: https://www.nccn.org/professionals/physician_gls/pdf/testicular.pdf. Accessed April 17, 2020.
30. Pfister D, Haidl F, Paffenholz P, et al. Metastatic surgery in testis cancer. Curr Opin Urol 2016;26:590–5.
31. Puc HS, Heelan R, Mazumdar M, et al. Management of residual mass in advanced seminoma: results and recommendations from the Memorial Sloan-Kettering Cancer Center. J Clin Oncol 1996;14:454–60.
32. Bachner M, Loriot Y, Gross-Goupil M, et al. 2-18fluoro-deoxy-D-glucose positron emission tomography (FDG-PET) for postchemotherapy seminoma residual lesions: a retrospective validation of the SEMPET trial. Ann Oncol 2012;23:59–64.
33. van Dijk MR, Steyerberg EW, Habbema JDF. Survival of non-seminomatous germ cell cancer patients according to the IGCC classification: An update based on meta-analysis. Eur J Cancer 2006;42:820–6.
34. Riggs SB, Burgess EF, Gaston KE, et al. Postchemotherapy surgery for germ cell tumors-what have we learned in 35 years? Oncologist 2014;19:498–506.
35. Hahn TL, Jacobson L, Einhorn LH, et al. Hepatic resection of metastatic testicular carcinoma: a further update. Ann Surg Oncol 1999;6:640–4.
36. Rivoire M, Elias D, De Cian F, et al. Multimodality treatment of patients with liver metastases from germ cell tumors: the role of surgery. Cancer 2001;92:578–87.
37. You YN, Leibovitch BC, Que FG. Hepatic metastasectomy for testicular germ cell tumors: is it worth it? J Gastrointest Surg 2009;13:595–601.
38. Cetin K, Beebe-Dimmer JL, Fryzek JP, et al. Recent time trends in the epidemiology of stage IV prostate cancer in the United States: analysis of data from the surveillance, epidemiology, and end results program. Urology 2010;75: 1396–404.

39. So AI, Chi KN, Danielson B, et al. Canadian Urological Association-Canadian Urologic Oncology Group guideline on metastatic castration-naive and castration-sensitive prostate cancer. Can Urol Assoc J 2020;14:17–23.

40. Saad F, Aprikian A, Finelli A, et al. 2019 Canadian Urological Association (CUA)-Canadian Uro Oncology Group (CUOG) guideline: management of castration-resistant prostate cancer (CRPC). Can Urol Assoc J 2019;13:307–14.

41. Halabi S, Kelly WK, Ma H, et al. Meta-analysis evaluating the impact of site metastasis on overall survival in men with castration-resistant prostate cancer. J Clin Oncol 2016;34:1652–9.

42. Bubendorf L, Schöpfer A, Wagner U, et al. Metastatic patterns of prostate cancer: an autopsy study of 1,589 patients. Hum Pathol 2000;31:578–83.

43. Budnik J, Suri J, Bates JE, et al. Prognostic significance of sites of visceral metastatic disease in prostate cancer: a population-based study of 12,180 patients. Clin Genitourin Cancer 2019;17:260–7.

44. Gandaglia G, Karakiewicz PI, Briganti A, et al. Impact of site of metastases on survival in patients with metastatic prostate cancer. Eur Urol 2015;68:325–34.

45. Francini E, Gray KP, Xie W, et al. Time of metastatic disease presentation and volume of disease are prognostic for metastatic hormone sensitive prostate cancer (mHSPC). Prostate 2018;78:889–95.

46. Rao A, Vapiwala N, Schaeffer EM, et al. Oligometastatic prostate cancer: a shrinking subset or an opportunity for cure? Am Soc Clin Oncol Educ Book 2019;39:309–20.

47. Slaoui A, Albisinni S, Aoun F, et al. A systematic review of contemporary management of oligometastatic prostate cancer: fighting a challenge or tilting at windmills? World J Urol 2019;37:2343–53.

48. Hamner JB, Crowder C. Evolving role of hepatic resection for metastatic urologic malignancies. Am Surg 2017;83:628–32.

49. Battaglia A, Devos G, Decaestecker K, et al. Metastasectomy for visceral and skeletal oligorecurrent prostate cancer. World J Urol 2019;37:1543–9.

50. Wang SC, McCarthy LP, Mehdi S. Isolated hepatic metastasis from prostate carcinoma. Urol Case Rep 2017;10:51–3.

51. Kawai H, Shiba H, Kanehira M, et al. Successful resection of a solitary metastatic liver tumor from prostate cancer 15 years after radical prostatectomy: a case report. Surg Case Rep 2017;3:17.

52. Tilmans G, Navez J, Komuta M, et al. Solitary prostate cancer liver metastasis: an exceptional indication for liver resection. Acta Chir Belg 2020;1–5 [Epub ahead of print].

53. Lang H, Nussbaum KT, Weimann A, et al. Liver resection for non-colorectal, non-neuroendocrine hepatic metastases. Chirurg 1999;70:439–46.

54. Ahmed KA, Bamey BM, Davis BJ, et al. Stereotactic body radiation therapy in the treatment of oligometastatic prostate cancer. Front Oncol 2013;2:215.

55. Bellmunt J. Treatment of metastatic urothelial cancer of the bladder and urinary tract UpToDate. Philadelphia, PA, USA: Wolters Kluwer; 2020. Available at: https://www.uptodate.com/contents/treatment-of-metastatic-urothelial-cancer-of-the-bladder-and-urinary-tract. Accessed April 26, 2020.

56. Abufaraj M, Dalbagni G, Daneshmand S, et al. The role of surgery in metastatic bladder cancer: a systematic review. Eur Urol 2018;73:543–57.

57. Bianchi M, Roghmann F, Becker A, et al. Age-stratified distribution of metastatic sites in bladder cancer: a population-based analysis. Can Urol Assoc J 2014;8:e148–58.

58. Dong F, Shen Y, Gao F, et al. Prognostic value of site-specific metastases and therapeutic roles of surgery for patients with metastatic bladder cancer: a population-based study. Cancer Manag Res 2017;9:611–26.

59. Bajorin DF, Dodd PM, Mazumdar M, et al. Long-term survival in metastatic transitional-cell carcinoma and prognostic factors predicting outcome of therapy. J Clin Oncol 1999;17:3173–81.

60. Apolo AB, Ostrovnaya I, Halabi S, et al. Prognostic model for predicting survival of patients with metastatic urothelial cancer treated with cisplatin-based chemotherapy. J Natl Cancer Inst 2013;105:499–503.

61. von der Maase H, Hansen SW, Roberts JT, et al. Gemcitabine and cisplatin versus methotrexate, vinblastine, doxorubicin, and cisplatin in advanced or metastatic bladder cancer: results of a large, randomized, multinational, multicenter, phase III study. J Clin Oncol 2000;18:3068–77.

62. Heidenreich A, Wilop S, Pinkawa M, et al. Surgical resection of urological tumor metastases following medical treatment. Dtsch Arztebl Int 2012;109:631–7.

63. Patel V, Lorduy AC, Sterna A, et al. Survival after metastasectomy for metastatic urothelial carcinoma: a systematic review and meta-analysis. Bladder Cancer 2017;3:121–32.

64. O'Rourke TR, Tekkis P, Yeung S, et al. Long-term results of liver resection for non-colorectal, non-neuroendocrine metastases. Ann Surg Oncol 2008;15:207–18.

65. Lendoire J, Moro M, Andriani O, et al. Liver resection for non-colorectal, non-neuroendocrine metastases: analysis of a multicenter study from Argentina. HPB (Oxford) 2007;9:435–9.

66. Schmelzle M, Eisenberger CF, am Esch JS, et al. Non-colorectal, non-neuroendocrine, and non-sarcoma metastases of the liver: resection as a promising tool in the palliative management. Langenbecks Arch Surg 2010;395:227–34.

67. Iwamoto H, Izumi K, Shimura Y, et al. Metastasectomy improves survival in patients with metastatic urothelial carcinoma. Anticancer Res 2016;36:5557–62.

68. Brooks NA, Dahmoush L, Brown JA. Long-term disease-free survival after hepatic metastasectomy for urothelial carcinoma of the bladder: a case report and review of the literature. Clin Med Insights Urol 2015;8:7–10.

69. Groeschl RT, Nachmany I, Steel JL, et al. Hepatectomy for noncolorectal non-neuroendocrine metastatic cancer: a multi-institutional analysis. J Am Coll Surg 2012;214:769–77.

70. Tsang ME, Mahar AL, Martel G, et al. Assessing tools for management of noncolorectal nonneuroendocrine liver metastases: external validation of a prognostic model. J Surg Oncol 2018;118:1006–11.

71. Fitzgerald TL, Brinkley J, Banks S, et al. The benefits of liver resection for non-colorectal, non-neuroendocrine liver metastases: a systematic review. Langenbecks Arch Surg 2014;399:989–1000.

72. Neri F, Ercolani G, Di Gioia P, et al. Liver metastases from non-gastrointestinal non-neuroendocrine tumours: review of the literature. Updates Surg 2015;67:223–33.

73. Heng DY, Xie W, Regan MM, et al. Prognostic factors for overall survival in patients with metastatic renal cell carcinoma treated with vascular endothelial growth factor-targeted agents: results from a large, multicenter study. J Clin Oncol 2009;27:5794–9.

74. Puente Vazquez J, Alonso Gordoa T, Moreno J, et al. New challenges in kidney cancer management: integration of surgery and novel therapies. Curr Treat Options Oncol 2015;16:337.

75. Collette L, Sylvester RJ, Stenning SP, et al. Impact of the treating institution on survival of patients with "poor-prognosis" metastatic nonseminoma. J Natl Cancer Inst 1999;91:839–46.
76. Sengeløv L, Kamby C, von der Maase H. Metastatic urothelial cancer: evaluation of prognostic factors and change in prognosis during the last twenty years. Eur Urol 2001;39:634–42.
77. Stevens DJ, Sooriakumaran P. Oligometastatic prostate cancer. Curr Treat Options Oncol 2016;17:62.

An Overview of Liver Directed Locoregional Therapies

Diederik J. Höppener, MD[a], Dirk J. Grünhagen, MD, PhD[a],
Alexander M.M. Eggermont, MD, PhD[b],
Astrid A.M. van der Veldt, MD, PhD[c],
Cornelis Verhoef, MD, PhD, FEBS[a],*

KEYWORDS

- Liver metastasis • Uveal melanoma • Cutaneous melanoma • Mucosal melanoma
- Systematic review • Surgery • Local therapy • Liver directed therapy

KEY POINTS

- A minority of patients diagnosed with melanoma liver metastasis are eligible for local therapy with curative intent (approximately 5%).
- For cutaneous melanoma liver metastasis, systemic therapy with immune checkpoint inhibition or targeted therapy should be considered as first-line treatment of choice.
- Uveal melanoma is the only melanoma liver metastasis type with data to support complete local/surgical intervention (5-year overall survival approximately 30%).
- Aggressive strategies with surgical tumor load reduction and adjuvant therapy in uveal melanoma have not been shown to improve survival.
- No recommendations for any liver-directed regional therapy in the treatment of mucosal melanoma liver metastasis can be made.

INTRODUCTION

Besides the skin, malignant melanomas also can originate within the uveal tract and from mucosal surfaces.[1,2] Malignant melanoma of cutaneous, uveal, and mucosal origin should be regarded as separate entities, each with distinct biology, epidemiology, and disease characteristics.[1,2] Of the malignant melanomas, cutaneous melanoma is the most common (227/1,000,000/y [**Fig. 1**A]). When cutaneous melanoma

[a] Department of Surgical Oncology and Gastrointestinal Surgery, Erasmus MC Cancer Institute, Dr. Molewaterplein 40, 3015 GD, Rotterdam, the Netherlands; [b] Princess Máxima Center for Pediatric Oncology, Heidelberglaan 25, 3584 CS, Utrecht, the Netherlands; [c] Department of Medical Oncology, Erasmus MC Cancer Institute, Dr. Molewaterplein 40, 3015 GD, Rotterdam, the Netherlands
* Corresponding author. Dr. Molewaterplein 40, Rotterdam 3015 GD, the Netherlands.
E-mail address: c.verhoef@erasmusmc.nl

Surg Oncol Clin N Am 30 (2021) 103–123
https://doi.org/10.1016/j.soc.2020.09.001   **surgonc.theclinics.com**

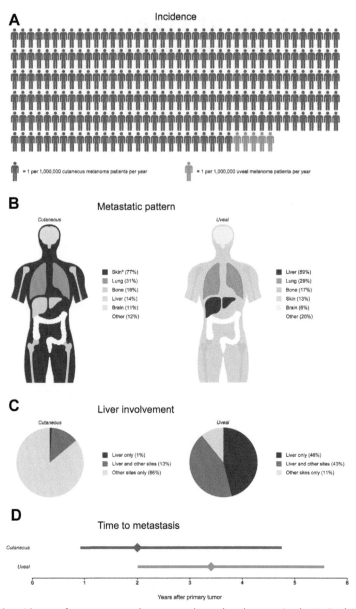

Fig. 1. (A) Incidence of cutaneous melanoma and uveal melanoma in the United States. (B) Metastatic pattern of cutaneous[3] and uveal[5] melanoma (C) Degree of liver involvement in metastatic cutaneous[3] and uveal[5] melanoma. (D) Time to metastasis in cutaneous[4] and uveal[6] melanoma. The diamond shape represents the median and the line represents the corresponding interquartile range. [a] Including subcutaneous tissue and regional lymph nodes.

metastasizes, it most often (77%) is to the locoregional skin and approximately 14% to the liver (**Fig. 1**B).[3] Liver metastases from cutaneous melanoma almost always are seen in combination with metastases at other sites (13%) and only rarely are confined to the liver (1% [**Fig. 1**C]).[3] The median time to metastasis of cutaneous melanoma is 2 years (**Fig. 1D**).[4] Compared with cutaneous melanoma, uveal melanoma is rare (5.1/1,000,000/y [**Fig. 1A**]). Uveal melanoma often metastasizes to the liver, which is involved in 89% of patients with metastatic uveal melanoma and represents the only site of metastasis in 46% (**Fig. 1B, C**).[5] The median time to metastasis of uveal melanoma is 3.4 years (**Fig. 1D**).[6] If uveal melanoma is rare, mucosal melanoma is extremely rare (2.3/1,000,000/y).[2] Mucosal melanoma has a metastatic pattern more comparable to cutaneous melanoma, with the lung the most frequent metastatic site (40%).[7] Metastases in the liver are seen in approximately 36% of metastatic mucosal melanoma patients, with 26% of patients presenting with liver-only metastases.[7] The median time to metastasis of mucosal melanoma is 3.5 years.[8] This article provides a systematic review (**Fig. 2**) of all liver-directed locoregional therapies, including surgical resection for melanoma liver metastases (MLMs), and briefly discusses current efficacy of systemic therapy in order to aid evidence-based clinical decision making in the surgical oncologists' and clinicians' practice.

PARTIAL LIVER RESECTION
Treatment Specifics

The study details, demographics, and treatment specifics of 37 studies investigating surgical treatment of MLMs are reported in Supplementary Data [Table 1].[9–45] Based on 12 studies that reported the complete diagnostic work-up,[12,14,15,21,23,25,26,28,32,35,36,41] a total of 5859 patients were diagnosed with MLMs. Of 5859 patients, 343 patients (6%) diagnosed with MLMs eventually were treated with curative intent resection (Rx). An important reason for patients not undergoing Rx was extrahepatic disease and more extensive liver involvement discovered during surgery compared with preoperative assessments, especially miliary disease in patients with MLMs from uveal origin. Large heterogeneity existed between studies concerning preoperative and postoperative treatment strategies; systemic therapy of any

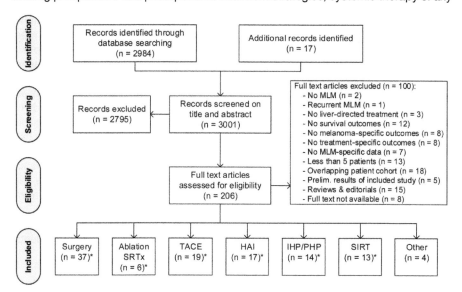

Fig. 2. Overview and flowchart of the article screening and selection process. Prelim, preliminary. * Three studies reported on multiple treatments: one on surgery and HAI, one on surgery and ablation, and one on TACE, SIRT, and IHP.

kind (SYS), hepatic arterial infusion chemotherapy (HAI), and/or transarterial chemoembolization (TACE) were administered both preoperatively and postoperatively across studies. Concurrent ablation was not often utilized (overall 9%, range 0%–31%), whereas major hepatectomy frequently was performed (overall 44%, range 0%–85%).

Outcomes

All 37 studies investigated Rx for MLMs,[9–45] with 7 studies additionally reporting on debulking for MLMs Supplementary Data [Table 2].[11,14,15,25,27,28,43] A total of 947 patients treated with Rx are described, 302 (32%) with MLMs from cutaneous, 489 (52%) with MLMs from uveal, 3 (<1%) with MLMs from mucosal, and 16 (2%) with MLMs from unknown primary origin. In the remaining 137 (14%) patients treated with Rx, MLM origin was not (clearly) reported. The 7 studies reporting on debulking describe a total of 221 patients, 6 (3%) patients with MLMs from cutaneous and 187 (86%) patients with MLMs from uveal origin; MLM origin was not (clearly) reported for 28 (13%) patients. This discrepancy in MLM origin between patients treated with Rx and debulking can be attributed to debulking (with adjuvant HAI/SYS) being standard of care treatment of disseminated liver disease in 2 dedicated uveal melanoma centers, whose series together account for all 187 patients with MLMs from uveal origin treated with debulking. Complete microscopic resection of all MLMs (R0) was achieved in 83% (range 40%-100%) of patients treated with Rx. Perioperative mortality and morbidity after surgical treatment of MLMs (both Rx and debulking) were approximately 2% (range 0%–8%) and 14% (range 0%–36%), respectively. In the patients rendered free of disease after Rx, recurrent disease was observed in a majority of patients (overall 75%, range 40%–100%). Median progression-free survival (PFS) (range of medians) for Rx was 12 (range 5–20) months. Median overall survival (OS) was 26 (range 10–100) months after Rx versus 11 (range 5–18) months after debulking. All but 1 of the studies that reported a median OS of greater than 36 months after Rx were small, highly selected series of less than 20 patients.[14,18,21,26,28,40,44] The study by Groeschl and colleagues,[30] which reported a median OS of 39 months in 31 patients, is a pooled multicenter retrospective analysis of 4 major liver centers, making it highly unlikely that 20 or more patients were treated in a single center. Three of the 4 studies comparing Rx to SYS/best supportive care (BSC) reported improved survival after Rx,[32,35,36] with the study that did not find a survival benefit comparing only 5 patients treated with Rx to 12 treated with SYS/BSC.[13] Similarly, all studies that compared Rx to debulking with or without adjuvant HAI or SYS reported an improved survival for Rx.[11,14,15,25,27,28,43] The only study that directly compared Rx (with HAI), debulking with HAI and SYS/BSC found OS for Rx (with HAI) to be significantly improved compared with the other treatments, with no difference observed between debulking with HAI and SYS/BSC.[15] Four studies directly compared patients with MLMs from cutaneous and uveal origin, with 3 reporting no survival differences between cutaneous and uveal origin[17,33,38] and 1 suggesting improved survival for patients with MLMs from uveal origin.[20] Lastly, 30 of the 37 studies reported long-term survivors (longer than 5 years) after Rx, suggesting possibility of cure.[9,11,12,14–20,23–26,28–31,33,35–45]

Individual patient survival data could be extracted from 14 studies for 99 patients treated with Rx for MLMs and are shown in **Fig. 3**.

ABLATION AND STEREOTACTIC RADIATION THERAPY

The study details, treatment specifics, and outcomes of 6 studies investigating ablation and stereotactic radiation therapy (SRTx) as treatment of MLMs are reported in

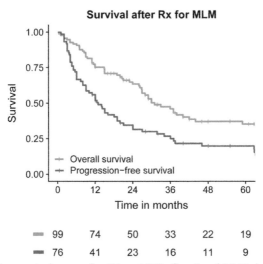

Fig. 3. Kaplan-Meier survival curves for OS and PFS after Rx of MLMs based on individual patient data of 99 patients extracted from 14 studies. PFS data were available for 76 patients.

Supplementary Data [Table 3].[38,46–50] There were 5 retrospective cohort studies and 1 prospective phase Ib/II trial.[50] One study investigated SRTx[49]; the other 5 reported on ablation, all of which treated patients using radiofrequency ablation (RFA)[38,46–48,50]; 2studies also treated patients using cryoablation,[38,48] and 1 study also used microwave ablation.[38] In all the retrospective series, complete treatment of all known (liver) lesions was performed using ablation, SRTx, or Rx (2 patients),[38,46–49] whereas in the prospective phase Ib/II trial by Rozeman and colleagues[50] only 1 liver lesion was treated by RFA and patients subsequently received 4 courses of systemic ipilimumab at varying dosages (0.3 mg/kg, 3 mg/kg, or 10 mg/kg). In this trial it was hypothesized that through an abscopal effect of treating a single MLM with RFA the efficacy of systemic ipilimumab therapy could increase. A total of 134 patients treated with ablation or SRTx are described, 55 (41%) of whom had MLMs from cutaneous and 79 (59%) uveal origin. No treatment-related mortality was reported. Treatment-related morbidity was approximately 20% (range 0%–42%), with the highest morbidity rate of 42% reported in the prospective phase Ib/II trial of RFA plus systemic ipilimumab.[50] Median PFS and OS were 7 (range 3–11) months and 19 (range 11–46) months, respectively. Reported survival was higher in the retrospective studies compared with the prospective phase Ib/II trial of RFA plus systemic ipilimumab. The trial correspondingly concluded that "Combining RFA with ipilimumab 3 mg/kg was well tolerated, but showed very limited clinical activity in uveal melanoma."[50] Akyuz and colleagues[46] directly compared ablation (and laparoscopic Rx in 2 patients) to systemic chemotherapy and found OS to be significantly improved in the patients treated with ablation. Doussot and colleagues[38] directly compared ablation with Rx (see results in Supplementary Data [Table 2] and demonstrated comparable survival outcomes.

TRANSARTERIAL CHEMOEMBOLIZATION

The study details, treatment specifics, and outcomes of 19 studies investigating TACE as treatment of MLMs are reported in Supplementary Data [Table 4].[51–69] There were

15 retrospective cohort studies,[51–53,56,57,59–66,68,69] 2 prospective cohort studies,[55,67] 1 pilot study[58] and 1 prospective phase II trial.[54] The most common chemotherapeutic agent used was cisplatin, which was used in 10 studies,[51–53,56–60,68,69] 2 of which combined cisplatin with doxorubicin and mitomycin C,[56,69] another combined cisplatin with dacarbazine,[53] and 1 study used either fotemustine or cisplatin.[59] Of the other 9 studies, 3 used mitomycin C,[55,62,63] 1 of which combined mitomycin C with doxorubicine[63]; 2 used 1,3-bis(2-chloroethyl)-1-nitrosourea (BCNU)[54,65]; and either fotemustine,[61] drug-eluting beads loaded with irinotecan (DEBIRI),[64] CPT-11,[66] or drug-eluting beads loaded with doxorubicin (DEBDOX)[67] was used in the remaining 4 studies. TACE was combined with SYS in 2 studies,[52,66] and 1 study combined TACE with HAI in 10 patients.[60] In total, 591 patients are described who underwent treatment with TACE for MLMs, a great majority of whom had MLMs of uveal origin (n = 539 [91%]), with only 52 patients (9%) with MLMs from cutaneous origin. Treatment-related mortality and morbidity were approximately 2% (range 0%–7%) and 28% (range 0%–67%), respectively. Response was seen in approximately 28% of patients (range 0%–67%). The 3 studies that reported a response rate of greater than 50% all treated 20 patients or fewer.[53,58,67] Two of these studies used cisplatin,[53,58] and 1 study treated patients with DEBDOX.[67] One study described 14 patients treated with DEBIRI and reported a response rate of 0%.[64] Median PFS and OS were 4 (range 2–9) months and 9 (range 5–28) months, respectively. Two studies directly compared TACE with SYS and reported no discernible survival difference between treatments.[52,64] Valpione and colleagues[66] retrospectively compared TACE with CPT-11 combined with SYS to "other first line regimens" and found a marginally improved OS for TACE (P = .050).

HEPATIC ARTERIAL INFUSION CHEMOTHERAPY

The study details, treatment specifics, and outcomes of 17 studies investigating HAI as treatment of MLMs are reported in Supplementary Data [Table 5].[27,70–85] There were 9 retrospective cohort studies,[27,71,76,77,79–81,83,84] 2 prospective pilot studies,[70,73] 5 prospective phase (I and) II trials,[72,74,75,78,85] and 1 randomized controlled trial (RCT).[82] Fotemustine was the most common drug and was used in 8 studies,[73,74,76–78,80,82,83] including the RCT.[82] One phase II trial combined fotemustine with systemic interferon alfa (IFN-α) and interleukin-2 (IL-2).[74] Another phase II trial combined fotemustine with dacarbazine followed by sequential adoptive cell therapy (ACT), systemic IL-2, and granulocyte-macrophage colony-stimulating factor (GM-CSF).[78] Three studies treated patients intra-arterially with cisplatin,[72,75,79] 1 combined with bland embolization[75] and another with vinblastine and dacarbazine.[79] Melphalan was used in 2 studies,[81,84] dacarbazine alone in 1,[70] and there was 1 phase I/II trial that used nab-paclitaxel.[85] For 2 studies, the drugs were not specified (including 1 conference abstract).[27,71] A proportion of the patients treated with HAI also underwent debulking in 2 studies.[27,76] In total, 483 patients treated with HAI for MLMs are described. Primary melanoma origin was cutaneous for 39 patients (8%), uveal for 415 patients (86%), mucosal for 5 patients (1%), and unknown for 7 patients (1%). For 17 patients (4%), primary melanoma origin was not reported. Treatment-related mortality and morbidity were 2% (range 0%–21%) and 25% (range 13%–38%), respectively. The study with the highest mortality (21%) reported no procedure-related morbidity within the 14 patients treated; however, 3 patients died within 30 days.[84] The response rate for HAI was 21% (range 7%–38%). The study with the highest response rate (38%) treated 8 patients with intra-arterial cisplatin, of which 3 responded.[72] Contrastingly, only 9 of the 86 patients (11%) randomized to HAI with fotemustine responded in the RCT (11%).[82] Median PFS and OS were 6 (range 3–9) months and 13 (range 3–21) months, respectively. One prospective phase II trial directly compared HAI with fotemustine and systemic IFN-α and IL-2 to SYS with fotemustine, IFN-α, and IL-2 and found no survival difference between treatments.[74] The only RCT randomized 171 patients to either HAI with fotemustine (n = 86) or SYS with fotemustine (n = 85) and did not find an improvement in OS, despite a better response rate and PFS observed in the patients treated with HAI.[82] Accrual was stopped prematurely based on a futility OS analysis.[82]

ISOLATED HEPATIC PERFUSION AND PERCUTANEOUS HEPATIC PERFUSION

The study details, treatment specifics, and outcomes of 14 studies investigating hepatic perfusion as treatment of MLMs are reported in Supplementary Data [Table 6].[69,86–98] There were 11 retrospective cohort studies,[69,88–94,96–98] 1 prospective phase I trial,[86] 1 prospective phase II trial,[87] and 1 phase III RCT.[95] All studies used melphalan as active drug in their perfusate.[69,86–98] One phase I trial combined melphalan with cisplatin[86] and there was a phase II trial that combined melphalan with tumor necrosis factor alfa (TNF-α).[87] In 1 retrospective series, either cisplatin or TNF-α also was added in a small number of patients.[93] Hepatic perfusion was performed operatively (ie, isolated hepatic perfusion [IHP]) in 7 studies[86–91,94] and percutaneously in the other 7,[69,92,93,95–98] including the phase III RCT.[95] In total, 364 patients treated with IHP/percutaneous hepatic perfusion (PHP) for MLMs are described. Origin of MLM was cutaneous in 20 patients (5%), uveal in 331 patients (91%), mucosal in 2 patients (<1%), and unknown in 1 patient (<1%). Primary melanoma origin was not reported for 10 patients (3%). Treatment-related mortality and morbidity were 6% (range 0%–30%) and 33% (9%–68%), respectively. The highest treatment-related mortality was observed in a small phase I trial of 10 patients published in 1994, of whom 3 died (30%).[86] Another retrospective cohort study of 27 patients reported a mortality rate of 22% (6 patients).[89] The response rate for IHP/PHP was 53% (range 10%–60%). Apart from 1 phase I trial with a response rate of 10%,[86] all other 11 studies that reported response had a response rate greater or equal to 33%.[87–93,95–98] Median PFS and OS were 8 (range 5–11) months and 11 (range 5–27) months, respectively. All 3 studies that reported a median OS of 20 months or longer were retrospective cohort studies.[69,93,98] One phase II trial directly compared IHP with melphalan to IHP with melphalan and TNF-α and reported a longer duration of response in the TNF-α group.[87] The randomized phase III trial included 93 patients, which were randomized to either PHP with melphalan (n = 44) or best alternative care (n = 49).[95] Despite a longer (hepatic) PFS and higher response rate in patients treated with PHP, no difference in OS was observed.[95] The investigators contribute this lack in OS difference to the 57% of patients in the best alternative care group that crossed over to PHP with melphalan after progression after their initial treatment.[95]

SELECTIVE INTERNAL RADIATION THERAPY

The study details, treatment specifics, and outcomes of 13 studies investigating selective internal radiation therapy (SIRT) as treatment of MLMs are reported in Supplementary Data [Table 7].[69,99–110] There were 12 retrospective cohort studies[69,99–107,109,110] and 1 prospective phase II trial.[108] All studies performed SIRT with yttrium 90 (Y90)-labeled microspheres. Two studies combined SIRT Y90 with systemic immunotherapy.[107,109] In total, 287 patients treated with SIRT Y90 for MLMs are described, which were of cutaneous origin in 23 patients (8%), of uveal origin in 259 patients (90%), of mucosal origin in 3 patients (1%), and the origin was unknown for

2 (<1%). Treatment-related mortality and morbidity were 2% (range 0%–13%) and 13% (range 0%–32%), respectively. The study that reported the highest mortality rate of 13% was a small retrospective cohort study with only 8 patients, of whom 1 died.[103] The response rate to SIRT Y90 was 26% (range 0%–77%). The 2 studies that reported exceptionally high response rates of 62%[101] and 77%[99] were both small retrospective series with 13 or fewer patients. Contrastingly, the largest retrospective series of 71 patients reported a response rate of 8%.[104] Median PFS and OS were 5 (range 1–15) months and 11 (range 4–26) months, respectively. The longest median OS of 26 months was observed in a small retrospective series of 12 patients treated with SIRT Y90 and systemic immunotherapy.[109] That same study also analyzed 12 patients who received only SIRT Y90 and reported an improved survival in the patients treated with SIRT Y90 plus systemic immunotherapy.[109] Two retrospective studies directly compared SIRT Y90 to SYS[106] or BSC.[105] Although both reported improved survival for SIRT Y90, the patients receiving SYS or BSC were treated in the same centers during the same period and, therefore, by default were not considered for or refused SIRT Y90.[105,106] Furthermore the patients treated with SIRT Y90 or BSC all were patients with progressive disease after prior SYS.[105] The prospective phase II trial compared SIRT Y90 in treatment-naïve patients (n = 23) to SIRT Y90 in patients with progressive disease after immunoembolization.[108] A difference in neither response rate nor survival was observed between the 2 groups. The trial, therefore, concluded that SIRT Y90 is safe and effective as either first-line or second-line treatment of MLMs of uveal origin.[108]

OTHER LOCOREGIONAL THERAPIES

The study details, treatment specifics, and outcomes of 4 studies investigating other locoregional treatments for MLMs are reported in Supplementary Data [Table 8].[111–114] There are no series about liver transplantation for unresectable MLMs, although an open nonrandomized clinical trial investigating liver transplantation for uveal MLMs has been registered (NCT01311466, clinicaltrials.gov) and reportedly recruited 2 patients from 2011 to 2017.

SYSTEMIC THERAPY
Systemic Therapy in Metastatic Cutaneous Melanoma

Until recently, dacarbazine was the chemotherapeutic agent used most often. Large clinical trials investigating dacarbazine monotherapy reported response rates of approximately 7%, with median survival times of just 6 months.[115,116] Combining dacarbazine with other agents did not improve clinical response or survival.[117–119] In 2010, ipilimumab, a CTLA-4 inhibitor, was proved to prolong survival in previously treated patients with metastatic cutaneous melanoma, with a response rate of 11% and a median survival of 10 months.[120] Besides prolonging survival, treatment with ipilimumab also produced durable responses with long-term survivors; pooled analysis of 1861 patients treated with ipilimumab showed overall survival plateauing at 20% from 3 years on, all the way up to 10 years.[121] In 2014, nivolumab and pembrolizumab, 2 anti–PD-1 antibodies, were approved for the treatment of metastatic melanoma. In a randomized phase III study of 834 advanced cutaneous melanoma patients, pembrolizumab proved superior to ipilimumab in terms of PFS and OS, with less toxicity.[122] Combining CTLA-4 and PD-1 checkpoint inhibitors has proved even more effective. In a randomized phase III trial, 945 patients with unresectable or metastatic cutaneous melanoma were randomized 1:1:1 to either first-line nivolumab, nivolumab plus ipilimumab, or ipilimumab.[123,124] Recent 5-year results demonstrated a striking 5-year PFS and OS for combination therapy of

36% and 52%, respectively, compared with 29% and 44%, respectively, for nivolumab and 8% and 26%, respectively, for ipilimumab.[125] Importantly, reported results are best in the BRAF-mutant patients, with 5-year OS rates of 60% for combination therapy, 46% for nivolumab, and 30% for ipilimumab.[125] Preliminary results for the combination of pembrolizumab and ipilimumab report similar efficacy.[126] Immune checkpoint inhibitors also have proved efficacy in the adjuvant setting, with adjuvant nivolumab demonstrating better performance than ipilimumab in resected stage III or stage IV cutaneous melanoma.[127] Combination therapy, however, again proves superior with recent results reporting a significantly improved 2-year recurrence-free survival of 70% for adjuvant nivolumab with ipilimumab in resected stage IV cutaneous melanoma versus 42% for nivolumab monotherapy and 14% for placebo.[128] In parallel, BRAF inhibitors (dabrafenib, encorafenib, and vemurafenib) and MEK inhibitors (trametinib, binimetinib, and cobimetinib) also have demonstrated considerable efficacy in BRAF-mutated patients with metastatic cutaneous melanoma, which are present in approximately 50%. Similarly to checkpoint inhibitors, BRAF and MEK inhibitors demonstrated superior survival compared with dacarbazine[129] and proved most effective when combined.[130–133] Results may be inferior (cave selection bias) compared with combination immune checkpoint inhibitor therapy, with reported 5-year PFS and OS rates of combined BRAF and MEK inhibitors of 19% and 34%, respectively.[134]

Systemic Therapy in Metastatic Uveal Melanoma

Similarly to metastatic cutaneous melanoma, dacarbazine long has been considered the standard and still is used as comparative treatment in contemporary clinical trials[135,136] Results of dacarbazine in the treatment of metastatic uveal melanoma are poor, with objective response seldom to never observed and a median OS of 9 months in clinical trial populations.[135,136] Several combinations with dacarbazine have been investigated, as well as other (combinations of) conventional chemotherapeutics, and several kinase inhibitors, but none definitively improved efficacy.[135–142] The CTLA-4 checkpoint inhibitors ipilumumab and tremelimumab both have been studied in metastatic uveal melanoma but both did not considerably improve survival; median OS was 7 months for ipilimumab[143,144] and 13 months for tremelimumab.[145] Concerning the combined treatment of nivolumab and ipilimumab, preliminary results report a median OS of 13 months, but final results from phase II studies have yet to be published.[146] A recent meta-analysis has pooled the individual patient data of many of these phase II trials, including several trials investigating liver-directed therapies, in order to create benchmarks for PFS and OS for future trials.[147] In total, individual patient data of 29 trials were included, resulting in a total of 912 patients.[147] Median PFS and OS were 3 months and 10 months, respectively, with a 1-year OS rate of 43%. These outcomes represent the benchmark against which (future) therapies for metastatic uveal melanoma should be gauged.[147]

Systemic Therapy in Metastatic Mucosal Melanoma

There is a high paucity of evidence concerning the systemic treatment of metastatic mucosal melanoma. Only retrospective cohort series and pooled analyses have been published. Reported response rates with (a combination of) dacarbazine-based chemotherapy range from 8% to 26%, with a median OS of 10 months to 12 months.[148,149] In contrast to uveal melanoma, there is evidence to suggest efficacy of immune checkpoint inhibitors in metastatic mucosal melanoma, with a reported response rate of 23% and a median PFS of 3 months for nivolumab monotherapy and 37% and 6 months, respectively, for nivolumab and ipilimumab combination therapy.[150,151] There is as yet no report on OS in these patients.

CONSIDERATIONS

The current body of evidence of liver-directed locoregional therapies for MLMs consists of 106 studies each describing 5 or more patients (see **Fig. 2**).[9–50,51–71,72–100,101–114] Most were retrospective cohort studies with the majority performed prior to immune checkpoint inhibitor systemic therapy. There currently are 3 prospective RCTs published, which almost exclusively included metastatic uveal melanoma patients.[82,95,114] All 3 RCTs failed to definitively demonstrate a survival benefit of liver-directed regional therapies.[82,95,114] Objectively the best results for any liver-directed therapy were seen when all MLMs were treated using local therapies, either with complete surgical resection or using ablative techniques. Herein, complete removal or ablation of all metastatic disease remains key, because multiple studies showed no discernible clinical benefit after surgical reduction of tumor load and subsequent adjuvant therapy.[11,14,15,25,27,28,43,50] Although many of these patients have recurrence of disease after curative treatment, repeat local treatment has been described and, therefore, should be considered in eligible patients.[152] In the 37 studies investigating surgical treatment of MLMs, 5 reported patients underwent repeat resection or ablation.[12,28,30,36,42] The absence of randomized data comparing complete local therapy remains impeding. All specialized centers performing these complex liver-directed therapies most certainly also perform surgical treatment of MLMs. This makes it highly likely that all patients eligible for complete local therapy for MLMs are by default not included in any of the studies investigating other liver-directed therapies. This selection bias likely overstates results observed for complete local treatment. Malignant melanoma of cutaneous, uveal, and mucosal origin should be regarded as separate entities, each with distinct biology.

Cutaneous Melanoma Liver Metastases

Compared with uveal MLMs, there are few studies that specifically evaluated liver-directed therapies for cutaneous MLMs. Although there are several studies investigating the surgical management, ablation, and radiotherapy of cutaneous MLMs (see Supplementary Data [Tables 1–3]), only 3 studies of other liver-directed therapies either had a majority of patients with cutaneous MLM,[69] or specifically reported results for patients with primary cutaneous melanoma.[60,77] Of these, 1 studied TACE,[60] another studied HAI,[77] and the third evaluated both TACE and PHP.[69] Reported results of these liver-directed therapies are poor compared with combination treatment with ipilimumab and nivolumab.[123–125] Granted, not all patients had metastatic disease or even visceral metastases in the prospective studies investigating checkpoint inhibitors and targeted therapies.[120–126,128–134,153,154] The reported 5-year PFS and OS rates for ipilimumab and nivolumab combination therapy of 32% and 52%, respectively,[123–125] in part achieved in patients with visceral cutaneous melanoma metastases, are however unparalleled compared with previous systemic therapies, liver-directed therapies, and even complete surgical resection (see Supplementary Data [Table 2], **Fig. 3**). Isolated (resectable) hepatic metastases in cutaneous melanoma are exceedingly rare (see **Fig. 1**).[3] They are so rare that in principle other metastatic sites always are part of the problem and so in principle systemic therapy always is considered as first-line treatment. Patients with cutaneous MLMs, therefore, always should be referred to a medical oncologist. The most effective systemic treatment of metastatic cutaneous melanoma is combination therapy with ipilimumab and nivolumab and is the treatment of choice in the absence of contraindications for immune checkpoint inhibitor systemic therapy. In some patients, solitary progression may become the target of a surgical salvage approach. If patients with isolated cutaneous

MLMs are considered for surgical resection, adjuvant systemic treatment with immune checkpoint inhibition should be part of the treatment course.[127,128] Future studies are needed to investigate whether the combination of (aggressive) surgical treatment and immune checkpoint inhibition can improve survival further.

Uveal Melanoma Liver Metastases

Studies investigating liver-directed locoregional therapies for MLMs almost exclusively were performed in patients with primary uveal melanoma. This can be attributed to the unique hepatotropic metastatic behavior of uveal melanoma[5] (see **Fig. 1**), with the hepatic metastases a driver of survival and poor results obtained with systemic therapy,[147] which has prompted many liver-directed therapies to focus on this rare disease. Uveal MLMs are the only MLM type with data to support complete local/surgical intervention and might be considered for selective patients in which a complete resection/ablation can be achieved. Herein it is important to recognize that in approximately half of all surgically explored (uveal) MLM patients, complete local treatment proves impossible (see Supplementary Data [Table 1]), meaning large uncertainty lies in a percutaneous approach. Aggressive strategies with combined reduction of tumor load and subsequent adjuvant therapy have not been shown to improve survival.[11,14,15,25,27,28,43] Novel immune checkpoint inhibitors have shown little to no clinical activity in metastatic uveal melanoma, although results of combined ipilimumab and nivolumab still are expected.[146] Despite the consistently higher response rates observed for IHP or PHP,[95] no single liver-directed or systemic therapy has proved superior effectiveness.[147] Treatment decisions in patients with metastatic uveal melanoma not eligible for complete local treatment, therefore, should be based more on a center's own experience and patient preference.

Mucosal Melanoma Liver Metastases

Only 13 patients with MLMs from mucosal origin are described in all 106 studies combined with no single study reporting specific outcomes for these patients. Based on current evidence, no recommendations for any liver-directed regional therapy in the treatment of MLMs from mucosal origin can be made. Although evidence is limited, immune checkpoint inhibitions should be the treatment of choice in metastatic mucosal melanoma, either as first-line treatment or possibly in the adjuvant setting.[150,151]

THE MEDICAL ONCOLOGIST'S PERSPECTIVE

Because the introduction of immune checkpoint inhibition and targeted therapy has significantly improved the survival of patients with advanced cutaneous melanoma, surgical treatment of advanced cutaneous MLMs has become complementary, whereas surgical treatment still is the cornerstone of the treatment of uveal MLMs. In an era of novel systemic therapies, surgical treatment can complement systemic therapy for cutaneous MLMs. In particular, local treatment of cutaneous MLMs can be considered for oligoprogression, which is defined as progressive disease at a limited number of disease sites after an initial response to systemic therapy.[155] Local treatment of oligoprogressive MLMs may eliminate drug resistant clones, thereby achieving stable disease or even complete response. After treatment with immune checkpoint inhibitors, pseudoprogression also can mimic oligoprogression. Pseudoprogression is a phenomenon in which metastases show an increase in size on imaging due to T-cell infiltration, which can be confirmed by a surgical biopsy.[156] On the other hand, surgical treatment may support the efficacy of systemic therapy by debulking large or symptomatic MLMs. Because low tumor burden, which is reflected by low serum lactate dehydrogenase, is associated with better outcome of patients with cutaneous melanoma during immune checkpoint inhibition,[157] surgical debulking may facilitate tumor response to these drugs.[158] Although the combination of surgical treatment of cutaneous MLMs and immune checkpoint inhibition has not yet been investigated prospectively, surgeons increasingly are consulted to complement systemic therapy with surgical treatment. Because immune checkpoint inhibitors have shown improved OS of greater than 10 years in patients with metastatic cutaneous melanoma,[121,125] treatment is shifting slightly from palliative toward more curative intent. This paradigm shift in the treatment of cutaneous metastatic melanoma requires a multidisciplinary approach, involving experienced radiologists, dermatologists, medical oncologists, radiotherapists, and surgeons.

DISCLOSURE

Authors have nothing to disclose.

SUPPLEMENTARY DATA

Supplemental Information can be found online at https://doi.org/10.1016/j.soc.2020.09.001.

REFERENCES

1. Eggermont AM, Spatz A, Robert C. Cutaneous melanoma. Lancet 2014; 383(9919):816–27.
2. Bishop KD, Olszewski AJ. Epidemiology and survival outcomes of ocular and mucosal melanomas: a population-based analysis. Int J Cancer 2014;134(12): 2961–71.
3. Tas F, Erturk K. Recurrence behavior in early-stage cutaneous melanoma: pattern, timing, survival, and influencing factors. Melanoma Res 2017;27(2): 134–9.
4. Mervic L. Time course and pattern of metastasis of cutaneous melanoma differ between men and women. PLoS One 2012;7(3):e32955.
5. Diener-West M, Reynolds SM, Agugliaro DJ, et al. Development of metastatic disease after enrollment in the COMS trials for treatment of choroidal melanoma: Collaborative Ocular Melanoma Study Group Report No. 26. Arch Ophthalmol 2005;123(12):1639–43.
6. Lane AM, Kim IK, Gragoudas ES. Survival Rates in Patients After Treatment for Metastasis From Uveal Melanoma. JAMA Ophthalmol 2018;136(9):981–6.
7. Lian B, Cui CL, Zhou L, et al. The natural history and patterns of metastases from mucosal melanoma: an analysis of 706 prospectively-followed patients. Ann Oncol 2017;28(4):868–73.
8. Heppt MV, Roesch A, Weide B, et al. Prognostic factors and treatment outcomes in 444 patients with mucosal melanoma. Eur J Cancer 2017;81:36–44.
9. Foster JH. Survival after liver resection for secondary tumors. Am J Surg 1978; 135(3):389–94.
10. Elias D, Cavalcanti de Albuquerque A, Eggenspieler P, et al. Resection of liver metastases from a noncolorectal primary: indications and results based on 147 monocentric patients. J Am Coll Surg 1998;187(5):487–93.
11. Lang H, Nussbaum KT, Weimann A, et al. Ergebnisse der Resektion nichtcolorectaler nichtneuroendokriner Lebermetastasen. Chirurg 1999;70(4):439–46.

12. Aoyama T, Mastrangelo MJ, Berd D, et al. Protracted survival after resection of metastatic uveal melanoma. Cancer 2000;89(7):1561–8.

13. Meyer T, Merkel S, Goehl J, et al. Surgical therapy for distant metastases of malignant melanoma. Cancer 2000;89(9):1983–91.

14. Rose DM, Essner R, Hughes TM, et al. Surgical resection for metastatic melanoma to the liver: the John Wayne Cancer Institute and Sydney Melanoma Unit experience. Arch Surg 2001;136(8):950–5.

15. Rivoire M, Kodjikian L, Baldo S, et al. Treatment of liver metastases from uveal melanoma. Ann Surg Oncol 2005;12(6):422–8.

16. Weitz J, Blumgart LH, Fong Y, et al. Partial hepatectomy for metastases from noncolorectal, nonneuroendocrine carcinoma. Ann Surg 2005;241(2):269–76.

17. Adam R, Chiche L, Aloia T, et al. Hepatic resection for noncolorectal nonendocrine liver metastases: analysis of 1,452 patients and development of a prognostic model. Ann Surg 2006;244(4):524–35.

18. Crook TB, Jones OM, John TG, et al. Hepatic resection for malignant melanoma. Eur J Surg Oncol 2006;32(3):315–7.

19. Kim J, Mori T, Chen SL, et al. Chemokine receptor CXCR4 expression in patients with melanoma and colorectal cancer liver metastases and the association with disease outcome. Ann Surg 2006;244(1):113–20.

20. Pawlik TM, Zorzi D, Abdalla EK, et al. Hepatic resection for metastatic melanoma: distinct patterns of recurrence and prognosis for ocular versus cutaneous disease. Ann Surg Oncol 2006;13(5):712–20.

21. Herman P, Machado MA, Montagnini AL, et al. Selected patients with metastatic melanoma may benefit from liver resection. World J Surg 2007;31(1):171–4.

22. Lendoire J, Moro M, Andriani O, et al. Liver resection for non-colorectal, non-neuroendocrine metastases: analysis of a multicenter study from Argentina. HPB (Oxford) 2007;9(6):435–9.

23. Frenkel S, Nir I, Hendler K, et al. Long-term survival of uveal melanoma patients after surgery for liver metastases. Br J Ophthalmol 2009;93(8):1042–6.

24. Lehner F, Ramackers W, Bektas H, et al. Leberresektion bei nicht kolorektalen, nicht neuroendokrinen Lebermetastasen-ist die Resektion im Rahmen des "onko-chirurgischen" Therapiekonzeptes gerechtfertigt? Zentralbl Chir 2009; 134(5):430–6.

25. Mariani P, Piperno-Neumann S, Servois V, et al. Surgical management of liver metastases from uveal melanoma: 16 years' experience at the Institut Curie. Eur J Surg Oncol 2009;35(11):1192–7.

26. Chua TC, Saxena A, Morris DL. Surgical metastasectomy in AJCC stage IV M1c melanoma patients with gastrointestinal and liver metastases. Ann Acad Med Singapore 2010;39(8):634–9.

27. Pilati PL, Mammano E, Tessari E, et al. Multimodal treatments for liver metastases from melanoma: Experience of a single institution. Ann Surg Oncol 2010; 17:S83.

28. Ripley RT, Davis JL, Klapper JA, et al. Liver resection for metastatic melanoma with postoperative tumor-infiltrating lymphocyte therapy. Ann Surg Oncol 2010; 17(1):163–70.

29. Caralt M, Marti J, Cortes J, et al. Outcome of patients following hepatic resection for metastatic cutaneous and ocular melanoma. J Hepatobiliary Pancreat Sci 2011;18(2):268–75.

30. Groeschl RT, Nachmany I, Steel JL, et al. Hepatectomy for noncolorectal non-neuroendocrine metastatic cancer: a multi-institutional analysis. J Am Coll Surg 2012;214(5):769–77.

31. de Ridder J, van Walsum M, Verhoef C, et al. Dutch Liver Working G. Hepatic resection for metastatic melanoma in The Netherlands: survival and prognostic factors. Melanoma Res 2013;23(1):27–32.

32. Marshall E, Romaniuk C, Ghaneh P, et al. MRI in the detection of hepatic metastases from high-risk uveal melanoma: a prospective study in 188 patients. Br J Ophthalmol 2013;97(2):159–63.

33. Ryu SW, Saw R, Scolyer RA, et al. Liver resection for metastatic melanoma: equivalent survival for cutaneous and ocular primaries. J Surg Oncol 2013; 108(2):129–35.

34. Yang XY, Xie F, Tao R, et al. Treatment of liver metastases from uveal melanoma: a retrospective single-center analysis. Hepatobiliary Pancreat Dis Int 2013; 12(6):602–6.

35. Faries MB, Leung A, Morton DL, et al. A 20-year experience of hepatic resection for melanoma: is there an expanding role? J Am Coll Surg 2014;219(1):62–8.

36. Gomez D, Wetherill C, Cheong J, et al. The Liverpool uveal melanoma liver metastases pathway: outcome following liver resection. J Surg Oncol 2014;109(6): 542–7.

37. Hau HM, Tautenhahn HM, Schoenberg MB, et al. Liver resection in multimodal concepts improves survival of metastatic melanoma: a single-centre case-matched control study. Anticancer Res 2014;34(11):6633–9.

38. Doussot A, Nardin C, Takaki H, et al. Liver resection and ablation for metastatic melanoma: A single center experience. J Surg Oncol 2015;111(8):962–8.

39. Hoffmann K, Bulut S, Tekbas A, et al. Is Hepatic Resection for Non-colorectal, Non-neuroendocrine Liver Metastases Justified? Ann Surg Oncol 2015; 22(Suppl 3):S1083–92.

40. Martel G, Hawel J, Rekman J, et al. Liver resection for non-colorectal, non-carcinoid, non-sarcoma metastases: a multicenter study. PLoS One 2015;10(3): e0120569.

41. Mariani P, Almubarak MM, Kollen M, et al. Radiofrequency ablation and surgical resection of liver metastases from uveal melanoma. Eur J Surg Oncol 2016; 42(5):706–12.

42. Aghayan DL, Kazaryan AM, Fretland AA, et al. Laparoscopic liver resection for metastatic melanoma. Surg Endosc 2018;32(3):1470–7.

43. Barnhill R, Vermeulen P, Daelemans S, et al. Replacement and desmoplastic histopathological growth patterns: A pilot study of prediction of outcome in patients with uveal melanoma liver metastases. J Pathol Clin Res 2018;4(4): 227–40.

44. Labgaa I, Slankamenac K, Schadde E, et al. Liver resection for metastases not of colorectal, neuroendocrine, sarcomatous, or ovarian (NCNSO) origin: A multicentric study. Am J Surg 2018;215(1):125–30.

45. Barnhill R, van Dam PJ, Vermeulen P, et al. Replacement and desmoplastic histopathological growth patterns in cutaneous melanoma liver metastases: frequency, characteristics, and robust prognostic value. J Pathol Clin Res 2020; 6(3):195–206.

46. Akyuz M, Yazici P, Dural C, et al. Laparoscopic management of liver metastases from uveal melanoma. Surg Endosc 2016;30(6):2567–71.

47. Bale R, Schullian P, Schmuth M, et al. Stereotactic Radiofrequency Ablation for Metastatic Melanoma to the Liver. Cardiovasc Intervent Radiol 2016;39(8): 1128–35.

48. White ML, Atwell TD, Kurup AN, et al. Recurrence and Survival Outcomes After Percutaneous Thermal Ablation of Oligometastatic Melanoma. Mayo Clin Proc 2016;91(3):288–96.
49. Franceschini D, Franzese C, De Rose F, et al. Role of extra cranial stereotactic body radiation therapy in the management of Stage IV melanoma. Br J Radiol 2017;90(1077):20170257.
50. Rozeman EA, Prevoo W, Meier MAJ, et al. Phase Ib/II trial testing combined radiofrequency ablation and ipilimumab in uveal melanoma (SECIRA-UM). Melanoma Res 2020;30(3):252–60.
51. Mavligit GM, Charnsangavej C, Carrasco CH, et al. Regression of ocular melanoma metastatic to the liver after hepatic arterial chemoembolization with cisplatin and polyvinyl sponge. JAMA 1988;260(7):974–6.
52. Bedikian AY, Legha SS, Mavligit G, et al. Treatment of uveal melanoma metastatic to the liver: a review of the M. D. Anderson Cancer Center experience and prognostic factors. Cancer 1995;76(9):1665–70.
53. Morassut S, Fiorentini G, Balestreri L, et al. Chemoembolization of liver metastases from ocular melanoma: Preliminary results. Reg Cancer Treat 1995;8(3–4): 173–6.
54. Patel K, Sullivan K, Berd D, et al. Chemoembolization of the hepatic artery with BCNU for metastatic uveal melanoma: results of a phase II study. Melanoma Res 2005;15(4):297–304.
55. Vogl T, Eichler K, Zangos S, et al. Preliminary experience with transarterial chemoembolization (TACE) in liver metastases of uveal malignant melanoma: local tumor control and survival. J Cancer Res Clin Oncol 2007;133(3):177–84.
56. Dayani PN, Gould JE, Brown DB, et al. Hepatic metastasis from uveal melanoma: angiographic pattern predictive of survival after hepatic arterial chemoembolization. Arch Ophthalmol 2009;127(5):628–32.
57. Gupta S, Bedikian AY, Ahrar J, et al. Hepatic artery chemoembolization in patients with ocular melanoma metastatic to the liver: response, survival, and prognostic factors. Am J Clin Oncol 2010;33(5):474–80.
58. Huppert PE, Fierlbeck G, Pereira P, et al. Transarterial chemoembolization of liver metastases in patients with uveal melanoma. Eur J Radiol 2010;74(3): e38–44.
59. Schuster R, Lindner M, Wacker F, et al. Transarterial chemoembolization of liver metastases from uveal melanoma after failure of systemic therapy: toxicity and outcome. Melanoma Res 2010;20(3):191–6.
60. Ahrar J, Gupta S, Ensor J, et al. Response, survival, and prognostic factors after hepatic arterial chemoembolization in patients with liver metastases from cutaneous melanoma. Cancer Invest 2011;29(1):49–55.
61. Edelhauser G, Schicher N, Berzaczy D, et al. Fotemustine chemoembolization of hepatic metastases from uveal melanoma: a retrospective single-center analysis. AJR Am J Roentgenol 2012;199(6):1387–92.
62. Farshid P, Darvishi A, Naguib N, et al. Repetitive chemoembolization of hypovascular liver metastases from the most common primary sites. Future Oncol 2013;9(3):419–26.
63. Duran R, Chapiro J, Frangakis C, et al. Uveal Melanoma Metastatic to the Liver: The Role of Quantitative Volumetric Contrast-Enhanced MR Imaging in the Assessment of Early Tumor Response after Transarterial Chemoembolization. Transl Oncol 2014;7(4):447–55.
64. Carling U, Dorenberg EJ, Haugvik SP, et al. Transarterial Chemoembolization of Liver Metastases from Uveal Melanoma Using Irinotecan-Loaded Beads:

Treatment Response and Complications. Cardiovasc Intervent Radiol 2015; 38(6):1532–41.

65. Gonsalves CF, Eschelman DJ, Thornburg B, et al. Uveal Melanoma Metastatic to the Liver: Chemoembolization With 1,3-Bis-(2-Chloroethyl)-1-Nitrosourea. AJR Am J Roentgenol 2015;205(2):429–33.

66. Valpione S, Aliberti C, Parrozzani R, et al. A retrospective analysis of 141 patients with liver metastases from uveal melanoma: a two-cohort study comparing transarterial chemoembolization with CPT-11 charged microbeads and historical treatments. Melanoma Res 2015;25(2):164–8.

67. Rostas J, Tam A, Sato T, et al. Image-Guided Transarterial Chemoembolization With Drug-Eluting Beads Loaded with Doxorubicin (DEBDOX) for Unresectable Hepatic Metastases from Melanoma: Technique and Outcomes. Cardiovasc Intervent Radiol 2017;40(9):1392–400.

68. Shibayama Y, Namikawa K, Sone M, et al. Efficacy and toxicity of transarterial chemoembolization therapy using cisplatin and gelatin sponge in patients with liver metastases from uveal melanoma in an Asian population. Int J Clin Oncol 2017;22(3):577–84.

69. Abbott AM, Doepker MP, Kim Y, et al. Hepatic Progression-free and Overall Survival After Regional Therapy to the Liver for Metastatic Melanoma. Am J Clin Oncol 2018;41(8):747–53.

70. Storm FK, Kaiser LR, Goodnight JE, et al. Thermochemotherapy for melanoma metastases in liver. Cancer 1982;49(6):1243–8.

71. Stehlin JS Jr, de Ipolyi PD, Greeff PJ, et al. Treatment of cancer of the liver. Twenty years' experience with infusion and resection in 414 patients. Ann Surg 1988;208(1):23–35.

72. Cantore M, Fiorentini G, Aitini E, et al. Intra-arterial hepatic carboplatin-based chemotherapy for ocular melanoma metastatic to the liver. Report of a phase II study. Tumori 1994;80(1):37–9.

73. Egerer G, Lehnert T, Max R, et al. Pilot study of hepatic intraarterial fotemustine chemotherapy for liver metastases from uveal melanoma: a single-center experience with seven patients. Int J Clin Oncol 2001;6(1):25–8.

74. Becker JC, Terheyden P, Kampgen E, et al. Treatment of disseminated ocular melanoma with sequential fotemustine, interferon alpha, and interleukin 2. Br J Cancer 2002;87(8):840–5.

75. Agarwala SS, Panikkar R, Kirkwood JM. Phase I/II randomized trial of intrahepatic arterial infusion chemotherapy with cisplatin and chemoembolization with cisplatin and polyvinyl sponge in patients with ocular melanoma metastatic to the liver. Melanoma Res 2004;14(3):217–22.

76. Peters S, Voelter V, Zografos L, et al. Intra-arterial hepatic fotemustine for the treatment of liver metastases from uveal melanoma: experience in 101 patients. Ann Oncol 2006;17(4):578–83.

77. Siegel R, Hauschild A, Kettelhack C, et al. Hepatic arterial Fotemustine chemotherapy in patients with liver metastases from cutaneous melanoma is as effective as in ocular melanoma. Eur J Surg Oncol 2007;33(5):627–32.

78. Cui CL, Chi ZH, Yuan XQ, et al. [Hepatic intra-arterial bio-chemotherapy for the treatment of melanoma patients with liver metastasis: a phase II clinical study]. Ai Zheng 2008;27(8):845–50.

79. Melichar B, Voboril Z, Lojik M, et al. Liver metastases from uveal melanoma: clinical experience of hepatic arterial infusion of cisplatin, vinblastine and dacarbazine. Hepatogastroenterology 2009;56(93):1157–62.

80. Farolfi A, Ridolfi L, Guidoboni M, et al. Liver metastases from melanoma: hepatic intra-arterial chemotherapy. A retrospective study. J Chemother 2011;23(5): 300–5.

81. Heusner TA, Antoch G, Wittkowski-Sterczewski A, et al. Transarterial hepatic chemoperfusion of uveal melanoma metastases: survival and response to treatment. Rofo 2011;183(12):1151–60.

82. Leyvraz S, Piperno-Neumann S, Suciu S, et al. Hepatic intra-arterial versus intravenous fotemustine in patients with liver metastases from uveal melanoma (EORTC 18021): a multicentric randomized trial. Ann Oncol 2014;25(3):742–6.

83. Itchins M, Ascierto PA, Menzies AM, et al. A multireferral centre retrospective cohort analysis on the experience in treatment of metastatic uveal melanoma and utilization of sequential liver-directed treatment and immunotherapy. Melanoma Res 2017;27(3):243–50.

84. Boone BA, Perkins S, Bandi R, et al. Hepatic artery infusion of melphalan in patients with liver metastases from ocular melanoma. J Surg Oncol 2018;117(5): 940–6.

85. Vera-Aguilera J, Bedikian AY, Bassett RL, et al. Phase I/II Study of Hepatic Arterial Infusion of Nab-paclitaxel in Patients With Metastatic Melanoma to the Liver. Am J Clin Oncol 2018;41(11):1132–6.

86. Hafstrom LR, Holmberg SB, Naredi PL, et al. Isolated hyperthermic liver perfusion with chemotherapy for liver malignancy. Surg Oncol 1994;3(2):103–8.

87. Alexander HR, Libutti SK, Bartlett DL, et al. A phase I-II study of isolated hepatic perfusion using melphalan with or without tumor necrosis factor for patients with ocular melanoma metastatic to liver. Clin Cancer Res 2000;6(8):3062–70.

88. Alexander HR Jr, Libutti SK, Pingpank JF, et al. Hyperthermic isolated hepatic perfusion using melphalan for patients with ocular melanoma metastatic to liver. Clin Cancer Res 2003;9(17):6343–9.

89. Rizell M, Mattson J, Cahlin C, et al. Isolated hepatic perfusion for liver metastases of malignant melanoma. Melanoma Res 2008;18(2):120–6.

90. van Iersel LB, Hoekman EJ, Gelderblom H, et al. Isolated hepatic perfusion with 200 mg melphalan for advanced noncolorectal liver metastases. Ann Surg Oncol 2008;15(7):1891–8.

91. Varghese S, Xu H, Bartlett D, et al. Isolated hepatic perfusion with high-dose melphalan results in immediate alterations in tumor gene expression in patients with metastatic ocular melanoma. Ann Surg Oncol 2010;17(7):1870–7.

92. Forster MR, Rashid OM, Perez MC, et al. Chemosaturation with percutaneous hepatic perfusion for unresectable metastatic melanoma or sarcoma to the liver: a single institution experience. J Surg Oncol 2014;109(5):434–9.

93. Ben-Shabat I, Belgrano V, Ny L, et al. Long-Term Follow-Up Evaluation of 68 Patients with Uveal Melanoma Liver Metastases Treated with Isolated Hepatic Perfusion. Ann Surg Oncol 2016;23(4):1327–34.

94. de Leede EM, Burgmans MC, Kapiteijn E, et al. Isolated (hypoxic) hepatic perfusion with high-dose chemotherapy in patients with unresectable liver metastases of uveal melanoma: results from two experienced centres. Melanoma Res 2016;26(6):588–94.

95. Hughes MS, Zager J, Faries M, et al. Results of a Randomized Controlled Multicenter Phase III Trial of Percutaneous Hepatic Perfusion Compared with Best Available Care for Patients with Melanoma Liver Metastases. Ann Surg Oncol 2016;23(4):1309–19.

96. Vogl TJ, Koch SA, Lotz G, et al. Percutaneous Isolated Hepatic Perfusion as a Treatment for Isolated Hepatic Metastases of Uveal Melanoma: Patient Outcome

and Safety in a Multi-centre Study. Cardiovasc Intervent Radiol 2017;40(6): 864–72.

97. Karydis I, Gangi A, Wheater MJ, et al. Percutaneous hepatic perfusion with melphalan in uveal melanoma: A safe and effective treatment modality in an orphan disease. J Surg Oncol 2018;117(6):1170–8.

98. Artzner C, Mossakowski O, Hefferman G, et al. Chemosaturation with percutaneous hepatic perfusion of melphalan for liver-dominant metastatic uveal melanoma: a single center experience. Cancer Imaging 2019;19(1):31.

99. Kennedy AS, Nutting C, Jakobs T, et al. A first report of radioembolization for hepatic metastases from ocular melanoma. Cancer Invest 2009;27(6):682–90.

100. Piduru SM, Schuster DM, Barron BJ, et al. Prognostic value of 18f-fluorodeoxy-glucose positron emission tomography-computed tomography in predicting survival in patients with unresectable metastatic melanoma to the liver undergoing yttrium-90 radioembolization. J Vasc Interv Radiol 2012;23(7):943–8.

101. Klingenstein A, Haug AR, Zech CJ, et al. Radioembolization as locoregional therapy of hepatic metastases in uveal melanoma patients. Cardiovasc Intervent Radiol 2013;36(1):158–65.

102. Memon K, Kuzel TM, Vouche M, et al. Hepatic yttrium-90 radioembolization for metastatic melanoma: a single-center experience. Melanoma Res 2014;24(3): 244–51.

103. Schelhorn J, Richly H, Ruhlmann M, et al. A single-center experience in radio-embolization as salvage therapy of hepatic metastases of uveal melanoma. Acta Radiol Open 2015;4(4). 2047981615570417.

104. Eldredge-Hindy H, Ohri N, Anne PR, et al. Yttrium-90 Microsphere Brachyther-apy for Liver Metastases From Uveal Melanoma: Clinical Outcomes and the Predictive Value of Fluorodeoxyglucose Positron Emission Tomography. Am J Clin Oncol 2016;39(2):189–95.

105. Xing M, Prajapati HJ, Dhanasekaran R, et al. Selective Internal Yttrium-90 Radio-embolization Therapy (90Y-SIRT) Versus Best Supportive Care in Patients With Unresectable Metastatic Melanoma to the Liver Refractory to Systemic Therapy: Safety and Efficacy Cohort Study. Am J Clin Oncol 2017;40(1):27–34.

106. Tulokas S, Maenpaa H, Peltola E, et al. Selective internal radiation therapy (SIRT) as treatment for hepatic metastases of uveal melanoma: a Finnish nation-wide retrospective experience. Acta Oncol 2018;57(10):1373–80.

107. Zheng J, Irani Z, Lawrence D, et al. Combined Effects of Yttrium-90 Transarterial Radioembolization around Immunotherapy for Hepatic Metastases from Uveal Melanoma: A Preliminary Retrospective Case Series. J Vasc Interv Radiol 2018;29(10):1369–75.

108. Gonsalves CF, Eschelman DJ, Adamo RD, et al. A Prospective Phase II Trial of Radioembolization for Treatment of Uveal Melanoma Hepatic Metastasis. Radiology 2019;293(1):223–31.

109. Levey AO, Elsayed M, Lawson DH, et al. Predictors of Overall and Progression-Free Survival in Patients with Ocular Melanoma Metastatic to the Liver Undergoing Y90 Radioembolization. Cardiovasc Intervent Radiol 2020;43(2):254–63.

110. Ponti A, Denys A, Digklia A, et al. First-Line Selective Internal Radiation Therapy in Patients with Uveal Melanoma Metastatic to the Liver. J Nucl Med 2020;61(3): 350–6.

111. Sato T, Eschelman DJ, Gonsalves CF, et al. Immunoembolization of malignant liver tumors, including uveal melanoma, using granulocyte-macrophage colony-stimulating factor. J Clin Oncol 2008;26(33):5436–42.

112. Alvarez-Downing MM, Inchauste SM, Dudley ME, et al. Minimally invasive liver resection to obtain tumor-infiltrating lymphocytes for adoptive cell therapy in patients with metastatic melanoma. World J Surg Oncol 2012;10:113.
113. Eichler K, Zangos S, Gruber-Rouh T, et al. MR-guided laser-induced thermotherapy (LITT) in patients with liver metastases of uveal melanoma. J Eur Acad Dermatol Venereol 2014;28(12):1756–60.
114. Valsecchi ME, Terai M, Eschelman DJ, et al. Double-blinded, randomized phase II study using embolization with or without granulocyte-macrophage colony-stimulating factor in uveal melanoma with hepatic metastases. J Vasc Interv Radiol 2015;26(4):523–32.e2.
115. Middleton MR, Grob JJ, Aaronson N, et al. Randomized phase III study of temozolomide versus dacarbazine in the treatment of patients with advanced metastatic malignant melanoma. J Clin Oncol 2000;18(1):158–66.
116. Avril MF, Aamdal S, Grob JJ, et al. Fotemustine compared with dacarbazine in patients with disseminated malignant melanoma: a phase III study. J Clin Oncol 2004;22(6):1118–25.
117. Rusthoven JJ, Quirt IC, Iscoe NA, et al. Randomized, double-blind, placebo-controlled trial comparing the response rates of carmustine, dacarbazine, and cisplatin with and without tamoxifen in patients with metastatic melanoma. National Cancer Institute of Canada Clinical Trials Group. J Clin Oncol 1996; 14(7):2083–90.
118. Falkson CI, Ibrahim J, Kirkwood JM, et al. Phase III trial of dacarbazine versus dacarbazine with interferon alpha-2b versus dacarbazine with tamoxifen versus dacarbazine with interferon alpha-2b and tamoxifen in patients with metastatic malignant melanoma: an Eastern Cooperative Oncology Group study. J Clin Oncol 1998;16(5):1743–51.
119. Agarwala SS, Ferri W, Gooding W, et al. A phase III randomized trial of dacarbazine and carboplatin with and without tamoxifen in the treatment of patients with metastatic melanoma. Cancer 1999;85(9):1979–84.
120. Hodi FS, O'Day SJ, McDermott DF, et al. Improved Survival with Ipilimumab in Patients with Metastatic Melanoma. N Engl J Med 2010;363(8):711–23.
121. Schadendorf D, Hodi FS, Robert C, et al. Pooled Analysis of Long-Term Survival Data From Phase II and Phase III Trials of Ipilimumab in Unresectable or Metastatic Melanoma. J Clin Oncol 2015;33(17):1889–94.
122. Robert C, Schachter J, Long GV, et al. Pembrolizumab versus Ipilimumab in Advanced Melanoma. N Engl J Med 2015;372(26):2521–32.
123. Larkin J, Chiarion-Sileni V, Gonzalez R, et al. Combined Nivolumab and Ipilimumab or Monotherapy in Untreated Melanoma. N Engl J Med 2015;373(1):23–34.
124. Wolchok JD, Chiarion-Sileni V, Gonzalez R, et al. Overall Survival with Combined Nivolumab and Ipilimumab in Advanced Melanoma. N Engl J Med 2017; 377(14):1345–56.
125. Larkin J, Chiarion-Sileni V, Gonzalez R, et al. Five-Year Survival with Combined Nivolumab and Ipilimumab in Advanced Melanoma. N Engl J Med 2019; 381(16):1535–46.
126. Long GV, Atkinson V, Cebon JS, et al. Standard-dose pembrolizumab in combination with reduced-dose ipilimumab for patients with advanced melanoma (KEYNOTE-029): an open-label, phase 1b trial. Lancet Oncol 2017;18(9): 1202–10.
127. Weber J, Mandala M, Del Vecchio M, et al. Adjuvant Nivolumab versus Ipilimumab in Resected Stage III or IV Melanoma. N Engl J Med 2017;377(19): 1824–35.

128. Zimmer L, Livingstone E, Hassel JC, et al. Adjuvant nivolumab plus ipilimumab or nivolumab monotherapy versus placebo in patients with resected stage IV melanoma with no evidence of disease (IMMUNED): a randomised, double-blind, placebo-controlled, phase 2 trial. Lancet 2020;395(10236):1558–68.

129. Chapman PB, Hauschild A, Robert C, et al. Improved Survival with Vemurafenib in Melanoma with BRAF V600E Mutation. N Engl J Med 2011;364(26):2507–16.

130. Larkin J, Ascierto PA, Dréno B, et al. Combined Vemurafenib and Cobimetinib in BRAF-Mutated Melanoma. N Engl J Med 2014;371(20):1867–76.

131. Long GV, Stroyakovskiy D, Gogas H, et al. Combined BRAF and MEK Inhibition versus BRAF Inhibition Alone in Melanoma. N Engl J Med 2014;371(20):1877–88.

132. Robert C, Karaszewska B, Schachter J, et al. Improved Overall Survival in Melanoma with Combined Dabrafenib and Trametinib. N Engl J Med 2014;372(1):30–9.

133. Dummer R, Ascierto PA, Gogas HJ, et al. Encorafenib plus binimetinib versus vemurafenib or encorafenib in patients with BRAF-mutant melanoma (COLUMBUS): a multicentre, open-label, randomised phase 3 trial. Lancet Oncol 2018;19(5):603–15.

134. Robert C, Grob JJ, Stroyakovskiy D, et al. Five-Year Outcomes with Dabrafenib plus Trametinib in Metastatic Melanoma. N Engl J Med 2019;381(7):626–36.

135. Carvajal RD, Piperno-Neumann S, Kapiteijn E, et al. Selumetinib in Combination With Dacarbazine in Patients With Metastatic Uveal Melanoma: A Phase III, Multicenter, Randomized Trial (SUMIT). J Clin Oncol 2018;36(12):1232–9.

136. Carvajal RD, Sosman JA, Quevedo JF, et al. Effect of selumetinib vs chemotherapy on progression-free survival in uveal melanoma: a randomized clinical trial. JAMA 2014;311(23):2397–405.

137. Kivelä T, Suciu S, Hansson J, et al. Bleomycin, vincristine, lomustine and dacarbazine (BOLD) in combination with recombinant interferon alpha-2b for metastatic uveal melanoma. Eur J Cancer 2003;39(8):1115–20.

138. Piperno-Neumann S, Diallo A, Etienne-Grimaldi MC, et al. Phase II Trial of Bevacizumab in Combination With Temozolomide as First-Line Treatment in Patients With Metastatic Uveal Melanoma. Oncologist 2016;21(3):281–2.

139. Homsi J, Bedikian AY, Papadopoulos NE, et al. Phase 2 open-label study of weekly docosahexaenoic acid-paclitaxel in patients with metastatic uveal melanoma. Melanoma Res 2010;20(6):507–10.

140. Schmittel A, Schmidt-Hieber M, Martus P, et al. A randomized phase II trial of gemcitabine plus treosulfan versus treosulfan alone in patients with metastatic uveal melanoma. Ann Oncol 2006;17(12):1826–9.

141. Penel N, Delcambre C, Durando X, et al. O-Mel-Inib: A Cancéro-pôle Nord-Ouest multicenter phase II trial of high-dose Imatinib mesylate in metastatic uveal melanoma. Investig New Drugs 2008;26(6):561–5.

142. Bhatia S, Moon J, Margolin KA, et al. Phase II trial of sorafenib in combination with carboplatin and paclitaxel in patients with metastatic uveal melanoma: SWOG S0512. PLoS One 2012;7(11):e48787.

143. Piulats Rodriguez JM, Ochoa de Olza M, Codes M, et al. Phase II study evaluating ipilimumab as a single agent in the first-line treatment of adult patients (Pts) with metastatic uveal melanoma (MUM): The GEM-1 trial. J Clin Oncol 2014;32(15_suppl):9033.

144. Zimmer L, Vaubel J, Mohr P, et al. Phase II DeCOG-study of ipilimumab in pre-treated and treatment-naive patients with metastatic uveal melanoma. PLoS One 2015;10(3):e0118564.

145. Joshua AM, Monzon JG, Mihalcioiu C, et al. A phase 2 study of tremelimumab in patients with advanced uveal melanoma. Melanoma Res 2015;25(4):342–7.
146. Piulats Rodriguez JM, De La Cruz Merino L, Espinosa E, et al. 1247PD -Phase II multicenter, single arm, open label study of nivolumab in combination with ipilimumab in untreated patients with metastatic uveal melanoma (GEM1402.NCT02626962). Ann Oncol 2018;29:viii443.
147. Khoja L, Atenafu EG, Suciu S, et al. Meta-analysis in metastatic uveal melanoma to determine progression free and overall survival benchmarks: an international rare cancers initiative (IRCI) ocular melanoma study. Ann Oncol 2019;30(8): 1370–80.
148. Yi JH, Yi SY, Lee HR, et al. Dacarbazine-based chemotherapy as first-line treatment in noncutaneous metastatic melanoma: multicenter, retrospective analysis in Asia. Melanoma Res 2011;21(3):223–7.
149. Shoushtari AN, Bluth MJ, Goldman DA, et al. Clinical features and response to systemic therapy in a historical cohort of advanced or unresectable mucosal melanoma. Melanoma Res 2017;27(1):57–64.
150. D'Angelo SP, Larkin J, Sosman JA, et al. Efficacy and Safety of Nivolumab Alone or in Combination With Ipilimumab in Patients With Mucosal Melanoma: A Pooled Analysis. J Clin Oncol 2017;35(2):226–35.
151. Shoushtari AN, Munhoz RR, Kuk D, et al. The efficacy of anti-PD-1 agents in acral and mucosal melanoma. Cancer 2016;122(21):3354–62.
152. Servois V, Bouhadiba T, Dureau S, et al. Iterative treatment with surgery and radiofrequency ablation of uveal melanoma liver metastasis: Retrospective analysis of a series of very long-term survivors. Eur J Surg Oncol 2019;45(9): 1717–22.
153. Robert C, Long GV, Brady B, et al. Nivolumab in previously untreated melanoma without BRAF mutation. N Engl J Med 2015;372(4):320–30.
154. Weber JS, D'Angelo SP, Minor D, et al. Nivolumab versus chemotherapy in patients with advanced melanoma who progressed after anti-CTLA-4 treatment (CheckMate 037): a randomised, controlled, open-label, phase 3 trial. Lancet Oncol 2015;16(4):375–84.
155. Patel PH, Palma D, McDonald F, et al. The Dandelion Dilemma Revisited for Oligoprogression: Treat the Whole Lawn or Weed Selectively? Clin Oncol 2019; 31(12):824–33.
156. Chiou VL, Burotto M. Pseudoprogression and Immune-Related Response in Solid Tumors. J Clin Oncol 2015;33(31):3541–3.
157. Nosrati A, Tsai KK, Goldinger SM, et al. Evaluation of clinicopathological factors in PD-1 response: derivation and validation of a prediction scale for response to PD-1 monotherapy. Br J Cancer 2017;116(9):1141–7.
158. Poklepovic AS, Carvajal RD. Prognostic Value of Low Tumor Burden in Patients With Melanoma. Oncology (Williston Park) 2018;32(9):e90–6.

Is There a Role for Locoregional Therapies for Non-colorectal Gastrointestinal Malignancies?

Gilton Marques Fonseca, MD, PhD[a],
Maria Ignez Freitas Melro Braghiroli, MD[b],
Jaime Arthur Pirola Kruger, MD, PhD[a],
Fabricio Ferreira Coelho, MD, PhD[a], Paulo Herman, MD, PhD[a],*

KEYWORDS

- Metastases • Liver • Gastrointestinal cancer • Treatment • Hepatectomy

KEY POINTS

- There is no conclusive evidence supporting or refuting the role of locoregional therapies for non-colorectal non-neuroendocrine gastrointestinal liver metastases.
- Liver metastases from gastric cancer are the leading indication for hepatic resection among all gastrointestinal non-colorectal non-neuroendocrine tumors, with better results reported by Eastern countries.
- There is no consistent evidence to recommend locoregional therapies for pancreatic adenocarcinoma liver metastases and available guidelines do not recommend this approach.
- Regarding liver metastases from esophageal malignancy, ampullary and small bowel adenocarcinomas, the evidence is too scarce to define the role of locoregional therapies.
- Multidisciplinary approach and individualized ("case-by-case") analysis are essential to define the best candidates for locoregional therapies.

INTRODUCTION

The liver is the most common site of metastases from solid gastrointestinal tract tumors. The main route is likely hematogenous spread through the portal venous

[a] Digestive Surgery Division, Liver Surgery Unit, Department of Gastroenterology, University of Sao Paulo Medical School, Avenida Doutor Enéas de Carvalho Aguiar, 255, Instituto Central, 9° andar, Sala 9074, Cerqueira Cesar, São Paulo, São Paulo CEP: 05403-900, Brazil; [b] Instituto do Cancer do Estado de Sao Paulo (ICESP), University of Sao Paulo, and Rede D'Or Sao Paulo, Av. Dr. Arnaldo, 251 - São Paulo, SP, Brazil. CEP: 01246-000, Brazil
* Corresponding author.
E-mail address: pherman@uol.com.br

Surg Oncol Clin N Am 30 (2021) 125–142
https://doi.org/10.1016/j.soc.2020.08.004
surgonc.theclinics.com

system, which drains all venous flow from gastrointestinal organs to the liver. In general, liver metastases from solid tumors are considered to be disseminated systemic disease and liver-directed therapy should only be administered in the palliative setting in order to relieve symptoms related to the hepatic disease. However, in some situations liver metastases can be considered as a "locoregional disease" rather than disseminated systemic disease, based on the argument that the portal vein route confines metastatic disease to the abdominal cavity, the liver being a primary harbinger of metastatic spread.[1]

Among patients in whom hematogenous dissemination has occurred, therapy typically involves systemic chemotherapeutic agents. Despite being the dominant treatment modality in most cases, chemotherapy alone is not able to offer a chance of cure or even effective palliation for many patients. In the context of a multidisciplinary approach, a selected group of patients may benefit from locoregional therapies.

The most widely accepted locoregional therapy is resection. Other nonsurgical treatment options are discussed in more detail in other articles of this issue and are based on thermal ablation, radiotherapy, or intra-arterial targeted catheter infusion. Thermal ablation leads to cellular destruction and necrosis through extremes of heat or cold. An image-guided probe is inserted into the tumor transmitting a high-frequency alternating current (radiofrequency ablation [RFA]) or freezing cold (cryoablation) or electromagnetic frequencies (microwave ablation [MWA]).[2] Stereotactic body radiotherapy (SBRT) is an image-guided delivery of high-dose radiation in a hypofractionated treatment plan leading to its destruction. Intra-arterial locoregional therapies take advantage of the fact that the tumor blood supply originates from the hepatic arterial system, as opposed to the predominant portal venous supply in the non-tumoral liver parenchyma. Examples of intra-arterial therapies include hepatic artery infusion (HAI), which aims to increase effective dose concentration into the tumor by using chemotherapy with high hepatic metabolism; transarterial chemoembolization (TACE), a therapy that allows significantly higher concentrations of chemotherapeutic agents within the tumor with a delivery system that uses lipid-based drugs or drug-eluting beads; and transarterial radioembolization (TARE), which delivers targeted, high-energy radioactive particles (usually Yttrium-90, ^{90}Y) to the tumor for the induction of cytotoxic effects, while minimizing damage to the surrounding healthy liver parenchyma.[3]

Recently, the role of locoregional therapies, especially resection, for colorectal liver metastases has been widely studied with long-term survival rates reaching 40% to 50% after 5 years and 20% to 30% after 10 years.[4,5] However, when liver metastases are originated from other gastrointestinal organs, the role of resection and other locoregional treatments remains unclear. In a large series analyzing liver resection for non-colorectal non-neuroendocrine liver metastases (NCNNLM) evaluating 1452 patients, Adam and colleagues[6] reported gastrointestinal primary tumors as the second-largest subset of patients (n = 230), after breast cancer, with intermediate survival rates (overall 5-year survival of 31% and median survival of 26 months). Other nonsurgical locoregional therapies have also been studied in an attempt to establish the role of these treatments for NCNNLM, especially gastric cancer liver metastases.

This article summarizes and discusses the available evidence evaluating the benefits, risks, and indications of locoregional therapies for metastatic NCNNLM.

ESOPHAGEAL CANCER LIVER METASTASES

Esophageal cancer is the sixth most common cause of cancer-related deaths in the world.[7] There are 2 main histologic types of esophageal malignancy: squamous cell carcinoma, most common in the upper esophagus, whereas adenocarcinoma predominates in the lower part of the organ, being more common in Western countries.[8]

There are only a few case series and case reports reporting liver resection for esophageal cancer liver metastases.[9] Liver metastases from esophageal cancer have a worse prognosis after resection when compared with other gastrointestinal malignancies. In the largest series published, Sano and colleagues[10] reported 51 patients submitted to resection of liver metastases from esophageal cancer with a median survival of 15 months and 5-year overall survival (OS) of 15%. Adam and colleagues[6] evaluated 20 patients with liver metastases from esophageal cancer and 25 patients from gastroesophageal junction cancer who underwent liver resection, reporting a 3-year survival of 32% and 12%, and a median survival of 16 and 14 months, respectively. Other smaller case series with the number of patients ranging from 3 to 26 showed similar results[8,9,11–16]; most of them mixing adenocarcinoma and squamous cell carcinoma histologic types. Liu and colleagues[8] reported on a group of 26 patients with squamous cell carcinoma liver metastases submitted to resection and compared outcomes with a nonsurgical group (n = 43). The resected group had an associated 1-year and 2-year OS rates of 50.8% and 21.2%, respectively, which were significantly higher than the 31% and 7.1% survival rates of patients in the nonsurgical group.

Regarding other locoregional therapies, the evidence is even scarcer. For HAI, there are a few small case series from Japan. Iwahashi and colleagues[17] reported 4 cases of gastric and esophageal liver metastases treated with HAI chemotherapy including cisplatin and 5-fluorouracil (5-FU) plus hyperthermotherapy: All patients showed a partial response and 3 of them were alive after 17 months. Nakajima and colleagues[18] reported 8 cases treated with arterial infusion of cisplatin plus 5-FU, showing an overall response of 50%, and complete response was observed in 2 patients.

The safety and effectiveness of MWA plus chemotherapy in esophageal cancer liver metastases was reported by Zhou and colleagues,[19] who evaluated 15 patients, who had an associated 3-year survival of 13.3% and a 2-year progression-free survival (PFS) of 13.3%. Recently, Wang and colleagues[20] reported 16 patients treated with cryoablation plus chemotherapy, reporting a technical success rate of 96% without any major complication. Again, the survival rate was poor, with 3-year survival of 18.8% and a 2-year PFS of 18.8%.

In terms of radiation, Omari and colleagues[21] studied 11 patients with metastases from esophageal squamous cell carcinoma treated with chemotherapy plus interstitial high-dose-rate brachytherapy using an ^{192}Iridium source. Five of the 11 patients had liver metastases, which were treated without severe adverse events. The results included all metastatic disease (liver, lung, lymph nodes, adrenal), with a median PFS of 3.4 months and OS of 13.7 months after radiation therapy. For SBRT, Milano and colleagues,[22] Egawa and colleagues[23] and Katano and colleagues,[24] reported OS ranging from 1 to 3 years in case reports, and only one of the patients had sustained local control.[24]

Radioembolization with Yttrium 90 (^{90}Y), was used for esophageal cancer liver metastases in small series including other tumors.[25–28] It is important to note that this treatment was proposed in the context of unresectable and chemorefractory disease. In a single study, tumor shrinkage was reported in one patient after radioembolization, allowing posterior liver resection, without recurrence after a 2-year follow-up.[28]

GASTRIC CANCER LIVER METASTASES

Gastric cancer has the sixth highest incidence and is the second most common cause of cancer-related death worldwide.[7] Hepatic metastases are diagnosed synchronously in 3% to 14% of patients with gastric cancer, and metachronously in up to 37% of patients after curative gastrectomy.[29] Liver metastases from gastric cancer are the leading indications for hepatic resection among gastrointestinal NCNNLM.[6,10]

The best evidence available addressing the impact of resection for gastric cancer liver metastases comes from meta-analyses[29–34] based on retrospective cohort studies and descriptive noncomparative studies since there are no randomized trials available. The first reports of resection for gastric cancer liver metastases came from single-institution case series describing 20 to 30 cases over the course of 2 decades, until multi-institutional studies that collected data from high-volume hospitals, especially from Eastern countries, reporting a 5-year survival rate near 30%.[35–39]

All meta-analyses of comparative studies favored resection in selected patients. Montagnani and colleagues[34] evaluated 33 observational studies involving 1304 patients submitted to liver resection for gastric cancer liver metastases and found a 5-year and 10-year OS of 22% (95% confidence interval [CI] 18%–26%) and 11% (95% CI 7%–18%), respectively (**Fig. 1**). Cui and colleagues,[33] in a more recent meta-analysis, obtained similar results analyzing 10 studies with 1287 patients (241 in the surgical group and 1046 in a nonsurgical group), showing that was associated with a decreased 5-year mortality (OR 0.13; 95% CI 0.07–0.24; P<.00001). Markar and colleagues[29] analyzed 9 studies with 679 patients: 235 in the resection group and 444

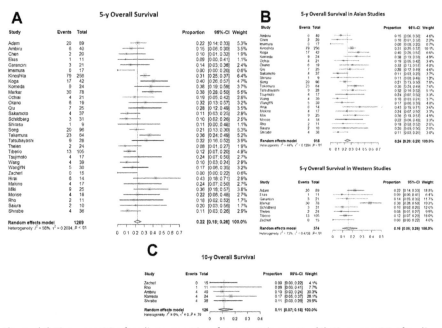

Fig. 1. (*A*) Five-year OS after liver resection from gastric cancer. (*B*) Five-year OS after liver resection from gastric cancer according to world region (Asian vs. Western studies). (*C*) Ten-year OS after liver resection from gastric cancer. (*From* Montagnani F, Crivelli F, Aprile G, et al. Long-term survival after liver metastasectomy in gastric cancer: Systematic review and meta-analysis of prognostic factors. Cancer Treat Rev 2018;69:11-20; with permission.)

in the nonresected group. In this study, liver resection was associated with an improved OS (hazard ratio [HR] 0.50; 95% CI 0.41–0.61; $P<.001$; $I^2 = 24.4\%$); with a median 1-year, 3-year, and 5-year survival of 68%, 31%, and 27%, respectively. Interestingly, studies from Eastern countries have reported better survival when compared with Western studies: 1-year (73% vs. 59%), 3-year (34% vs. 24.5%), and 5-year (27.3% vs. 16.5%), respectively. Liao and colleagues[32] also compared studies in Asian countries (5 studies, 117 patients) with those from Western countries (3 studies, 79 patients) and found that Asian cohorts had higher median 1-year (76% vs. 60%), 2-year (47% vs. 30%) and 3-year (39% vs. 23%) OS rates. One possible reason for these differences is that Western cohorts usually included patients in a more advanced stage of the disease, with a higher disease burden. Using the available evidence, the Japanese Gastric Cancer Treatment Guidelines[40] from the Japanese Gastric Cancer Association, states that "one cannot deny a possibility that liver resection results in long-term survival among highly selected patients."

In an effort to identify patients who may benefit from resection of gastric cancer liver metastases, several prognostic factors have been studied. Montagnani and colleagues[34] found the following factors associated with OS: (1) in the primary tumor: lower T stages, absence or limited nodal involvement, serosa or lymphatic or vascular involvement; (2) in the metastatic liver disease: single or fewer than 3 metastases, unilobar disease, diameter of the largest lesion less than 5 cm and negative margins. The study showed low or very low levels of heterogeneity, suggesting that the effects of these prognostic factors on OS were similar, despite differences in time, procedures, and patients.

Another question is about the role of preoperative or postoperative chemotherapy around the time of hepatic resection. Montagnani and colleagues,[34] in a meta-analysis of 12 studies encompassing 729 patients found a tendency toward a longer OS ($P = .08$) in patients submitted to postoperative chemotherapy. However, this matter remains debatable. The European Organization for Research and Treatment of Cancer, the Gastrointestinal Tract Cancer Group (GITCG) and the Japan Clinical Oncology Group Stomach Cancer Study Group conducted a survey with specialists from 18 countries in patients with resectable synchronous or metachronous gastric cancer liver metastases without evidence of extrahepatic metastases. Most of them (47.5%) preferred preoperative chemotherapy followed by the resection of primary (if in place) and liver metastases. In order to study this issue, the RENAISSANCE (AIO-FLOT5) trial (NCT02578368),[41] a randomized study, is being conducted comparing chemotherapy alone versus chemotherapy plus surgery in patients with limited metastases of gastric or esophagogastric junction cancer. The previous non-randomized trial (AIO-FLOT3), from the same German group,[42] demonstrated better results in patients who received neoadjuvant chemotherapy followed by resection using the same strategy.

The best level of evidence regarding ablation techniques for gastric cancer liver metastases comes from a recent systematic review with meta-analysis[43] evaluating 12 observational studies (10 with RFA ablation and 2 with MWA), with a 3-year and 5-year survival of 28%, and 19%, respectively, and a median survival of 23 months. The procedures were considered safe, with median 30-day morbidity of 6% (0%–23%) without mortality. Three studies compared ablative techniques with resection (**Fig. 2**A) and showed that patients submitted to resection had a significantly higher survival rate when compared with the ablation group (HR 0.81; 95% CI 0.75–0.88). However, when compared to systemic therapy, patients submitted to thermal ablation tended to have better survival rate, but without statistical significance (HR 2.12; 95% CI 0.77–3.47) in 4 studies (**Fig. 2**B). A meta-analysis of 7 studies confirmed an

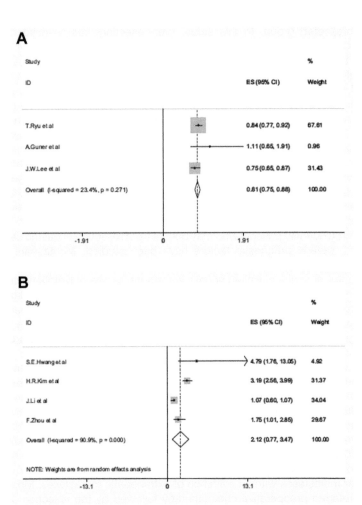

Fig. 2. Forrest plot showing the results of thermal ablation of gastric liver metastases when compared with (*A*) hepatic resection, (*B*) systemic chemotherapy. (*From* Tang K, Liu Y, Dong L, et al. Influence of thermal ablation of hepatic metastases from gastric adenocarcinoma on long-term survival: Systematic review and pooled analysis. Medicine [Baltimore] 2018;97(49):e13525; with permission.)

associated prolonged survival for ablating tumors smaller than 3 cm (HR 1.46; 95% CI 1.03–1.88; *P* = .002) and the benefits of systemic chemotherapy after thermal ablation (HR 2.14; 95% CI 1.05–3.23; *P* = .000). There is only 1 randomized study regarding cryotherapy versus resection for liver metastases,[44] evaluating metastases from multiple primary site tumors, including only 9 patients with gastric cancer (4 in the cryotherapy group and 5 in the surgical group). Beyond feasibility, the small number of treated patients precludes any definitive conclusion about the impact of the treatment on this specific tumor.

Apart from case reports, there is limited evidence for the use of HAI in liver metastases from gastric cancer. In 1999, Kumada and colleagues[45] analyzed the efficacy of HAI using 5-fluorouracil, epirubicin, and mitomycin C (FEM) in 63 patients with unresectable gastric cancer liver metastases, with an overall response rate of 55.6% and a median OS of 10.5 months. Seki and colleagues[46] also analyzed the efficacy of HAI-FEM as a second-line therapy, after the failure of systemic S-1 plus cisplatin treatment in 14 patients, with a response rate of 42.9% and complete response in 14.3%, reporting a median OS of 12.7 months. More recently, Fukami and colleagues[47] evaluated the role of adjuvant HAI-FEM regimen after liver resection for gastric cancer metastases in 14 patients. They found a 57% recurrence rate over a median follow-up of 29 months, with a 5-year OS rate higher than other series (43%). Further comparative studies are needed to define the role of HAI chemotherapy in gastric cancer liver metastases.

Regarding therapies based on radiation, studies on SBRT for gastric cancer liver metastases are only case reports[48] or as small parts of case series with tumors from other sites.[49–51] Data about radioembolization also comes from studies where gastric liver metastases are a small part of the series.[52–54] Therefore, it is not possible to define the role of SBRT in gastric cancer liver metastases.

PANCREATIC CANCER LIVER METASTASES

Pancreatic adenocarcinoma is projected to become the second leading cause of cancer-related death in 2030 in the United States. Currently, it is the third leading cause of cancer death, with OS in advanced stages ranging from 6 to 11 months.[55,56] Approximately 50% of the patients with pancreatic adenocarcinoma have metastatic disease at the time of diagnosis.[56] In selected metastatic patients with oligometastases and stable disease after chemotherapy, locoregional therapies have been studied, although there are no randomized controlled trials or evidence-based guidelines about its role or the best therapeutic strategy.[55]

Guidelines on the management of pancreatic adenocarcinoma do not specifically recommend liver resection for pancreatic adenocarcinoma liver metastases.[57] However, a recent systematic review[55] found 17 studies reporting resection for pancreatic liver metastases, with median OS ranging from 5.9 to 56 months. The largest series is mixed with interaortocaval lymph node resection[58] or other histologic subtypes of pancreatic cancers,[59] making the analysis of results difficult. In these studies, there is no pattern or consensus about patient selection for liver resection, regimens of adjuvant/neoadjuvant chemotherapy or timing for liver resection (synchronous or staged pancreatic and liver resection). Furthermore, there is no consensus about which patients are most likely to benefit from resection.

Interestingly, the best long-term results (median OS of 56 months) were reported by Frigerio and colleagues,[60] that selected patients with liver-only metastases, all submitted to neoadjuvant chemotherapy with complete disappearing of liver metastases. In this study, only the primary pancreatic tumor was resected, showing that the complete response to neoadjuvant chemotherapy was the main prognostic factor. This study suggests that one of the most important factors for selection may be the response to chemotherapy.[60,61]

There is considerable variation on prognostic factors among different studies. The most relevant prognostic factors appear to be response to preoperative chemotherapy, oligometastatic disease, and R0 resection.[55,61,62] In highly selected patients presenting with favorable prognostic factors, when compared with patients submitted to palliative chemotherapy only, resection of liver metastases is associated with better survival.

In patients with synchronous metastases, the timing of liver and pancreatic resection is also controversial. Some investigators report better outcomes with synchronous resection,[62,63] with median survivals ranging from 5.9 to 14.5 months and 5-year OS rates of up to 8.1%. Hackert and colleagues,[58] comparing 62 patients submitted to synchronous resection with 23 patients whose metastases were resected separately, showed similar long-term survival (respectively 10.6 months for synchronic vs. 14.8 months median survival, $P = .21$). Dunschede and colleagues[64] found no difference in survival in synchronous resection when compared with chemotherapy alone (median OS respectively 8 vs. 11 months), whereas the survival after metachronous resection increased to 31 months.

The mortality after pancreatic liver metastases resection ranges from 0% to 9%,[55,64,65] with high morbidity rates, reaching up to 68%,[66] in cases of synchronous resection. In fact, the studies comparing morbidity after synchronous or metachronous liver resection showed higher morbidity in synchronous resections. When compared with metachronous resection, the morbidity rates after synchronous resection were, respectively, 45% versus 22% according to Hackert and colleagues,[58] and 33% versus 0% according to Dunschede and colleagues.[64] De Jong and colleagues[59] reported higher morbidity after metachronous resection (40.6% vs. 26.3%), especially liver abscess, due to the biliary colonization following biliary-enteric anastomosis.

There has always been a concern that the use of ablative techniques for liver metastases in patients who have undergone a pancreatoduodenectomy or biliary-enteric anastomosis may lead to an increased risk of ablation zone abscess, secondary to ascending biliary contamination, with risk rates of 40% to 50%.[67,68] Although overall complication rates are low, specific reported complications include hepatic or extrahepatic injuries, pneumothorax, and hemorrhage with lower complication rates.[55] The first prospective single-arm study evaluating the role of RFA of pancreatic adenocarcinoma liver metastases was conducted by Park and colleagues[69] in 34 patients with ≤5 liver metastases, ≤3 cm diameter in size and no extrahepatic metastases, treated during pancreatic resection or after pancreatectomy. Three patients developed pleural effusion managed conservatively and one patient developed a liver abscess. The median survival after ablation was 18 months and 3-year OS after pancreatic resection was 32.4%. Another single-arm retrospective study[70] with 102 patients with similar characteristics showed a minor complication rate of 9.8%, all conservatively managed. The median OS and 1-year survival rate were, respectively, 11.4 months and 47.1%. Further comparative studies are necessary to establish the role and risks of RFA in these patients.

The use of SBRT in the treatment of pancreatic adenocarcinoma liver metastases is very limited. The role of SBRT is quite difficult to establish because the studies that have investigated its efficacy and safety in the treatment of liver metastasis did not focus on a specific primary site.[71–73] A phase II study of proton-based SBRT for liver metastases encompassing 89 patients with tumors from different histologies and sites (13 from pancreatic adenocarcinoma) showed that KRAS mutation was the strongest predictor of poor local control ($P = .02$) and tumors with both KRAS and TP53 mutation had higher radio resistance, with local control of 20%, compared with 69.2% in all other tumors ($P = .001$).[74]

Regarding radioembolization in pancreatic cancer liver metastasis, the largest series comes from a multicenter study[75] from 3 North American institutions with 33 patients whose tumors progressed despite systemic chemotherapy. Partial response was observed in 42% of patients, whereas 37% showed stable disease and 21% had progressive disease. Median OS after radioembolization and diagnosis of the primary tumor were, respectively, 8.1 and 20.8 months. The reported complications were ≤ grade 2, except for 2 patients with grade 3 side effects, which included abdominal distention/pain, fatigue, or ascites, that disappeared in a short time. Other studies showed more severe complications, such as radiation cholecystitis, gastric ulceration, liver abscess, cholangitis, ascites and death from treatment-related liver failure.[75–80]

Some investigators have studied the role of TACE in pancreatic adenocarcinoma liver metastases. Azizi and colleagues[81] reported 32 patients with pancreatic liver metastases without extrahepatic disease with a median OS from the first TACE of 16 months, increasing to 20 months in the subgroup with stable disease (72% of patients) or partial response (9.4% of patients). A more recent study[82] evaluated 18 patients with liver metastases from pancreatic adenocarcinoma submitted to TACE. The OS was 9.1 months and none of the patients developed a severe complication.

Finally, a retrospective study by Ouyang and colleagues[83] highlighted the importance of the multidisciplinary approach in these cases. They evaluated 184 patients with pancreatic adenocarcinoma liver metastases treated with systemic chemotherapy alone (n = 64) or systemic chemotherapy plus liver-directed therapy (n = 120). The groups had similar clinical characteristics and the liver-directed therapy group received different approaches, depending on the multidisciplinary decision. Median OS was 8.7 months in the group treated with liver-directed therapy and 6.3 months in the chemotherapy group ($P = .01$); the liver-directed approach was an independent favorable prognostic factor after multivariate analysis.

AMPULLARY CANCER LIVER METASTASES

The periampullary region is a complex anatomic area including the ampulla of Vater, distal bile duct, duodenum and the head of the pancreas. Despite the similarities of the surgical treatment for these tumors (pancreatoduodenectomy), their biological behavior is different. Periampullary tumors are classified histopathologically into intestinal type or pancreatobiliary type, with the intestinal type having a more favorable prognosis.[84] We have discussed pancreatic liver metastases in the previous section and now we will focus on the non-pancreatic ampullary tumors.

Adam and colleagues[6] reported 15 patients submitted to hepatic resection for ampullary liver metastases, with a 5-year survival and median survival of 46% and 38 months, respectively. de Jong and colleagues[85] evaluated 40 patients with periampullary liver metastases (pancreas head n = 20, ampulla of Vater n = 5, distal bile duct n = 5, duodenum n = 5) submitted to liver-directed therapy (resection and/or RFA). Median survival after liver resection of intestinal-type tumors (ampulla and duodenum) was 23 months with a 3-year survival of 33%, compared with 13 months and 3-year survival of 8% for patients with pancreaticobiliary type tumors ($P = .05$). The perioperative complication rate was 30%, with a mortality rate of 5%, without difference between synchronous or metachronous resection. Kurosaki and colleagues[86] evaluated 13 patients who underwent metachronous liver resection of metastases from periampullary tumors (papilla of Vater n = 6, distal bile duct n = 7) and found a 5-year OS rate of 45%. Patients with a single liver tumor and received adjuvant chemotherapy had an associated better survival. Three of 6 patients with primary tumor of the papilla of Vater were alive after 5 years, whereas only 1 of 7 patients with liver metastases of the distal bile duct.

Other locoregional therapies directed to ampullary liver metastases, such as percutaneous stereotactic image-guided MWA[87] and HAI[88] have been published in case reports or small case series that included other primary tumors. Thus, it is not possible to evaluate its prognostic significance.

SMALL BOWEL CANCER LIVER METASTASES

Small bowel tumors are rare, especially adenocarcinomas, and represent less than 5% of all gastrointestinal tumors.[89] There is a paucity of data regarding the results of locoregional therapies for liver metastases from small bowel adenocarcinomas. Adam and colleagues,[6] in a multicenter study with resected NCNNLM, reported 28 patients with primary tumors from the small bowel and 12 patients from the nonampullary duodenum. Patients with liver metastases from small bowel had the best prognosis after resection among all gastrointestinal tumors, with a 5-year survival of 49% and a median OS of 58 months, whereas duodenal tumors metastases resection had a 5-year and median OS of 21% and 34 months, respectively. Another recent study[10] with 1539 patients submitted to liver resection for NCNNLM evaluated the prognosis of 24 patients with duodenal carcinoma metastases and found a median OS of 66 months, with 5-year and 10-year OS of 57% and 27%, respectively. Rompteaux and colleagues[89] evaluated 34 patients from several French centers submitted to curative intent resection of metastases from small bowel adenocarcinoma, and 9 of them (29.4%) had isolated liver metastases resected. Median OS was 28.6 months and 41.2% of the patients were alive after 3-year follow-up. The factors associated with worse prognosis after resection were poor differentiation, R1 margins, and lymphatic invasion. Thus, the last National Comprehensive Cancer Network Practice Guidelines for treatment of small bowel adenocarcinoma recommends that "certain patients with small bowel adenocarcinoma and limited metastasis to visceral organs may be candidates for metastasectomy."[90]

There is a lack of evidence on other modalities of locoregional therapies for small bowel non-neuroendocrine malignancies and its role in the treatment of liver metastases.

SUMMARY

After thoroughly reviewing the results of several studies, the main practical question remains: is there a role for locoregional therapies for non-colorectal gastrointestinal liver metastases? There is no conclusive evidence of its real role. The higher benefit appears to be in selected patients with liver metastases from gastric, especially surgical resection, with a high number of systematic reviews and meta-analysis supporting it, followed by small bowel adenocarcinoma. The best results come from Eastern countries, where there is a higher incidence of gastric adenocarcinoma and a systematic screening program, which allows detecting patients with lower disease burden. Regarding pancreatic adenocarcinoma liver metastases, despite many groups studying its role, there is no consistent evidence to recommend any locoregional therapy in daily clinical practice and the guidelines do not recommend this approach. Regarding liver metastases from esophageal tumors and ampullary adenocarcinomas, the evidence is scarce for the role of locoregional therapies. Thus, this approach should be considered only in highly selected patients from high-volume specialized centers on a case-to-case basis and after multidisciplinary discussion.

There are many limitations in studies focusing on the role of locoregional therapies in gastrointestinal NCNNLM. First, there are not enough randomized trials evaluating this subject and many retrospective studies include metastases from different primary sites. Mixing different liver metastases with distinct biological behavior in the same study adds little information about the best approach and selection of patients, prognostic impact and the exact role of locoregional therapies. Further studies should focus on specific tumor sites and histologic subtypes to provide qualified clinical information on the management of these patients.

Another important point of discussion is that, as retrospective cohort studies, there is a strong patient selection bias, without clear and homogeneous selection criteria. Notwithstanding, when managing patients with advanced cancer and systemic disease, the response to chemotherapy should be the watershed that divides patients that may benefit from liver-directed therapies from those who would not. In this context, a multidisciplinary discussion is essential.

The famous statement from the surgical oncologist Blake Cady is more true than ever for locoregional therapies for gastrointestinal malignancies liver metastases: "Biology is King; selection of cases is Queen, and the technical details of surgical procedures are Princes and Princesses of the realm who frequently try to overthrow the powerful forces of the King and Queen."[91] We need to understand the biology of these tumors to select patients who will benefit most from locoregional therapies.

COMMENTARY: THE MEDICAL ONCOLOGIST POINT-OF-VIEW

From the clinical oncology perspective, specifically for the gastrointestinal oncology specialist, we have faced a great improvement in the treatment of gastrointestinal malignancies over the past decades. Looking specifically at colon cancer, we have learned that some patients with the metastatic disease can be cured with surgery. Indeed, it was made possible with the evolution of systemic therapies, the understanding of molecular patterns and prognostic factors and modern surgical approaches associated with the availability of ablative techniques.[92–94]

Based on these findings from colon cancer and advances on systemic treatment in other gastrointestinal malignancies, the question that emerged was if a curative perspective could be offered to patients with NCNNLM. As previously described in this article, the literature is unclear regarding the real benefit offered to these patients. Most data are provided by case series or meta-analysis including different tumor primaries. We should also be aware that published data tend to be biased by displaying only the highly selected and few successful cases. Despite that, in daily practice, we face patients that may benefit from a more aggressive approach and we should be attentive to potential candidates. Clinical disease behavior should be one of the most important indicators that a patient might benefit from surgery for metastasis. Patients with limited tumor burden that present with sustained response to systemic treatment, have good performance and are amenable to complete resection, might be considered for locoregional therapies including surgery. Multidisciplinary discussion is also an important step to make sure all possibilities are being contemplated and the proposed strategy is reasonable. It is also important to have a clear and open conversation with patients so that they have expectations aligned with the medical team.

Although we still have much to learn regarding molecular prediction models for gastrointestinal tumors, a few subgroups are worth discussing in more detail. For gastric cancer, the subgroup of patients with her-2 amplification treated with specific therapy demonstrate better responses and may be potential candidates for more aggressive locoregional approaches.[95] In pancreatic adenocarcinoma, we have recently incorporated the first targeted therapy for those with germline BRCA mutations. These patients tend to have good responses to platinum agents and after that, the disease is likely to be sensitive to the PARP inhibitor olaparib.[96] In this subgroup of individuals, when optimal responses are appreciated, local approaches can be considered. Finally, among all gastrointestinal tumors, those that are mismatch repair (MMR) deficient are recognized as being sensitive to immunotherapy. The response rate to this approach exceeds 50% and tends to be sustained.[97] It is worth mentioning that in patients with complete or nearly complete responses we might offer a more aggressive approach, but we do not have a clear answer if this offers any advantage over the maintenance of the systemic treatment that is, being effective.

In the near future, we should improve our knowledge of disease behavior based on molecular findings. Also, liquid biopsies might give us information on the presence of minimal disease. All the previously mentioned information gathered will aid to understand the benefit of surgical approaches.

CLINICS CARE POINTS

- Locoregional therapies for non-colorectal gastrointestinal liver metastases should be considered only in highly selected patients on a case-to-case basis and after multidisciplinary discussion, preferably in high-volume specialized centers, since there is no conclusive evidence of its real role.
- The understanding of tumor biology is crucial for an adequate selection of patients that would benefit from locoregional therapies.
- The most accepted and resolutive locoregional therapy is resection; nonsurgical treatment options are based on thermal ablation, radiotherapy, or intra-arterial targeted catheter infusion. Indications should be individualized.

DISCLOSURE

The authors declare no conflicts of interest.

REFERENCES

1. Choi EA, Abdalla EK. Patient selection and outcome of hepatectomy for noncolorectal non-neuroendocrine liver metastases. Surg Oncol Clin N Am 2007; 16(3):557–77, ix.

2. Simon CJ, Dupuy DE, Mayo-Smith WW. Microwave ablation: principles and applications. Radiographics 2005;25(Suppl 1):S69–83.

3. Xing M, Kooby DA, El-Rayes BF, et al. Locoregional therapies for metastatic colorectal carcinoma to the liver–an evidence-based review. J Surg Oncol 2014; 110(2):182–96.

4. Adam R, De Gramont A, Figueras J, et al. The oncosurgery approach to managing liver metastases from colorectal cancer: a multidisciplinary international consensus. Oncologist 2012;17(10):1225–39.

5. Kruger JAP, Fonseca GM, Makdissi FF, et al. Evolution in the surgical management of colorectal liver metastases: propensity score matching analysis (PSM) on the impact of specialized multidisciplinary care across two institutional eras. J Surg Oncol 2018;118(1):50–60.

6. Adam R, Chiche L, Aloia T, et al. Hepatic resection for noncolorectal nonendocrine liver metastases: analysis of 1,452 patients and development of a prognostic model. Ann Surg 2006;244(4):524–35.

7. Ferlay J, Colombet M, Soerjomataram I, et al. Estimating the global cancer incidence and mortality in 2018: GLOBOCAN sources and methods. Int J Cancer 2019;144(8):1941–53.

8. Liu J, Wei Z, Wang Y, et al. Hepatic resection for post-operative solitary liver metastasis from oesophageal squamous cell carcinoma. ANZ J Surg 2018; 88(4):E252–6.

9. Schizas D, Lazaridis II, Moris D, et al. The role of surgical treatment in isolated organ recurrence of esophageal cancer-a systematic review of the literature. World J Surg Oncol 2018;16(1):55.

10. Sano K, Yamamoto M, Mimura T, et al. Outcomes of 1,639 hepatectomies for non-colorectal non-neuroendocrine liver metastases: a multicenter analysis. J Hepatobiliary Pancreat Sci 2018;25(11):465–75.

11. Seesing MFJ, van der Veen A, Brenkman HJF, et al. Resection of hepatic and pulmonary metastasis from metastatic esophageal and gastric cancer: a nationwide study. Dis Esophagus 2019;32(12):doz034.

12. Huddy JR, Thomas RL, Worthington TR, et al. Liver metastases from esophageal carcinoma: is there a role for surgical resection? Dis Esophagus 2015;28(5): 483–7.

13. Ichida H, Imamura H, Yoshimoto J, et al. Pattern of postoperative recurrence and hepatic and/or pulmonary resection for liver and/or lung metastases from esophageal carcinoma. World J Surg 2013;37(2):398–407.

14. Andreou A, Vigano L, Zimmitti G, et al. Response to preoperative chemotherapy predicts survival in patients undergoing hepatectomy for liver metastases from gastric and esophageal cancer. J Gastrointest Surg 2014;18(11):1974–86.

15. Bresadola V, Rossetto A, Adani GL, et al. Liver resection for noncolorectal and nonneuroendocrine metastases: results of a study on 56 patients at a single institution. Tumori 2011;97(3):316–22.

16. Van Daele E, Scuderi V, Pape E, et al. Long-term survival after multimodality therapy including surgery for metastatic esophageal cancer. Acta Chir Belg 2018; 118(4):227–32.

17. Iwahashi M, Tanimura H, Nakamori M, et al. Clinical evaluation of hepatic arterial infusion of low dose-CDDP and 5-FU with hyperthermotherapy: a preliminary study for liver metastases from esophageal and gastric cancer. Hepatogastroenterology 1999;46(28):2504–10.

18. Nakajima Y, Nagai K, Kawano T, et al. Therapeutic strategy for postoperative liver metastasis from esophageal squamous cell carcinoma; clinical efficacy of and problem with hepatic arterial infusion chemotherapy. Hepatogastroenterology 2001;48(42):1652–5.

19. Zhou F, Yu X, Liang P, et al. Combined microwave ablation and systemic chemotherapy for liver metastases from oesophageal cancer: preliminary results and literature review. Int J Hyperthermia 2016;32(5):524–30.

20. Wang Y, Zhang WH, Chang X, et al. CT-guided percutaneous cryoablation combined with systemic chemotherapy for liver metastases from esophageal carcinoma: Initial experience. Cryobiology 2019;87:99–104.

21. Omari J, Heinze C, Wilck A, et al. Image-guided interstitial high-dose-rate brachytherapy in the treatment of metastatic esophageal squamous cell carcinoma. J Contemp Brachytherapy 2018;10(5):439–45.

22. Milano MT, Katz AW, Zhang H, et al. Oligometastases treated with stereotactic body radiotherapy: long-term follow-up of prospective study. Int J Radiat Oncol Biol Phys 2012;83(3):878–86.

23. Egawa T, Okubo Y, Kemmochi T, et al. A case of liver metastasis from esophageal cancer treated with stereotactic body radiation therapy. Gan To Kagaku Ryoho 2013;40(12):1850–2 [in Japanese].

24. Katano A, Yamashita H, Nakagawa K. Stereotactic body radiotherapy for oligorecurrence in the liver in a patient with esophageal carcinoma: a case report. Mol Clin Oncol 2017;7(6):1061–3.

25. Sato KT, Lewandowski RJ, Mulcahy MF, et al. Unresectable chemorefractory liver metastases: radioembolization with 90Y microspheres–safety, efficacy, and survival. Radiology 2008;247(2):507–15.

26. Cianni R, Urigo C, Notarianni E, et al. Radioembolisation using yttrium 90 (Y-90) in patients affected by unresectable hepatic metastases. Radiol Med 2010;115(4):619–33.

27. Fidelman N, Kerlan RK Jr, Hawkins RA, et al. Radioembolization with (90)Y glass microspheres for the treatment of unresectable metastatic liver disease from chemotherapy-refractory gastrointestinal cancers: final report of a prospective pilot study. J Gastrointest Oncol 2016;7(6):860–74.

28. Whitney R, Tatum C, Hahl M, et al. Safety of hepatic resection in metastatic disease to the liver after yttrium-90 therapy. J Surg Res 2011;166(2):236–40.

29. Markar SR, Mikhail S, Malietzis G, et al. Influence of surgical resection of hepatic metastases from gastric adenocarcinoma on long-term survival: systematic review and pooled analysis. Ann Surg 2016;263(6):1092–101.

30. Martella L, Bertozzi S, Londero AP, et al. Surgery for liver metastases from gastric cancer: a meta-analysis of observational studies. Medicine (Baltimore) 2015;94(31):e1113.

31. Petrelli F, Coinu A, Cabiddu M, et al. Hepatic resection for gastric cancer liver metastases: a systematic review and meta-analysis. J Surg Oncol 2015;111(8):1021–7.

32. Liao YY, Peng NF, Long D, et al. Hepatectomy for liver metastases from gastric cancer: a systematic review. BMC Surg 2017;17(1):14.

33. Cui JK, Liu M, Shang XK. Hepatectomy for liver metastasis of gastric cancer: a meta-analysis. Surg Innov 2019;26(6):692–7.

34. Montagnani F, Crivelli F, Aprile G, et al. Long-term survival after liver metastasectomy in gastric cancer: Systematic review and meta-analysis of prognostic factors. Cancer Treat Rev 2018;69:11–20.

35. Kodera Y. Surgery with curative intent for stage IV gastric cancer: Is it a reality of illusion? Ann Gastroenterol Surg 2018;2(5):339–47.

36. Oki E, Tokunaga S, Emi Y, et al. Surgical treatment of liver metastasis of gastric cancer: a retrospective multicenter cohort study (KSCC1302). Gastric Cancer 2016;19(3):968–76.

37. Kinoshita T, Saiura A, Esaki M, et al. Multicentre analysis of long-term outcome after surgical resection for gastric cancer liver metastases. Br J Surg 2015;102(1):102–7.

38. Guner A, Son T, Cho I, et al. Liver-directed treatments for liver metastasis from gastric adenocarcinoma: comparison between liver resection and radiofrequency ablation. Gastric Cancer 2016;19(3):951–60.

39. Tatsubayashi T, Tanizawa Y, Miki Y, et al. Treatment outcomes of hepatectomy for liver metastases of gastric cancer diagnosed using contrast-enhanced magnetic resonance imaging. Gastric Cancer 2017;20(2):387–93.

40. Japanese gastric cancer treatment guidelines 2014 (ver. 4). Gastric Cancer 2017;20(1):1–19.

41. Al-Batran SE, Goetze TO, Mueller DW, et al. The RENAISSANCE (AIO-FLOT5) trial: effect of chemotherapy alone vs. chemotherapy followed by surgical resection on survival and quality of life in patients with limited-metastatic adenocarcinoma of the stomach or esophagogastric junction - a phase III trial of the German AIO/CAO-V/CAOGI. BMC Cancer 2017;17(1):893.

42. Al-Batran SE, Homann N, Pauligk C, et al. Effect of neoadjuvant chemotherapy followed by surgical resection on survival in patients with limited metastatic

gastric or gastroesophageal junction cancer: the AIO-FLOT3 TRIAL. JAMA Oncol 2017;3(9):1237–44.

43. Tang K, Liu Y, Dong L, et al. Influence of thermal ablation of hepatic metastases from gastric adenocarcinoma on long-term survival: Systematic review and pooled analysis. Medicine (Baltimore) 2018;97(49):e13525.

44. Bala MM, Riemsma RP, Wolff R, et al. Cryotherapy for liver metastases. Cochrane Database Syst Rev 2019;(7):CD009058.

45. Kumada T, Arai Y, Itoh K, et al. Phase II study of combined administration of 5-fluorouracil, epirubicin and mitomycin-C by hepatic artery infusion in patients with liver metastases of gastric cancer. Oncology 1999;57(3):216–23.

46. Seki H, Ohi H, Ozaki T, et al. Hepatic arterial infusion chemotherapy using fluorouracil, epirubicin, and mitomycin C for patients with liver metastases from gastric cancer after treatment failure of systemic S-1 plus cisplatin. Acta Radiol 2016; 57(7):781–8.

47. Fukami Y, Kaneoka Y, Maeda A, et al. Adjuvant hepatic artery infusion chemotherapy after hemihepatectomy for gastric cancer liver metastases. Int J Surg 2017;46:79–84.

48. Lewis GD, Chiang SB, Butler EB, et al. The utility of positron emission tomography/computed tomography in target delineation for stereotactic body radiotherapy for liver metastasis from primary gastric cancer: an illustrative case report and literature review. J Gastrointest Oncol 2017;8(3):E39–42.

49. Goodman KA, Wiegner EA, Maturen KE, et al. Dose-escalation study of single-fraction stereotactic body radiotherapy for liver malignancies. Int J Radiat Oncol Biol Phys 2010;78(2):486–93.

50. Yamashita H, Onishi H, Matsumoto Y, et al. Local effect of stereotactic body radiotherapy for primary and metastatic liver tumors in 130 Japanese patients. Radiat Oncol 2014;9:112.

51. Berkovic P, Gulyban A, Nguyen PV, et al. Stereotactic robotic body radiotherapy for patients with unresectable hepatic oligorecurrence. Clin Colorectal Cancer 2017;16(4):349–57.e1.

52. Benson AB 3rd, Geschwind JF, Mulcahy MF, et al. Radioembolisation for liver metastases: results from a prospective 151 patient multi-institutional phase II study. Eur J Cancer 2013;49(15):3122–30.

53. Pieper CC, Willinek WA, Thomas D, et al. Incidence and risk factors of early arterial blood flow stasis during first radioembolization of primary and secondary liver malignancy using resin microspheres: an initial single-center analysis. Eur Radiol 2016;26(8):2779–89.

54. Prince JF, van den Bosch M, Nijsen JFW, et al. Efficacy of radioembolization with (166)Ho-microspheres in salvage patients with liver metastases: a phase 2 study. J Nucl Med 2018;59(4):582–8.

55. Ghidini M, Petrillo A, Salati M, et al. Surgery or locoregional approaches for hepatic oligometastatic pancreatic cancer: myth, hope, or reality? Cancers (Basel) 2019;11(8):1095.

56. Kandel P, Wallace MB, Stauffer J, et al. Survival of patients with oligometastatic pancreatic ductal adenocarcinoma treated with combined modality treatment including surgical resection: a pilot study. J Pancreat Cancer 2018;4(1):88–94.

57. Tempero MA, Malafa MP, Al-Hawary M, et al. Pancreatic adenocarcinoma, version 2.2017, NCCN clinical practice guidelines in oncology. J Natl Compr Canc Netw 2017;15(8):1028–61.

58. Hackert T, Niesen W, Hinz U, et al. Radical surgery of oligometastatic pancreatic cancer. Eur J Surg Oncol 2017;43(2):358–63.

59. De Jong MC, Farnell MB, Sclabas G, et al. Liver-directed therapy for hepatic metastases in patients undergoing pancreaticoduodenectomy: a dual-center analysis. Ann Surg 2010;252(1):142–8.
60. Frigerio I, Regi P, Giardino A, et al. Downstaging in stage IV pancreatic cancer: a new population eligible for surgery? Ann Surg Oncol 2017;24(8):2397–403.
61. Crippa S, Bittoni A, Sebastiani E, et al. Is there a role for surgical resection in patients with pancreatic cancer with liver metastases responding to chemotherapy? Eur J Surg Oncol 2016;42(10):1533–9.
62. Andreou A, Knitter S, Klein F, et al. The role of hepatectomy for synchronous liver metastases from pancreatic adenocarcinoma. Surg Oncol 2018;27(4):688–94.
63. Yang J, Zhang J, Lui W, et al. Patients with hepatic oligometastatic pancreatic body/tail ductal adenocarcinoma may benefit from synchronous resection. HPB (Oxford) 2019;22(1):91–101.
64. Dunschede F, Will L, von Langsdorf C, et al. Treatment of metachronous and simultaneous liver metastases of pancreatic cancer. Eur Surg Res 2010; 44(3–4):209–13.
65. Gleisner AL, Assumpcao L, Cameron JL, et al. Is resection of periampullary or pancreatic adenocarcinoma with synchronous hepatic metastasis justified? Cancer 2007;110(11):2484–92.
66. Tachezy M, Gebauer F, Janot M, et al. Synchronous resections of hepatic oligometastatic pancreatic cancer: Disputing a principle in a time of safe pancreatic operations in a retrospective multicenter analysis. Surgery 2016;160(1):136–44.
67. Elias D, Di Pietroantonio D, Gachot B, et al. Liver abscess after radiofrequency ablation of tumors in patients with a biliary tract procedure. Gastroenterol Clin Biol 2006;30(6–7):823–7.
68. Choi D, Lim HK, Kim MJ, et al. Liver abscess after percutaneous radiofrequency ablation for hepatocellular carcinomas: frequency and risk factors. AJR Am J Roentgenol 2005;184(6):1860–7.
69. Park JB, Kim YH, Kim J, et al. Radiofrequency ablation of liver metastasis in patients with locally controlled pancreatic ductal adenocarcinoma. J Vasc Interv Radiol 2012;23(5):635–41.
70. Hua YQ, Wang P, Zhu XY, et al. Radiofrequency ablation for hepatic oligometastatic pancreatic cancer: An analysis of safety and efficacy. Pancreatology 2017;17(6):967–73.
71. Yuan ZY, Meng MB, Liu CL, et al. Stereotactic body radiation therapy using the CyberKnife((R)) system for patients with liver metastases. Onco Targets Ther 2014;7:915–23.
72. Andratschke N, Alheid H, Allgauer M, et al. The SBRT database initiative of the German Society for Radiation Oncology (DEGRO): patterns of care and outcome analysis of stereotactic body radiotherapy (SBRT) for liver oligometastases in 474 patients with 623 metastases. BMC Cancer 2018;18(1):283.
73. Mahadevan A, Blanck O, Lanciano R, et al. Stereotactic Body Radiotherapy (SBRT) for liver metastasis - clinical outcomes from the international multi-institutional RSSearch(R) Patient Registry. Radiat Oncol 2018;13(1):26.
74. Hong TS, Wo JY, Borger DR, et al. Phase II study of proton-based stereotactic body radiation therapy for liver metastases: importance of tumor genotype. J Natl Cancer Inst 2017;109(9):1–8.
75. Kim AY, Frantz S, Brower J, et al. Radioembolization with Yttrium-90 microspheres for the treatment of liver metastases of pancreatic adenocarcinoma: a multicenter analysis. J Vasc Interv Radiol 2019;30(3):298–304.e2.

76. Cao C, Yan TD, Morris DL, et al. Radioembolization with Yttrium-90 microspheres for pancreatic cancer liver metastases: results from a pilot study. Tumori 2010; 96(6):955–8.
77. Michl M, Haug AR, Jakobs TF, et al. Radioembolization with Yttrium-90 microspheres (SIRT) in pancreatic cancer patients with liver metastases: efficacy, safety and prognostic factors. Oncology 2014;86(1):24–32.
78. Gibbs P, Do C, Lipton L, et al. Phase II trial of selective internal radiation therapy and systemic chemotherapy for liver-predominant metastases from pancreatic adenocarcinoma. BMC Cancer 2015;15:802.
79. Kim AY, Unger K, Wang H, et al. Incorporating Yttrium-90 trans-arterial radioembolization (TARE) in the treatment of metastatic pancreatic adenocarcioma: a single center experience. BMC Cancer 2016;16:492.
80. Michl M, Lehner S, Paprottka PM, et al. Use of PERCIST for prediction of progression-free and overall survival after radioembolization for liver metastases from pancreatic cancer. J Nucl Med 2016;57(3):355–60.
81. Azizi A, Naguib NN, Mbalisike E, et al. Liver metastases of pancreatic cancer: role of repetitive transarterial chemoembolization (TACE) on tumor response and survival. Pancreas 2011;40(8):1271–5.
82. Sun JH, Zhou TY, Zhang YL, et al. Efficacy of transcatheter arterial chemoembolization for liver metastases arising from pancreatic cancer. Oncotarget 2017; 8(24):39746–55.
83. Ouyang H, Ma W, Zhang T, et al. Systemic chemotherapy in combination with liver-directed therapy improves survival in patients with pancreatic adenocarcinoma and synchronous liver metastases. Pancreatology 2018;18(8):983–9.
84. Williams JL, Chan CK, Toste PA, et al. Association of histopathologic phenotype of periampullary adenocarcinomas with survival. JAMA Surg 2017;152(1):82–8.
85. de Jong MC, Tsai S, Cameron JL, et al. Safety and efficacy of curative intent surgery for peri-ampullary liver metastasis. J Surg Oncol 2010;102(3):256–63.
86. Kurosaki I, Minagawa M, Kitami C, et al. Hepatic resection for liver metastases from carcinomas of the distal bile duct and of the papilla of Vater. Langenbecks Arch Surg 2011;396(5):607–13.
87. Perrodin S, Lachenmayer A, Maurer M, et al. Percutaneous stereotactic image-guided microwave ablation for malignant liver lesions. Sci Rep 2019;9(1):13836.
88. Vitale FV, Romeo P, Luciani B, et al. Mitomycin-based hepatic arterial infusion chemotherapy for solitary ampullary cancer liver metastasis: an unusual treatment for an uncommon disease. J Oncol Pharm Pract 2015;21(5):396–9.
89. Rompteaux P, Gagniere J, Gornet JM, et al. Resection of small bowel adenocarcinoma metastases: Results of the ARCAD-NADEGE cohort study. Eur J Surg Oncol 2019;45(3):331–5.
90. Benson AB, Venook AP, Al-Hawary MM, et al. Small bowel adenocarcinoma, version 1.2020, NCCN Clinical Practice Guidelines in Oncology. J Natl Compr Canc Netw 2019;17(9):1109–33.
91. Cady B. Basic principles in surgical oncology. Arch Surg 1997;132(4):338–46.
92. Nordlinger B, Guiguet M, Vaillant JC, et al. Surgical resection of colorectal carcinoma metastases to the liver. A prognostic scoring system to improve case selection, based on 1568 patients. Association Francaise de Chirurgie. Cancer 1996; 77(7):1254–62.
93. Adam R, Avisar E, Ariche A, et al. Five-year survival following hepatic resection after neoadjuvant therapy for nonresectable colorectal. Ann Surg Oncol 2001; 8(4):347–53.

94. Morris EJ, Forman D, Thomas JD, et al. Surgical management and outcomes of colorectal cancer liver metastases. Br J Surg 2010;97(7):1110–8.

95. Bang YJ, Van Cutsem E, Feyereislova A, et al. Trastuzumab in combination with chemotherapy versus chemotherapy alone for treatment of HER2-positive advanced gastric or gastro-oesophageal junction cancer (ToGA): a phase 3, open-label, randomised controlled trial. Lancet 2010;376(9742):687–97.

96. Golan T, Hammel P, Reni M, et al. Maintenance olaparib for germline BRCA-mutated metastatic pancreatic cancer. N Engl J Med 2019;381(4):317–27.

97. Le DT, Durham JN, Smith KN, et al. Mismatch repair deficiency predicts response of solid tumors to PD-1 blockade. Science 2017;357(6349):409–13.

Intraarterial Chemotherapy for Liver Metastases

Louise C. Connell, MB BCH, BAO, BMedSc, Nancy E. Kemeny, MD*

KEYWORDS

- Hepatic arterial infusion chemotherapy • Colorectal cancer • Conversion to resection
- Intrahepatic cholangiocarcinoma • Survival

KEY POINTS

- The liver is the most common site for metastases from colorectal cancer, occurring in more than 60% of patients and represents the main prognostic driver.
- Colorectal cancer liver metastases (CRLM) management continues to evolve, with surgery as the preferred strategy. Less than 20% of patients, however, are resectable at presentation.
- Hepatic arterial infusion (HAI) chemotherapy is delivered with the goal of converting patients to resection, reducing recurrence risk, treating recurrent disease, and improving overall survival.
- In patients with unresectable CRLM, combination HAI with systemic chemotherapy can convert approximately 50% of patients to resection even in the setting of prior therapy.
- A 5-year overall survival rate of 78% has been shown when adjuvant HAI FUDR is combined with modern systemic chemotherapy in patients post liver resection.

INTRODUCTION

Colorectal cancer (CRC) *is one of* the leading cancers globally in terms of both incidence and cancer-related mortality.[1] There are approximately 150,000 new cases diagnosed annually, with an average 50,000 deaths per year, in the United States.[2]

Liver metastatic disease is the main prognostic driver for patients with CRC. Approximately 25% of patients will have synchronous liver metastases at initial diagnosis, and more than 50% will develop liver metastases during their lifetime.[3]

The liver is the most frequent and often the only site of metastatic disease in patients with CRC because venous drainage from the colon and rectum allows metastases to travel to the liver via the portal vein. Because the liver is the most common site of metastatic disease for patients with CRC, liver-directed therapies have been developed and increasingly incorporated in the treatment paradigm.

Department of Medicine, Gastrointestinal Oncology Service, Memorial Sloan Kettering Cancer Center, 300 East 66th Street, 10th floor, New York, NY 10065, USA
* Corresponding author.
E-mail address: kemenyn@mskcc.org

Surg Oncol Clin N Am 30 (2021) 143–158
https://doi.org/10.1016/j.soc.2020.08.005
1055-3207/21/© 2020 Elsevier Inc. All rights reserved.
surgonc.theclinics.com

The rationale for the use of hepatic arterial infusion (HAI) chemotherapy is based on the unique anatomy of the liver. Healthy liver tissue has a dual blood supply receiving most of its perfusion from the portal vein. Liver tumors, on the other hand, mainly derive their blood supply from the hepatic artery.[4] This characteristic is exploited to allow delivery of high concentrations of chemotherapy selectively into the liver metastases.

Management of colorectal liver metastases (CRLM) is an ever evolving and expanding field. Liver resection, where feasible, remains the only chance for cure in these patients and is the preferred definitive therapeutic approach. Most of the patients, approximately 85%, with CRLM, however, have unresectable disease at presentation with a 5-year survival of less than 10% when treated with systemic chemotherapy alone.[5,6] In such patients, the use of liver-directed chemotherapy via hepatic arterial infusion may be used in conjunction with systemic chemotherapy in an effort to reduce the burden of liver disease and convert to resection.

In those patients who are able to undergo complete resection, nearly 70% develop recurrent disease, typically within the 2 years, and 30% to 50% will recur within the liver alone.[7,8] HAI chemotherapy is used in this setting as an adjuvant treatment in conjunction with systemic chemotherapy to reduce the risk of recurrence.

This article summarizes the role of HAI chemotherapy in the treatment of metastatic CRC to the liver.

BACKGROUND OF HEPATIC ARTERIAL INFUSION

HAI chemotherapy takes advantage of the anatomic structure of the liver with its dual blood supply. Regional arterial supply to metastatic tumors allows for the delivery of high chemotherapy concentrations with minimal systemic toxicities.

One way to deliver HAI chemotherapy is via a catheter surgically inserted into the gastroduodenal artery and connected to a subcutaneously implanted pump, which is placed at laparotomy. Laparoscopic and robotic approaches have been used for implantation as less invasive strategies.[9] Other options for HAI administration is to use a hepatic arterial port or through a percutaneously placed catheter connected to an external pump.

The liver predominantly metabolizes certain drugs during the first pass through the hepatic arterial circulation, which results in high local concentrations of the drug with minimal systemic toxicity. The most suitable drugs for HAI are those with high total body clearance and short plasma half-life.[10,11]

Fluorouracil (5-FU) was the first agent to be used for HAI. Later floxuridine (FUDR), a prodrug of 5-FU, was found to have much higher concentration within tumor, with even fewer systemic side effects than 5-FU. FUDR is now the most widely used agent in internal pumps because of its short half-life and high first-pass metabolism rate and allows for increased concentration of the drug in hepatic tumors and very low concentrations systemically.[12]

More modern chemotherapy agents have also been used for HAI therapy, including irinotecan[13] and oxaliplatin.[14,15] These drugs have a lower first-pass hepatic extraction compared with FUDR and a different systemic toxicity profile. A study from China of 31 patients evaluated the use of HAI with irinotecan and oxaliplatin with bolus FUDR given only every 4 to 8 weeks, with a 61% response rate and a median survival of 24.8 months.[16] Irinotecan is not as effective due to a lack of a hepatic extraction advantage.[17]

The systemic toxicity rate with HAI FUDR is very low given the high extraction rate of 95%.[11,18] Toxicity from HAI FUDR therapy includes mainly biliary toxicity and gastric ulceration secondary to extrahepatic perfusion. Extrahepatic perfusion of FUDR into the gastrointestinal tract can cause diarrhea, pancreatitis and/or gastroduodenal ulceration.[19] Biliary toxicity is the most common side effect of HAI FUDR, seen as an elevation of the liver enzymes.[20] As a result, it is imperative to closely monitor liver function tests every 2 weeks during therapy and adjust the FUDR dose based on the liver enzymes (**Table 1**).

Dexamethasone can be combined with HAI FUDR to decrease the risk of biliary toxicity. A randomized study of HAI therapy with FUDR with or without dexamethasone in patients with liver metastatic CRC highlighted that hyperbilirubinemia occurs in about one-third of patients treated with FUDR therapy alone. The addition of dexamethasone reduced the incidence of hyperbilirubinemia from 30% to 9%. FUDR in combination with dexamethasone also improved the response rate.[21]

HAI therapy has very much evolved in the last 30 years in conjunction with improved surgical techniques and the emergence of modern systemic chemotherapy agents. In the United States, HAI therapy is now an acceptable first-line option for unresectable CRLM and is also a treatment option in the adjuvant setting after liver resection. However, it remains infrequently used, much of which can be explained by the level of resources needed to deliver this therapy, with specific technical expertise and knowledge as well as the requirement of a multidisciplinary team to manage treatment. Fortunately, the potential of HAI chemotherapy in the management of select patients with CRLM is increasingly being acknowledged, and new centers are appearing with specialist interest in this treatment modality across the world.[22,23]

HEPATIC ARTERIAL INFUSION AS ADJUVANT THERAPY AFTER LIVER RESECTION

Hepatic resection for colorectal liver metastases has improved 5-year survival rates.[24,25] The recurrence rate following liver resection for CRC metastases however

Table 1
Algorithm for hepatic arterial infusion floxuridine dose reduction

Liver Enzymes	Reference Value	% FUDR Dose
AST (at pump emptying or day of planned retreatment, whichever is higher)	0 to <2 x reference value	100%
	2 to <3 x reference value	80%
	3 to <4 x reference value	50%
	>4 x reference value	Hold
Alk Phos (at pump emptying or day of planned retreatment, whichever is higher)	0 to <1.2 x reference value	100%
	1.2 to <1.5 x reference value	50%
	>1.5 x reference value	Hold
Tbili (at pump emptying or day of planned retreatment, whichever is higher)	0 to <1.2 x reference value	100%
	1.2 to <1.5 x reference value	50%
	>1.5 x reference value	Hold

Recommencing FUDR Treatment After Hold		
Reason for Treatment Delay	FUDR Resumed When Value Has Returned to:	% FUDR Dose
AST elevation	2 x reference value	25% of last dose
Alk phos elevation	1.2 x reference value	25% of last dose
Tbili elevation	1.2 x reference value	25% of last dose

Abbreviations: Alk phos, alkaline phosphatase; AST, aspartate aminotransferase; Tbili, total bilirubin.

remains high, at 60% to 70%, usually occurring within 2 years, and 70% of recurrences occur in the liver.[26–28]

Adjuvant liver-directed therapy with HAI can target residual micrometastatic disease in the liver, to reduce the risk of hepatic recurrence and improve survival. Early on, 4 randomized trials compared adjuvant HAI therapy after resection of CRLM with either adjuvant systemic therapy or a no-treatment control arm. The results were mixed. Of these 4 studies, 3 showed a significant decrease in hepatic disease-free survival as well as overall survival (OS).[29–33] However, the study by Lorenz and colleagues, which compared adjuvant HAI with 5FU to no treatment, failed to show a survival benefit, and was terminated early.

In 2004, a Cochrane review of 7 randomized adjuvant HAI studies showed no OS improvement, and HAI was not recommended by the investigators based on this. The Cochrane review is now somewhat outdated. It incorporated a total of 592 patients from 7 randomized studies, published between 1990 and 2002, comparing adjuvant HAI with systemic therapy alone/observation. The studies used a variety of HAI therapies, including FUDR, 5-FU, and 5-FU/mitomycin. Only one of these studies incorporated a combination of adjuvant systemic (5-FU alone) chemotherapy and HAI in the investigational arm. The review demonstrated that a significant reduction in liver recurrence was observed in the HAI group; however, there was no OS advantage favoring the investigational approach, and HAI therapy was associated with greater toxicity.[34]

A more recent report in 2016 from Memorial Sloan Kettering Cancer Center (MSKCC) compared the long-term survival of 287 patients with resected CRLM that received adjuvant HAI and systemic therapy on 4 consecutive adjuvant protocols from 1991 to 2009. The patients were divided into 2 groups based on whether they received therapy before or after the year 2003, in an effort to reflect changes in the systemic chemotherapy combinations being used in the management of patients with CRC. The median follow-up for patients enrolled before 2003 was 15 years. In that group, the systemic chemotherapy consisted of 5-FU/leucovorin (LV) or irinotecan added to HAI. For patients enrolled after 2003, the median follow-up was 9 years and the median survival has not been reached. Systemic chemotherapy consisted of FOLFOX, FOLFIRI ± bevacizumab. The difference in the 3-year and 5-year overall survival between the 2 patient groups (after 2003 or before 2003) was 92% and 73% versus 78% and 56% ($P<.01$), respectively, demonstrating the excellent survival obtained with resection, HAI, and modern chemotherapy.[35]

Another recent publication from MSKCC looked at 2368 consecutive patients who underwent liver resection of colorectal metastases; 785 had HAI and 1583 did not. The HAI group of patients had a significantly higher disease burden (ie, significantly increased clinical risk score)[24] but still had a longer median survival of 67 versus 44 months for those treated with adjuvant systemic chemotherapy alone ($P<.01$).[36] The analysis that spanned for more than 21 years from 1992 through 2012 also assessed whether or not HAI therapy was administered with perioperative modern systemic chemotherapy as a subgroup analysis. The results showed prolonged 5-year OS for patients receiving HAI therapy, compared with those treated without HAI (52.9% vs. 37.9%, $P<.001$) and also greater 10-year OS (38.0% vs. 23.8%, $P<.001$).

Subgroup analysis demonstrated that independent of receiving modern systemic chemotherapy or not, and regardless of whether HAI was received in the preoperative or adjuvant setting, there remained a significantly associated greater OS in the HAI arm. For those who received preoperative modern systemic chemotherapy, median OS rates in the HAI arm and the no-HAI arm were 77 and 45 months, respectively.

For those who did not receive preoperative modern systemic chemotherapy, median OS rates in the HAI arm and the no-HAI arm were 55 and 43 months, respectively.

The use of HAI plus systemic chemotherapy in relation to a patient's KRAS mutational status has been reported. In 169 patients who underwent liver resection followed by adjuvant HAI FUDR and systemic chemotherapy, the 3-year overall survival was 95% versus 81% for KRAS wild-type (n = 118) and KRAS-mutated (n = 51) patients, respectively.[37]

Currently, there are 2 ongoing randomized clinical trials being conducted to further assess the role of adjuvant HAI after resection of CRLM. The first is a phase II trial, the so-called PUMP trial, which is being performed in the Netherlands that is planned to evaluate the efficacy of adjuvant HAI FUDR therapy in "low-risk" patients. Low risk for recurrence is defined as no more than 2 of 5 of the following factors: disease-free interval less than 12 months, node-positive CRC, more than 1 CRLM, largest liver metastasis more than 5 cm in diameter, serum carcinoembryonic antigen greater than 200 μg/L.[38] Patients are randomized to either resection without any adjuvant therapy or HAI pump placement at time of resection with 6 cycles of HAI FUDR. The primary endpoint of the study is progression-free survival (PFS). Secondary endpoints are OS, hepatic PFS, safety, quality of life, and cost-effectiveness. The aim of the study is to corroborate prior results at MSKCC for adjuvant HAI FUDR.[30]

A second study currently underway is a phase II/III trial, PACHA-01, which is comparing adjuvant systemic FOLFOX and HAI oxaliplatin + systemic 5-FU in patients deemed "high risk" for recurrence, defined as having 4 or more resected CRLM in patients who have undergone R0 or R1 resection and/or thermal ablation.[39] The primary objectives are to assess the 18-month hepatic recurrence-free survival in patients treated with HAI oxaliplatin + systemic 5-FU after curative intent surgery and demonstrate superiority in recurrence-free survival of HAI oxaliplatin compared with systemic oxaliplatin + 5-FU (FOLFOX).

HEPATIC ARTERIAL INFUSION IN THE METASTATIC SETTING

Early studies using HAI FUDR alone demonstrated increased objective response rates compared with systemic chemotherapy with intravenous FUDR or 5-FU alone (41 vs 14%, respectively; $P<.01$) but failed to show an overall survival advantage.[40] Using HAI 5-FU alone, lower response rates were seen (24%) with a median survival of 19.2 months.[41] In a randomized study comparing HAI plus systemic bolus 5-FU/LV (n = 40) or HAI alone (n = 36), increased survival was observed in the combined group (20 vs 14 months, $P = .0033$) but without a significant increase in response rate.[42]

More recently, evaluation of HAI with modern systemic agents such as irinotecan and oxaliplatin has been conducted. A study assessing HAI FUDR plus systemic irinotecan in previously treated patients led to a response rate of 74% and a median survival of 21 months.[43] Another study that evaluated HAI therapy with systemic oxaliplatin combined with irinotecan or 5-FU/LV (FOLFOX) demonstrated further improvement. Of those who received HAI FUDR plus oxaliplatin and irinotecan, 90% had a partial response and median survival was 35.8 months.[44] In a Chinese study, which included patients with extrahepatic disease, HAI FUDR plus systemic FOLFOX produced a response rate of 68.6% and a median survival of 25 months.[45]

In KRAS wild-type patients, systemic chemotherapy agents that target the epidermal growth factor (EGFR), such as cetuximab and panitumumab, can be used. In more recent studies in patients with KRAS wild-type tumors, the median survival has been reported to be as high as 30 months with modern systemic chemotherapy and cetuximab. In a review of 75 patients with unresectable liver metastases with known KRAS status treated with HAI and systemic chemotherapy, the median survival was 68 months for patients with KRAS wild-type tumors versus 29 months for patients with KRAS MUT (P<.003).[46]

For patients who fail first-line chemotherapy, modern systemic chemotherapy agents such as irinotecan alone,[47] irinotecan and cetuximab,[48] and FOLFOX[49] produce response rates ranging from 9% to 22% and a median survival of 14 months or less. In patients who fail first- and second-line chemotherapy, therapeutic options are very limited. Regorafenib and TAS102 in the refractory setting demonstrate response rates of 1% and 1.6%, respectively, and a median survival of 6.4 and 7.1 months, respectively.[50,51]

In a 2016 study of a heavily pretreated population of patients who had progressed after 5-FU/LV, oxaliplatin, and irinotecan therapies, the response rate was 33%, the median survival was 20 months, and the PFS was 6 months after using HAI plus systemic therapy. Nineteen of fifty-seven (33%) patients had a partial response and 31 (54%) had stable disease.[52]

CONVERTING UNRESECTABLE TO RESECTABLE LIVER DISEASE WITH HEPATIC ARTERIAL INFUSION

Most of the patients with colorectal liver metastases present with initially unresectable disease. In the absence of extrahepatic metastases, liver resection is a potentially curative, therapeutic option that has been proved to positively affect overall survival in this patient group.[25,53–56] Considering the improved outcomes observed in patients who undergo liver resection for CRLM, the goal of therapy for those with unresectable liver metastases should focus on optimizing the response rate to facilitate surgery. The correlation between response rate and resection rate is high in the setting of liver-confined colorectal metastases (r = 0.96, P = .002).[57]

In patients who are diagnosed with inoperable liver-limited disease, systemic chemotherapy can decrease tumor size and convert approximately 15% to 30% of unresectable patients to resectability, especially when targeted chemotherapy agents are used.[58,59]

However, even in the era of modern systemic chemotherapy, no significant improvement in prognosis has been observed with combinations such as FOLFOX, FOLFIRI, and FOLFOXIRI, as well as the use of targeted therapies including anti-EGFR for RAS wild-type tumors and antivascular endothelial growth factor (VEGF) agents. Response rates to first-line therapy in metastatic CRC range from 34% to 66%, whereas in the second-line therapy response rates remain low, typically ranging from 4% to 15%.[60] In patients with KRAS wild-type tumors, with the use of anti-EGFR therapy, higher responses up to 30% to 40% for second-line have been demonstrated.[61] Progression-free survival for first-line agents is 5.1 to 13 months and decreases to 1.7 to 7.3 months for second-line agents.[62] Therefore, liver-directed strategies such as HAI chemotherapy represents an attractive option for locoregional disease control and possible conversion to surgical resection for patients with higher-volume liver-dominant metastatic CRC to improve prognosis. Decisions regarding the management of CRLM should ideally be made by a hepatobiliary multidisciplinary team.[63]

The definition of resectability has become more complex and can be institution and surgeon dependent, making it difficult to compare data. Over time, the boundaries of hepatic resection have been pushed further, with improvements in surgical techniques. One core feature when determining operability is to ensure that the future liver remnant after surgery is sufficient to maintain adequate liver function. Most of the studies indicate that resected patients have outcomes similar to those patients with initially resectable colorectal liver metastases and that long-term survival and cure is possible.[64]

HAI alone was initially compared with available systemic chemotherapies for first-line use for unresectable CRLM. Superior response rates of HAI therapy were repeatedly demonstrated in multiple early prospective trials but this did not translate into consistent improvements in OS.[65–68] Initial randomized studies in the first-line setting that compared HAI FUDR monotherapy with systemic 5-FU in patients with unresectable CRLM led to overall response rates between 42% and 47% for the HAI groups versus 9% to 24% for the systemic chemotherapy arms.[66,69,70] HAI therapy with systemic chemotherapy was first studied by Safi and colleagues in 1989 in a phase I prospective study comparing HAI FUDR with HAI FUDR and systemic FUDR. The results of this study showed that addition of systemic FUDR to HAI FUDR therapy was well tolerated, with no significant difference in rates of toxicities between the 2 groups. However, no significant difference was found in response rate or extrahepatic recurrence.[71] Later phase I/II studies of HAI with modern systemic chemotherapy found this combination strategy to be safe and effective, with responses of 64% to 100% among patients with previously untreated, liver-limited, unresectable disease. In previously treated patients with CRLM, response rates of 74% to 85% have been observed with combination HAI and modern systemic chemotherapies.

Furthermore, a 2006 meta-analysis of randomized controlled trials comparing HAI and systemic chemotherapy in unresectable disease showed that there was no survival advantage to HAI alone.[72] There were several limitations to this analysis, however, including single-institution studies with small numbers of patients, outdated HAI chemotherapy regimens, and allowance for cross-over to HAI in patients who had initially failed systemic chemotherapy. To address these limitations, a multiinstitutional prospective randomized clinical trial, Cancer And Leukemia Group B (CALGB) 9481, investigated response rate in patients receiving HAI FUDR compared with systemic 5-FU only, with a significant improvement in survival demonstrated (24.4 vs. 20 months; $P = .0034$).[69]

In 2009, a study of 153 patients randomized to receive HAI FUDR alone or HAI FUDR and systemic 5-FU as first-line therapy demonstrated no difference in response (52.7% vs. 50.6%) and OS (18.0 vs. 19.1 months). Of the variables considered as predictors of tumor response, the only predictors of OS were response to therapy and lower tumor burden (<50% of liver parenchymal involvement). OS in patients with less than 50% liver involvement compared with greater than 50% was significantly greater (21.3 vs. 13.2 months).[73] These results suggest that HAI therapy can be more beneficial if likely responders can be identified through biomarkers such as gene mutational status.

As mentioned previously, with the introduction of oxaliplatin and irinotecan for systemic therapy in the late 1990s, a series of clinical trials tested the efficacy and safety of HAI in combination with modern agents.[74] A single-arm phase I study of 49 patients conducted by Kemeny and colleagues at MSKCC compared HAI FUDR/dexamethasone added to systemic oxaliplatin and irinotecan in patients with adverse prognostic characteristics (at least 5 hepatic lesions to be enrolled and 53% pretreated patients with systemic chemotherapy). Ninety-two percent of the 49 patients had a complete (8%) or partial (84%) response. Forty-seven percent of patients were able to proceed with liver resection with curative intent. Thirty-nine percent underwent R0 resection. In patients who were chemotherapy-naïve, the median survival was 50.8 months, and for patients who were previously treated the median survival was 35 months.[75] In 2010, Goere and colleagues[76] analyzed 87 patients who received HAI oxaliplatin with systemic 5-FU and leucovorin, as second-line therapy, and 24% (21/87) of patients were converted to resection, with 5-year OS of 56%. Further studies continue to consistently show high response rates up to 76% and conversion to resection up to 52% using various combinations of HAI with modern agents[77–80] (**Table 2**).

HAI has also demonstrated antitumor activity and improved survival in patients with refractory CRC. In 39 patients progressing on oxaliplatin therapy and then treated with HAI FUDR/Dex plus systemic irinotecan, the response rate was 44%, with 18% of these patients ultimately undergoing resection or ablation.[81] In patients treated with HAI oxaliplatin via a port and systemic 5-FU/LV, of which 75% were previously treated, 19% of patients were converted from unresectable to resectable.[15] Another study with 54 patients who were all previously treated with prior systemic FOLFIRI or FOLFOX, HAI oxaliplatin via an intrahepatic arterial catheter connected to a subcutaneous port and systemic 5-FU/LV resulted in 18% conversion to resection.[82]

The addition of biological agents such as bevacizumab to liver-directed and combination systemic chemotherapy has also been studied. Increased biliary toxicity was observed when concurrent administration of systemic bevacizumab was used. The addition of bevacizumab did not improve response rates or conversion rates to liver resection.[83] A prospective study by D'Angelica and colleagues[77] of 49 patients with advanced, unresectable liver-limited CRC treated with HAI and best systemic chemotherapy yielded a response rate of 76%. The conversion rate to liver resection was 47% at 6 months after treatment start, and of note, 65% of the study population had been previously treated with systemic chemotherapy. Median overall survival for all patients was 38 months.

There was a low rate of surgical complications after liver resection, with only one individual experiencing a grade 3 adverse event (a biloma requiring percutaneous

Table 2
Recent studies of hepatic artery infusion chemotherapy with systemic therapy for unresectable colorectal cancer liver metastases

Author	Study Design	Sample Size	HAI Drug	Systemic	Response Rate	Conversion to Resection
D'Angelica et al,[77] 2015[a]	Phase II	49	FUDR	Oxaliplatin/ irinotecan/ bevacizumab or irinotecan/ 5-FU/LV/ bevacizumab	76%	47%
Levi et al,[78] 2016	Phase II	64	Irinotecan/ oxaliplatin/ 5-FU	Cetuximab	40.6%	29.7%
Lim et al,[79] 2017	Retrospective	61	Oxaliplatin	5-FU/LV or 5-FU/ bevacizumab or 5-FU/ anti-EGFR	21.3%	16.4%
Pak et al,[80] 2018[a]	Phase II	64	FUDR	Oxaliplatin/ irinotecan or 5-FU/LV/ irinotecan/ bevacizumab	73%	52%

[a] Same trial including an update and expansion.
Data from Refs.[77–80]

drainage). A high degree of biliary complications was evident in the first 24 patients who also received concurrent systemic bevacizumab. Bevacizumab was discontinued for the following 25 patients who were enrolled. The conversion to resection was the only factor associated with longer OS and PFS.

A landmark analysis confirmed a higher 3-year OS among patients who underwent liver resection compared with those that remained unresectable (80% vs 26%). At a median follow-up of 39 months (32–65 months), 10 of the 49 patients (20%) had no evidence of disease.[77] An updated analysis of this study with a median follow-up among survivors of 63 months reported a 52% conversion to resection at a median of 5 months, an overall survival of 37.4 months, and 5-year survival of 36%.[84]

OTHER INDICATIONS FOR HEPATIC ARTERIAL INFUSION—INTRAHEPATIC CHOLANGIOCARCINOMA

HAI chemotherapy in combination with systemic chemotherapy has also been proved as an effective and safe treatment in patients with unresectable intrahepatic cholangiocarcinoma with locally advanced or metastatic disease confined to the liver.

Intrahepatic cholangiocarcinoma (ICC) is rare but increasing in incidence and mortality.[85,86] Most patients with ICC present with either unresectable or distant metastatic disease, for which the prognosis is poor.[87,88] Most patients with advanced ICC present with disease confined to the liver that is unresectable owing to tumor location and/or multifocal involvement. Even in patients with resectable disease, 60% of patients develop recurrent disease.[87,89] Currently, the standard systemic therapy for ICC remains platinum-based chemotherapy in combination with gemcitabine, with marginal improvement in median OS to 11.7 months.[90,91]

Results with HAI chemotherapy have been encouraging in this patient group, with evidence supporting its use dating back over 30 years ago.[92] In a phase II trial, 34 unresectable patients (26 ICC; 8 hepatocellular carcinoma [HCC]) received HAI FUDR with an objective response rate of 47% and 1 patient with initially unresectable ICC proceeded to resection. Median PFS was 7.4 months, and disease-specific survival was 29 months.[93] Similar outcomes were observed in a subsequent study, in which 22 patients (18 ICC; 4 HCC) were treated with HAI FUDR plus bevacizumab. In this trial, median PFS and OS were 8.5 and 31.1 months, respectively. However, this study was prematurely terminated owing to increased biliary toxicity associated with bevacizumab[94] In a retrospective review of 78 ICC patients, who underwent treatment with combined HAI FUDR and systemic chemotherapy, the OS was superior compared with patients who received systemic treatment alone (30.8 vs 18.4 months, respectively; $P<.001$).[95] More recently, a multicenter phase II trial assessing HAI FUDR combined with systemic gemcitabine and oxaliplatin (GemOx) in unresectable IHC was published by Cercek and colleagues.[96] A response rate of 58% and an excellent disease control rate of 84% in the primary tumor was demonstrated at 6 months. More recently, the combination of intraarterial 5-FU and oxaliplatin also showed some activity in a phase II trial in which 37 patients with locally advanced biliary tract malignancies (32 ICC; 1 extrahepatic cholangiocarcinoma; 4 gallbladder cancer) were included. In this trial, the response rate, PFS, and OS were 16%, 6.5 months, and 13.5 months, respectively.[97]

SUMMARY

CRC is a major public health problem throughout the world, and the liver is the most common site of metastatic spread and the main driver in terms of prognosis in most of the patients. Great advances have been made with the use of liver-directed therapies such as HAI chemotherapy when incorporated into the treatment paradigm. The role of HAI chemotherapy in CRLM is now well established by numerous prospective and retrospective studies.

In patients with unresectable metastases to the liver, HAI can be used with systemic chemotherapy to achieve increased response rates even in patients after progression on first- and second-line chemotherapy. Results show an increased response and conversion to resection offering the patients the chance for cure with the use of HAI and systemic therapy versus systemic therapy alone. In patients who receive HAI in the adjuvant setting after liver surgrey, HAI therapy given with systemic chemotherapy can increase disease-free survival and hepatic disease-free survival. In summary, HAI with systemic chemotherapy is a reasonable treatment option in select patients with oligometastatic disease to the liver in order to achieve improved outcomes.

Administration and delivery of HAI therapy can certainly be complex, which explains in large part its relatively infrequent use in the global oncology community to date. It is important to stress the value and inherent need of a dedicated multidisciplinary infrastructure incorporating all aspects of HAI management such as surgical, medical, radiologic, and nursing to run a successful HAI program. In recent years, the potential of HAI therapy is being increasingly acknowledged and more centers in the United States and Europe are emerging as advocates in the field, with several phase II and phase III trials underway currently.

Future directions in the field will entail refinements in the patient selection process, including the identification of those patients likely to benefit from HAI through the identification of molecular markers as well as the inclusion of increasing data of molecularly driven systemic therapies into clinical trial design. Furthermore, a key component to progressing the field is the establishment of multiinstitutional registries comparing combination hepatic arterial infusion regimens with not only systemic chemotherapy alone but also with alternative liver-directed treatment approaches (eg, yttrium-90 radioembolization and transarterial chemoembolization) increasingly used in CRLM, in an effort to improve survival, in a patient group with an inherently poor prognosis.

DISCLOSURE

N.E. Kemeny has received research funding from Amgen. L.C. Connell has nothing to disclose.

CLINICS CARE POINTS

- Hepatic arterial infusional (HAI) should be administered in combination with systemic chemotherapy within the context of a dedicated multidisciplinary program.
- Combination therapy is possible, especially due to the high hepatic extraction rates of floxuridine (FUDR), and is indicated to ensure intrahepatic and extrahepatic control of disease.
- HAI-FUDR should not be combined with bevacizumab, as it is associated with significantly worse biliary toxicity when combined with HAI-FUDR.
- The addition of dexamethasone (Dex) to FUDR has been shown to significantly decrease FUDR-related biliary toxicity.
- Combination therapy with HAI-FUDR and systemic chemotherapy is associated with high response rates both in the first-line and in the refractory disease setting, with high rates of conversion to complete resection.

REFERENCES

1. Torre LA, Bray F, Siegel RL, et al. Global Cancer Statistics, 2012. CA Cancer J Clin 2015;65:87–108.
2. Siegel RL, Miller KD, Goding Sauer A, et al. Colorectal cancer statistics, 2020. CA Cancer J Clin 2020. https://doi.org/10.3322/caac.21601.
3. Pozzo C, Barone C, Kemeny N. Advances in neoadjuvant therapy for colorectal cancer with liver metastases. Cancer Treat Rev 2008;34:293–301.
4. Breedis C, Young G. The blood supply of neoplasms in the liver. Am J Pathol 1954;30:969–77.
5. Scheele J, Stangle R, Altendorf-Hofmann A. Hepatic metastases from colorectal carcinoma: impact of surgi- cal resection on the natural history. Br J Surg 1990; 77:1241–6.
6. Sanoff HK, Sargent DJ, Campbell ME, et al. Five-year data and prog- nostic factor analysis of oxaliplatin and irinotecan combinations for advanced colorectal cancer: N9741. J Clin Oncol 2008;26:5721–7.
7. D'Angelica M, Kornprat P, Gonen M, et al. Effect on outcome of recurrence patterns after hepatectomy for colorectal metastases. Ann Surg Oncol 2011;18: 1096–103.
8. Chan KM, Wu TH, Cheng CH, et al. Prognostic significance of the number of tumors and aggressive surgical approach in colorectal cancer hepatic metastasis. World J Surg Oncol 2014;12:155.
9. Qadan M, D'Angelica MI, Kemeny NE, et al. Robotic hepatic arterial infusion pump placement. HPB (Oxford) 2017;19:429–35.
10. Kemeny NE. Treatment of metastatic colon cancer: "the times they are A-changing". J Clin Oncol 2013;31:1913–6.
11. Ensminger WD, Rosowsky A, Raso V, et al. A clinical-pharmacological evaluation of hepatic arterial infusions of 5-fluoro-2'-deoxyuridine and 5-fluorouracil. Cancer Res 1978;38:3784–92.
12. Ensminger WD, Gyves JW. Clinical pharmacology of hepatic arterial chemotherapy. Semin Oncol 1983;10:176–82.
13. van Riel JM, van Groeningen CJ, Kedde MA, et al. Continuous administration of irinotecan by hepatic arterial infusion: a phase I and pharmacokinetic study. Clin Cancer Res 2002;8:405–12.
14. Dzodic R, Gomez-Abuin G, Rougier P, et al. Pharmacokinetic advantage of intra-arterial hepatic oxaliplatin administration: comparative results with cisplatin using a rabbit VX2 tumor model. Anticancer Drugs 2004;15:647–50.
15. Ducreux M, Ychou M, Laplanche A, et al. gastrointestinal group of the Federation Nationale des Centres de Lutte Contre le Cancer: Hepatic arterial oxaliplatin infusion plus intravenous chemotherapy in colorectal cancer with inoperable hepatic metastases: a trial of the gas- trointestinal group of the Federation Nationale des Centres de Lutte Contre le Cancer. J Clin Oncol 2005;23:4881–7.
16. Chen Y, Wang X, Yan Z, et al. Hepatic arterial infusion with irinotecan, oxaliplatin, and floxuridine plus systemic chemotherapy as first-line treat- ment of unresectable liver metastases from colorectal cancer. Onkologie 2012;35:480–4.
17. van Riel JM, van Groeningen CJ, de Greve J, et al. Continuous infusion of he patic arterial irinotecan in pretreated patients with colorectal cancer metastatic to the liver. Ann Oncol 2004;15:59–63.
18. Collins JM. Pharmacologic rationale for regional drug delivery. J Clin Oncol 1984; 2:498–504.

19. Gluck WL, Akwari OE, Kelvin FM, et al. A reversible enteropathy complicating continuous hepatic artery infusion chemotherapy with 5-fluoro-2-deoxyuridine. Cancer 1985;56:2424–7.

20. Cohen AD, Kemeny NE. An update on hepatic arterial infusion chemotherapy for colorectal cancer. Oncologist 2003;8:553–66.

21. Kemeny N, Seiter K, Niedzwiecki D, et al. A randomized trial of intrahepatic infusion of fluorodeoxyuridine with dexamethasone versus fluorodeoxyur- idine alone in the treatment of metastatic colorectal cancer. Cancer 1992;69:327–34.

22. Karanicolas PJ, Ko YJ. Hepatic arterial infusion for unresectable liver metastases from colorectal cancer: the dawn of a new era? Ann Surg Oncol 2017;24:6–7.

23. Dhir M, Jones HL, Shuai Y, et al. Hepatic arterial infusion in combination with modern systemic chemotherapy is associated with improved survival compared with modern systemic chemotherapy alone in patients with isolated unresectable colorectal liver metastases: a case-control study. Ann Surg Oncol 2017;24:150–8.

24. Fong Y, Fortner J, Sun RL, et al. Clinical score for predicting recurrence after hepatic resection for metastatic colorectal cancer: analysis of 1001 consecutive cases. Ann Surg 1999;230:309–18 [discussion: 318–21].

25. Rees M, Tekkis PP, Welsh FK, et al. Evaluation of long-term survival after hepatic resection for metastatic colorectal cancer: a multifactorial model of 929 patients. Ann Surg 2008;247:125–35.

26. Ye LC, Liu TS, Ren L, et al. Randomized controlled trial of cetuximab plus chemotherapy for patients with KRAS wild-type unresectable colorectal liver-limited metastases. J Clin Oncol 2013;31:1931–8.

27. Muratore A, Polastri R, Bouzari H, et al. Repeat hepatectomy for colorectal liver metastases: a worthwhile operation? J Surg Oncol 2001;76:127–32.

28. Topal B, Kaufman L, Aerts R, et al. Patterns of failure following curative resection of colorectal liver metastases. Eur J Surg Oncol 2003;29:248–53.

29. Kemeny MM, Adak S, Gray B, et al. Combined-modality treatment for resectable metastatic colorectal carcinoma to the liver: surgical resection of hepatic metastases in combination with continuous infusion of chemotherapy–an intergroup study. J Clin Oncol 2002;20:1499–505.

30. Kemeny N, Huang Y, Cohen AM, et al. Hepatic arterial infusion of chemotherapy after resection of hepatic metastases from colorectal cancer. N Engl J Med 1999; 341:2039–48.

31. Kemeny NE, Gonen M. Hepatic arterial infusion after liver resection. N Engl J Med 2005;352:734–5.

32. Lygidakis NJ, Sgourakis G, Vlachos L, et al. Metastatic liver disease of colorectal origin: the value of locoregional immunochemotherapy combined with systemic chemotherapy following liver resection. Results Prospective Randomized Study. Hepatogastroenterology 2001;48:1685–91.

33. Lorenz M, Muller HH, Schramm H, et al. Randomized trial of surgery versus surgery followed by adjuvant hepatic arterial infusion with 5-fluorouracil and folinic acid for liver metastases of colorectal cancer. German Cooperative on Liver Metastases (Arbeitsgruppe Lebermetastasen). Ann Surg 1998;228:756–62.

34. Nelson R, Freels S. Hepatic artery adjuvant chemotherapy for patients having resection or ablation of colorectal cancer metastatic to the liver. Cochrane Database Syst Rev 2004;(2):CD003770.

35. Kemeny NE, Chou JF, Boucher TM, et al. Updated long-term survival for patients with metastatic colorectal cancer treated with liver resection followed by hepatic arterial infusion and systemic chemotherapy. J Surg Oncol 2016;113:477–84.

36. Groot Koerkamp B, Sadot E, Kemeny NE, et al. Perioperative hepatic arterial infusion pump chemotherapy Q:1; 2 Is associated with longer survival after resection of colorectal liver metastases: a propensity score analysis of 2,368 consecutive patients. J Clin Oncol 2017;35:1938–44.

37. Kemeny NE, Chou JF, Capanu M, et al. KRAS mutation influences recurrence patterns in patients undergoing hepatic resection of colorectal metastases. Cancer 2014;120:3965–71.

38. Buisman FE, Homs MYV, Grunhagen DJ, et al. Adjuvant hepatic arterial infusion pump chemotherapy and resection versus resection alone in patients with low-risk resectable colorectal liver metastases - the multicenter randomized controlled PUMP trial. BMC Cancer 2019;19:327.

39. Goere D, Pignon JP, Gelli M, et al. Postoperative hepatic arterial chemotherapy in high-risk patients as adjuvant treatment after resection of colorectal liver metastases - a randomized phase II/III trial - PACHA-01 (NCT02494973). BMC Cancer 2018;18:787.

40. Meta-Analysis Group in Cancer, Piedbois P, Buyse M, Kemeny N, et al. Reappraisal of hepatic arterial infusion in the treat- ment of nonresectable liver metastases from colorectal cancer. J Natl Cancer Inst 1996;88:252–8.

41. Arai Y, Aoyama A, Inaba Y, et al. Phase II study on hepatic arterial infusion chemotherapy using percutaneous catheter placement techniques for liver metastases from colorectal cancer (JFMC28 study). Asia Pac J Clin Oncol 2015; 11:41–8.

42. Fiorentini G, Cantore M, Rossi S, et al. Hepatic arterial chemotherapy in combination with systemic chemotherapy compared with hepatic arterial chemotherapy alone for liver metastases from colorectal cancer: results of a multi-centric randomized study. In Vivo 2006;20:707–9.

43. Kemeny N, Gonen M, Sullivan D, et al. Phase I study of hepatic arterial in- fusion of floxuridine and dexamethasone with systemic irinotecan for unresectable hepatic metastases from colorectal cancer. J Clin Oncol 2001;19:2687–95.

44. Kemeny N, Jarnagin W, Paty P, et al. Phase I trial of systemic oxaliplatin combination chemotherapy with hepatic arterial infusion in patients with unresectable liver metastases from colorectal cancer. J Clin Oncol 2005;23:4888–96.

45. Li C, Gu Y, Zhao M, et al. Phase I trial of hepatic arterial infusion (HAI) of floxuridine with modified oxaliplatin, 5-fluorouracil and leucovorin (m-FOLFOX6) in Chinese patients with unresectable liver metastases from colorectal cancer. Cancer Chemother Pharmacol 2014;74:1079–87.

46. Connell L, Chou JF, Boucher TM, et al. Relevance of CEA and LDH in relation to KRAS status in patients with unresectable colorectal liver metastases. J Clin Oncol 2016;34(suppl 4). abstr 762.

47. Rothenberg ML, Eckardt JR, Kuhn JG, et al. Phase II trial of irinotecan in patients with progressive or rapidly recurrent colorectal cancer. J Clin Oncol 1996;14: 1128–35.

48. Cunningham D, Humblet Y, Siena S, et al. Cetuximab monotherapy and cetuximab plus irinotecan in irinotecan-refractory metastatic colorectal cancer. N Engl J Med 2004;351:337–45.

49. Rothenberg ML, Oza AM, Bigelow RH, et al. Superiority of oxaliplatin and fluorouracil-leucovorin compared with either therapy alone in patients with progressive colo- rectal cancer after irinotecan and fluorouracil-leucovorin: interim results of a phase III trial. J Clin Oncol 2003;21:2059–69.

50. Grothey A, Van Cutsem E, Sobrero A, et al. CORRECT Study Group: Regorafenib monotherapy for previously treated metastatic colorectal cancer (CORRECT): an

international, multicentre, randomised, placebo-controlled, phase 3 trial. Lancet 2013;381:303–12.

51. Mayer RJ, Van Cutsem E, Falcone A, et al, RE- COURSE Study Group. Randomized trial of TAS-102 for refractory metastatic colorectal cancer. N Engl J Med 2015;372:1909–19.

52. Cercek A, Boucher TM, Gluskin J, et al. Response rates of hepatic arterial infusion pump therapy in patients with metastatic colorec- tal cancer liver metastases refractory to all standard therapies. J Surg Oncol 2016;114:655–63.

53. Tomlinson JS, Jarnagin WR, DeMatteo RP, et al. Actual 10-year survival after resection of colorectal liver metastases defines cure. J Clin Oncol 2007;25: 4575–80.

54. Wei AC, Greig PD, Grant D, et al. Survival after hepatic resection for colorectal metastases: a 10-year experience. Ann Surg Oncol 2006;13:668–76.

55. de Jong MC, Pulitano C, Ribero D, et al. Rates and patterns of recurrence following curative intent surgery for colorectal liver metastasis: an international multi-institutional analysis of 1669 patients. Ann Surg 2009;250:440–8.

56. Morris EJ, Forman D, Thomas JD, et al. Surgical management and outcomes of colorectal cancer liver metastases. Br J Surg 2010;97:1110–8.

57. Folprecht G, Grothey A, Alberts S, et al. Neoadjuvant treatment of unresectable colorectal liver metastases: correlation between tumour response and resection rates. Ann Oncol 2005;16:1311–9.

58. Barone C, Nuzzo G, Cassano A, et al. Final analysis of colorectal cancer patients treated with irinotecan and 5-fluorouracil plus folinic acid ne- oadjuvant chemotherapy for unresectable liver metastases. Br J Cancer 2007;97:1035–9.

59. Tabernero J, Van Cutsem E, Díaz-Rubio E, et al. Phase II trial of cetuximab in combination with fluorouracil, leucovorin, and oxaliplatin in the first-line treatment of metastatic colorectal cancer. J Clin Oncol 2007;25:5225–32.

60. Tournigand C, André T, Achille E, et al. FOLFIRI followed by FOLFOX6 or the reverse sequence in advanced colorectal cancer: a randomized GERCOR study. J Clin Oncol 2004 Jan 15;22(2):229–37.

61. Peeters M, Price TJ, Cervantes A, et al. Randomized phase III study of panitumumab with fluorouracil, leucovorin, and irinotecan (FOLFIRI) compared with FOLFIRI alone as second-line treatment in patients with metastatic colorectal cancer. J Clin Oncol 2010;28:4706–13.

62. Holch J, Stintzing S, Heinemann V. Treatment of Metastatic Colorectal Cancer: Standard of Care and Future Perspectives. Visc Med 2016;32:178–83.

63. Adam R, Pascal G, Castaing D, et al. Tumor progression while on chemotherapy: a contraindication to liver resection for multiple colorectal metastases? Ann Surg 2004;240:1052–61 [discussion: 61–64].

64. Lam VW, Spiro C, Laurence JM, et al. A systematic review of clinical response and survival outcomes of downsizing systemic chemotherapy and rescue liver surgery in patients with initially unresectable colorectal liver metastases. Ann Surg Oncol 2012;19:1292–301.

65. Kemeny N, Daly J, Reichman B, et al. Intrahepatic or systemic infusion of fluorodeoxyuridine in patients with liver metastases from colorectal carcinoma. A randomized trial. Ann Intern Med 1987;107:459–65.

66. Hohn DC, Stagg RJ, Friedman MA, et al. A randomized trial of continuous intravenous versus hepatic intraarterial floxuridine in patients with colorectal cancer metastatic to the liver: the Northern California Oncology Group trial. J Clin Oncol 1989;7:1646–54.

67. Martin JK Jr, O'Connell MJ, Wieand HS, et al. Intra-arterial floxuridine vs systemic fluorouracil for hepatic metastases from colorectal cancer. A randomized trial. Arch Surg 1990;125:1022–7.
68. Kerr DJ, McArdle CS, Ledermann J, et al. Intrahepatic arterial versus intravenous fluorouracil and folinic acid for colorectal cancer liver metastases: a multicentre randomised trial. Lancet 2003;361:368–73.
69. Kemeny NE, Niedzwiecki D, Hollis DR, et al. Hepatic arterial infusion versus systemic therapy for hepatic metastases from colorectal cancer: a randomized trial of efficacy, quality of life, and molecular markers (CALGB 9481). J Clin Oncol 2006;24:1395–403.
70. Rougier P, Laplanche A, Huguier M, et al. Hepatic arterial infusion of floxuridine in patients with liver metastases from colorectal carcinoma: long-term results of a prospective randomized trial. J Clin Oncol 1992;10:1112–8.
71. Safi F, Bittner R, Roscher R, et al. Regional chemotherapy for hepatic metastases of colorectal carcinoma (continuous intraarterial versus continuous intraarterial/intravenous therapy). Results of a controlled clinical trial. Cancer 1989;64:379–87.
72. Mocellin S, Pilati P, Lise M, et al. Meta-analysis of hepatic arterial infusion for unresectable liver metastases from colorectal cancer: the end of an era? J Clin Oncol 2007;25:5649–54.
73. Pilati P, Mammano E, Mocellin S, et al. Hepatic arterial infusion for unresectable colorectal liver metastases combined or not with systemic chemotherapy. Anticancer Res 2009;29:4139–44.
74. Datta J, Narayan RR, Kemeny NE, et al. Role of Hepatic Artery Infusion Chemotherapy in Treatment of Initially Unresectable Colorectal Liver Metastases: A Review. JAMA Surg 2019;154(8):768–76.
75. Kemeny NE, Melendez FD, Capanu M, et al. Conversion to resectability using hepatic artery infusion plus systemic chemotherapy for the treatment of unresectable liver metastases from colorectal carcinoma. J Clin Oncol 2009;27:3465–71.
76. Goere D, Deshaies I, de Baere T, et al. Prolonged survival of initially unresectable hepatic colorectal cancer patients treated with hepatic arterial infusion of oxaliplatin followed by radical surgery of metastases. Ann Surg 2010;251:686–91.
77. D'Angelica MI, Correa-Gallego C, Paty PB, et al. Phase II trial of hepatic artery infusional and systemic chemotherapy for patients with unresectable hepatic metastases from colorectal cancer: conversion to resection and long-term outcomes. Ann Surg 2015;261:353–60.
78. Levi FA, Boige V, Hebbar M, et al. Conversion to resection of liver metastases from colorectal cancer with hepatic artery infusion of combined chemotherapy and systemic cetuximab in multicenter trial OPTILIV. Ann Oncol 2016;27:267–74.
79. Lim A, Le Sourd S, Senellart H, et al. Hepatic Arterial Infusion Chemotherapy for Unresectable Liver Metastases of Colorectal Cancer: A Multicenter Retrospective Study. Clin Colorectal Cancer 2017;16:308–15.
80. Pak LM, Kemeny NE, Capanu M, et al. Prospective phase II trial of combination hepatic artery infusion and systemic chemotherapy for unresectable colorectal liver metastases: Long term results and curative potential. J Surg Oncol 2018;117:634–43.
81. Gallagher DJ, Raggio G, Capanu M, et al. Hepatic arterial infusion plus systemic irinotecan in patients with unresectable hepatic metastases from colorectal cancer previously treated with systemic oxaliplatin: a retrospective analysis. Ann Oncol 2007;18:1995–9.

82. Boige V, Malka D, Elias D, et al. Hepatic arterial infusion of oxaliplatin and intravenous LV5FU2 in unresectable liver metastases from colorec- tal cancer after systemic chemotherapy failure. Ann Surg Oncol 2008;15:219–26.
83. Cercek A, D'Angelica M, Power D, et al. Floxuridine hepatic arterial infusion associated biliary toxicity is increased by concurrent administration of systemic bevacizumab. Ann Surg Oncol 2014;21:479–86.
84. Ma LW, Kemeny NE, Capanu M, et al. Prospective phase II trial of combina- tion hepatic artery and systemic chemotherapy for un- resectable colorectal liver metastases: long term results and curative potential. J Am Coll Surg 2016;223: S78–9.
85. Saha SK, Zhu AX, Fuchs CS, et al. Forty-year trends in cholangiocarcinoma incidence in the US: intrahepatic disease on the rise. Oncologist 2016;21(5):594–9.
86. Mavros MN, Economopoulos KP, Alexiou VG, et al. Treatment and prognosis for patients with intrahepatic cholangiocarcinoma: systematic review and meta-analysis. JAMA Surg 2014;149(6):565–74.
87. Spolverato G, Kim Y, Alexandrescu S, et al. Management and Outcomes of Patients with Recurrent Intrahepatic Cholangiocarcinoma Following Previous Curative-Intent Surgical Resection. Ann Surg Oncol 2016;23(1):235–43.
88. Weber SM, Jarnagin WR, Klimstra D, et al. Intrahepatic cholangiocarcinoma: resectability, recurrence pattern, and outcomes. J Am Coll Surg 2001;193(4): 384–91.
89. Doussot A, Gönen M, Wiggers JK, et al. Recurrence patterns and disease-free survival after resection of intrahepatic cholangiocarcinoma: preoperative and postoperative prognostic models. J Am Coll Surg 2016;223(3):493–505.e2.
90. Valle J, Wasan H, Palmer DH, et al, ABC-02 Trial Investigators. Cisplatin plus gemcitabine versus gemcitabine for biliary tract cancer. N Engl J Med 2010; 362(14):1273–81.
91. André T, Tournigand C, Rosmorduc O, et al, GERCOR Group. Gemcitabine combined with oxaliplatin (GEMOX) in advanced biliary tract adenocarcinoma: a GERCOR study. Ann Oncol 2004;15(9):1339–43.
92. Seeger J, Woodcock TM, Blumenreich MS, et al. Hepatic perfusion with FUdR utilizing an implantable system in patients with liver primary cancer or metastatic cancer confined to the liver. Cancer Invest 1989;7(1):1–6.
93. Jarnagin WR, Schwartz LH, Gultekin DH, et al. Regional chemotherapy for unresectable primary liver cancer: results of a phase II clinical trial and assessment of DCE-MRI as a biomarker of survival. Ann Oncol 2009;20(9):1589–95.
94. Kemeny NE, Schwartz L, Gonen M, et al. Treating primary liver cancer with hepatic arterial infusion of floxuridine and dexamethasone: does the addition of systemic bevacizumab improve results. Oncology 2011;80(3–4):153–9.
95. Konstantinidis IT, Groot Koerkamp B, Do RK, et al. Unresectable intrahepatic cholangiocarcinoma: systemic plus hepatic arterial infusion chemotherapy is associated with longer survival in comparison with systemic chemotherapy alone. Cancer 2016;122(5):758–65.
96. Cercek A, Kemeny NE, Boerner T, et al. A bi-institutional phase II study of hepatic arterial infusion (HAI) with floxuridine (FUDR) and dexamethasone (Dex) combined with systemic gemcitabine and oxaliplatin (GemOx) for unresectable intrahepatic cholangiocarcinoma (ICC). J Clin Oncol 2018;36(15_suppl):4092.
97. Sinn M, Nicolaou A, Gebauer B, et al. Hepatic arterial infusion with oxaliplatin and 5-FU/folinic acid for advanced biliary tract cancer: a phase II study. Dig Dis Sci 2013;58(8):2399–405.

External Beam Radiation Therapy for Liver Metastases

Paul B. Romesser, MD[a,b], Brian P. Neal, PhD[c],
Christopher H. Crane, MD[a],*

KEYWORDS

- External beam radiation • Liver metastasis • Ablative radiation • Stereotactic body
- Radiation therapy • Proton therapy • Tumor control probability
- Moderate hypofractionation

KEY POINTS

- Whole-liver radiation is safe only up to 30 Gy with conventional fractionation, and at best this dose achieves short-term palliation.
- Modern conformal radiotherapy techniques provide necessary technology to safely deliver high-dose radiation to small liver volumes.
- Ablative doses of radiation are well tolerated and effective for small liver metastases.
- The safe delivery of ablative radiation can be challenging in patients with large liver metastases due to the limitations of healthy normal liver parenchyma and the proximity of radiosensitive gastrointestinal organs, such as the stomach, duodenum and colon.
- Controlling respiratory motion, the use of image guidance, and increasing the number of radiation fractions sometimes are necessary to safely deliver ablative doses in the more challenging cases.

INTRODUCTION

Metastatic lesions to the liver arise commonly in many solid organ malignancies and are asymptomatic most of the time. Depending on the disease burden, liver metastases can cause pain, anorexia, or more severe consequences, such as morbidity and mortality from venous or biliary obstruction, leading to hepatic parenchymal loss and hepatic insufficiency.[1] Historically, the development of metastasis to the liver was

Funding: P.B. Romesser and C.H. Crane are supported by a NIH/ NCI Cancer Center Support Grant (P30 CA008748).
[a] Department of Radiation Oncology, Memorial Sloan Kettering Cancer Center, 1275 York Avenue, Box #22, New York, NY 10065, USA; [b] Early Drug Development Service, Department of Medicine, Memorial Sloan Kettering Cancer Center, 1275 York Avenue, Box #22, New York, NY 10065, USA; [c] Medical Physics, ProCure Proton Therapy Center, 103 Cedar Grove Lane, Somerset, NJ 08873, USA
* Corresponding author.
E-mail address: Cranec1@mskcc.org

Surg Oncol Clin N Am 30 (2021) 159–173
https://doi.org/10.1016/j.soc.2020.08.006
surgonc.theclinics.com

considered incurable, and systemic therapy was the only option considered.[2] With the recognition of the value of liver-directed therapies over the past 2 decades, the treatment paradigm for metastatic disease to the liver has changed dramatically, especially in patients with liver confined oligometastatic disease.[3]

Oligometastasis is an intermediate state of limited metastatic spread that exists before the manifestation of widely metastatic systemic disease.[4] Given improved staging, largely driven through better imaging modalities, a greater proportion of patients now are identified early in the metastatic spectrum. For example, a large number of patients with metastatic colorectal cancer, including those with de novo metastases at the time of diagnosis or those who develop stage IV disease after curative intent therapy for early stage disease, often are found to have metastases in limited distinct anatomic locations.[5,6] Although the exact number and location of metastatic lesions constituting the oligometastatic state remain actively debated, there is strong evidence that a subset of these patients can have prolonged survival with local therapies directed at the metastatic tumors.

Initial data supporting the use of local therapy to treat oligometastatic disease was first derived from surgical metastasectomy series. These series demonstrated that cure was possible in patients with oligometastatic colorectal cancer who underwent resection of liver and/or lung metastases.[7–14] A large population-based study in the United Kingdom demonstrated that the 5-year survival of patients with oligometastatic colorectal cancer who underwent liver resection was comparable to that of patients with stage III colorectal cancer (44.2% [95% CI, 42.4%–46.1%] versus 42.2% [95% CI, 41.7%–42.7%], respectively).[8] Surgery remains the gold standard for treating liver metastases in colorectal cancer and in selected patients with oligometastatic indolent noncolorectal cancers.[2] A large multi-institutional retrospective study from France reported promising long-term survival (approximately 25% at 10 years) in 1452 patients with noncolorectal liver metastases treated with surgical metastasectomy.[15]

Unfortunately, only a minority of patients will be appropriate for surgical metastasectomy (approximately 20%–30%), due to unfavorable disease distribution within the liver, comorbidities precluding surgery or the presence of extrahepatic disease.[16] Although there has been significant improvement in progression-free survival and overall survival over the past 2 decades with systemic therapies, the vast majority of patients remains incurable.[17] A notable exception to this is the improvement in survival for patients with metastatic melanoma, lung cancer, and tumors harboring mismatch repair deficiencies treated with immune checkpoint blockade therapy.[18,19] Although the survival for patients with metastatic colorectal cancer has improved gradually over the last 2 decades, from a median survival of less than 12 months to more than 30 months, with incremental advances in chemotherapy regimens and the addition of immunotherapy for mismatch repair-deficient colorectal cancer, the majority of these patients cannot be cured except for a subset with liver and/or lung isolated disease that is potentially curable with resection.[7–14,17,20] Thus, there has been significant interest in developing alternatives to surgical metastasectomy.

Patients who have tumors that are unsuitable for surgical metastasectomy for technical or medical reasons may be treated with radiofrequency ablation (RFA), microwave ablation, cryotherapy, and/or high-intensity focal ultrasound.[21] In patients with surgically unresectable colorectal cancer with limited metastatic disease RFA has been demonstrated to prolong progression-free survival and overall survival compared with systemic chemotherapy alone in a randomized phase II trial (European Organisation for Research and Treatment of Cancer 40004).[22,23] An American Society of Clinical Oncology review on RFA for colorectal liver metastases found a large variability in 5-year survival rates (approximately 15%–55%) and local tumor recurrence rates (approximately 3%–60%).[24] Tumor size of 3 cm or greater or location close to large vessels was associated with reduced local control, whereas multiple and extrahepatic metastases were associated with poor survival.[24,25]

These ablative options generally are safe, convenient, and cost effective and achieve high tumor control rates in appropriately selected patients, which justifies their use as a second option to surgery in patients with small liver metastases.[24] Stereotactic ablative radiotherapy (SABR) is a complementary treatment option. The primary difference between them is that SABR offers selective cell killing, which provides a better therapeutic index for cases where resection and thermal ablation are not recommended. The selectivity comes from the ability of normal tissues to repair sublethal DNA damage caused by ionizing radiation between treatment fractions. This ability is enhanced by increasing the number of fractions that may be necessary to lower the toxicity risk if gastrointestinal organs are nearby. Even if standard ablative doses are given in 5 fractions (50 Gy, 100 Gy biological effective dose [BED]) permanent injury to the vessels and of the biliary tree are rare. Motion management, image guidance, and proton therapy are technological advances in the planning and technical delivery of external beam radiation therapy that allow ablative doses to be delivered even in the most challenging tumors metastatic to the liver.

WHOLE-LIVER RADIATION: LIMITATIONS AND CONTROVERSIES

Historically, treatment of liver metastases with external beam radiation therapy was reserved for patients with symptomatic disease requiring palliation of symptoms. Low-dose whole-liver radiation, even in a single fraction, has been shown to rapidly palliate symptoms and improve quality of life in a high percentage of patients.[25–28] Although effective for palliation, whole-liver radiation is ineffective at eradicating metastatic disease, given the low tolerance of the whole liver to high-dose irradiation.

Radiation-induced liver disease (RILD) was first reported in the 1960s by Ingold and colleagues at Stanford University, who identified liver hepatitis in 12 patients who underwent liver irradiation to doses between 30 and 60 Gy.[29,30] RILD is a veno-occlusive process, which induces an increase in pressure of the portal system and manifests as a clinical syndrome of fatigue, elevated liver enzymes (in particular alkaline phosphatase over liver transaminases), tender anicteric hepatomegaly, and ascites.[31,32] The severity of RILD varies depending on the received dose, volume of liver irradiated, and underlying liver dysfunction with some patients developing fulminant liver failure.[32] Treatment is supportive largely with diuretics for fluid retention, paracentesis for ascites, steroids for reducing hepatic congestion, and anticoagulation to decrease the risk of thrombosis.

Because there are no effective therapies for RILD efforts have largely focused on mitigating the risk of developing RILD. As the risk of RILD is correlated with the dose and volume of liver irradiated, the Quantitative Analyses of Normal Tissue Effects in the Clinic (QUANTEC) published recommendations that whole-liver radiation should be restricted to 30 Gy in 2-Gy fractions or 21 Gy in 3-Gy fractions to limit the risk of RILD to less than 5%.[33] The realization that the whole liver could be treated safely only up to 30 Gy in conventional fractionation, and that at best this dose achieves short-term palliation, led many to conclude that the role of radiation therapy in the treatment of intrahepatic malignancies and metastases was quite limited.[31]

ABLATIVE LIVER RADIATION
Liver Dose Constraints and Dose Limiting Toxicities

The development of conformal radiotherapy techniques, including 3-dimensional conformal radiotherapy and intensity-modulated radiation therapy (IMRT), provided the necessary technology to deliver high dose radiation to a small volume of the liver. Although the tolerance of the whole liver to radiotherapy is low, partial volumes can tolerate very high radiation dose provided a sufficient volume of healthy liver parenchyma is spared.[33] The University of Michigan conducted a series of prospective studies with increasing dose to partial liver volumes and demonstrated that high doses were safe to partial liver volumes and that there was an apparent dose response.[34–40] Dose volume guidelines were empirically estimated from partial hepatectomy series and subsequently prospectively validated.[34–40] The QUANTEC practice guidelines for liver SABR recommend limiting 700 cm^3 of functional liver parenchyma, to less than 15 Gy in 3 to 5 fractions and limiting the mean dose to the liver to less than 15 Gy in 3 fractions and less than 20 Gy in 6 fractions for patients without underlying liver disease.[33] In doing so, the risk of RILD or liver decompensation is extremely low. Several reports have noted that patients with advanced cirrhosis or liver decompensation are at a higher risk of RILD.[41–43] Thus, it is critical to optimize the medical management of cirrhosis and/or liver decompensation prior to initiating radiation therapy. Given a higher risk of RILD and liver decompensation in patients with underlying liver disease, more stringent liver constraints are recommended.[37–40]

Dose Response and Clinical Outcomes for Stereotactic Ablative Radiotherapy of Liver Metastases

Liver-directed external beam radiation has been demonstrated to be well tolerated and effective for the ablation of metastatic tumors to the liver. The first report of high dose focal radiation to the liver using a stereotactic technique came from the Karolinska institute in the 1990's and reported on the first 42 lesions of the lung, liver, and retroperitoneal space in 31 patients treated with extracranial stereotactic radiation therapy.[44] This report established the efficacy and safety of highly conformal liver stereotactic radiation with 80% local control during a follow up period of 1.5 months to 30 months. Subsequently, investigators at the University of Heidelberg evaluated single fraction radiation in a dose escalation scheme starting at 14 Gy and increasing to 26 Gy to the liver in 37 patients with 55 liver metastases.[45] They reported no significant toxicity and a local control rate of 67% at 18 months for all patients. The investigators went on to report that the local control rate significantly correlated with radiation dose, with patients treated with 22 Gy to 26 Gy having 81% tumor control at 18 months compared with 0% at 18 months for tumors treated in the 14-Gy to 20-Gy range. Additional other groups have reported on the safety and efficacy of SABR for liver metastases, with local tumor control rates of 70% to 95% at 2 years (**Table 1**).[45–55] Investigators from the University of Colorado evaluated the safety and efficacy of SABR for the treatment of liver metastases in the first phase I/II trial in the United States.[56] In the initial phase I report, there was no dose limiting toxicity in patients with 3 or fewer liver metastases, measuring less than 6 cm, treated with SABR to 36 Gy to 60 Gy in 12 to 20 Gy fractions.[47,56] In the subsequent combined multi-institutional report of the phase I/II study, 47 patients with 63 liver metastases were treated, of whom 38 patients were treated to the phase I escalated dose of 60-Gy in 20-Gy fractions. The 2-year local control was 92% for all lesions and 100% for lesions measuring less than 3 cm in size.[47] Importantly, only 1 patient experienced grade 3 or higher toxicity, demonstrating the safety of liver SABR.[47] More recently,

Table 1
Selected prospective trials for liver stereotactic ablative radiotherapy

Study, Year Published	Study Type	Patient, no.	Lesion, mp.	Lesion Size	Primary Histology	Dose (Gy)/ Fractionation	BED (a/ b = 10)	Local Control	Overall Survival	Toxicity
Herfarth et al,[45] 2001	Phase I/II, single center	37	60	<6 cm, 1–132 cm³	Mixed	14–26/1	33–94	71% @ 1 y	72% @ 1 y	
Méndez Romero et al,[46] 2006	Phase I/II, single center	17	39	<7 cm, 1–322 cm³	Mixed	37.5/3	84	100% @ 1 y 86% @ 2 y	85% @ 1 y 62% @ 2 y	12% G3 Liver
Rusthoven et al,[47] 2009	Phase I/II multicenter	47	63	<6 cm, 1–98 cm³	Mixed	36–60/3	79–180	95% @ 1 y 92% @ 2 y	30% @ 2 y	1.5% G3 (dermatitis)
Lee et al,[48] 2009	Phase I, dose escalation	68	142	≤8 cm, 1.2–3090 cm³	Mixed	28–60/6	41–120	71% @ 1 y	47% @ 1.5 y	10% G3+
Rule et al,[49] 2011	Phase I, dose escalation	27	37	<8 cm, 9–247 cm³	Mixed	30/3–50/5–60/5	60–132	100%, 89%, 56%ª @ 2 y	50%, 67%, 56%ª @ 2 y	4% G3 Liver
Comito et al,[50] 2014	Observational	42	52	<6 cm, 20–24 cm³	Colorectal	75/3	263	95% @ 1 y 85% @ 2 y	85% @ 1 y 65% @ 2 y	60% G2, 0% G3
Scorsetti et al,[51] 2015	Phase 2, single arm	42	52	<6 cm, 2–134 cm³	Colorectal	75/3	263	95% @ 1 y 91% @ 2 y 85% @ 3 y	65% @ 2 y	25% G2 Liver, 0% G3
Goodman et al,[52] 2010	Phase I, dose escalation	26	40	<5 cm, 1–147 cm³	Mixed	18–30/1	50–120	77% @ 1 y	50% @ 2 y	8% GI bleeding
Meyer et al,[53] 2016	Phase I, dose escalation	14	17	4–79 cm³	Mixed	35–40/1	158–200	100% @ 2.5 y	78% @ 2 y	6% G2
Scorsetti et al,[54] 2018	Phase 2, single arm	61	76	<6 cm, 2–134 cm³	Mixed	75/3	263	94% @ 1 y 78% @ 3 y 78% @ 5 y	85% @ 1 y 31% @ 3 y 18% @ 5 y	2% G3 chest wall pain
Dawson et al,[55] 2019	Phase I, multicenter dose escalation	26	37	≤8 cm, 23–438 cm³	Mixed	35–50/10	47–75	NR	NR	7.7% G3 GI

Abbreviations: G2, grade 2; G3, grade 3; GI, gastrointestinal; Gy, gray; NR, not reported.
ª 60 Gy/12 Gy per fraction, 50 Gy/10 Gy per fraction, and 30 Gy/10 Gy per fraction dose cohorts.
Data from Refs.[45–55]

large cooperative group reports have further demonstrated the safety and feasibility of SABR for the treatment of liver metastases in the multi-institutional setting.[55,57]

Several studies have evaluated the potential prognostic factors for local control in patients with metastatic liver tumors treated with radiation therapy. One of the largest reports on 427 patients with 568 metastases from 25 academic and community-based centers found that higher dose (BED >100 Gy) and smaller tumors (<4 cm^3) had significantly improved local control rates that seemingly translated to a significant improvement in survival. This dose response effect was further evaluated in a tumor control probability analysis of 3719 metastases from a total of 62 published studies treated with 89 different treatment prescriptions.[58] Treatment to a BED of approximately 80 Gy or higher was sufficient in the model to achieve 90% tumor control at 1 year, but a BED of approximately 100 Gy or higher was necessary to maintain 90% tumor control at 2 years. Unfortunately, the model was unable to account for tumor size, which as previously discussed is a likely confounder for local tumor control after SABR.[59]

Treatment Planning Consideration for Liver Stereotactic Ablative Radiotherapy

The delivery of high-dose conformal radiation to the liver permits focal ablative therapy but has the potential for serious acute and late toxicity, particularly if the delivered dose does not accurately reflect the intended treatment plan. Thus, in the planning and execution of ablative liver radiation it is important to highlight several specific challenges. Standard planning for SABR typically includes a multiphase contrast computed tomography (CT) simulation scan in the treatment position. Simulation CT scans can be appropriately timed to coordinate with the portal-venous or delayed venous phases for optimal contrast differentiation between the tumor and underlying liver enhancement to facilitate target delineation. Because metastatic tumors to the liver often are hypovascular, the portal-venous phase is most commonly preferred, in which the metastatic lesion appear hypodense compared with the liver parenchyma. If poorly visualized, multimodality imaging by the use of magnetic resonance imaging, preferred, or PET can help improve the ability to accurately define metastatic targets.[25,60,61]

Respiratory motion must be controlled, or at a minimum the range of motion must be accounted for during radiation treatment delivery in the upper abdomen. The predominant motion is in the cranio-caudal direction due to diaphragmatic movement.[62] The degree of intrafraction motion can be significant, particularly near the dome, with liver excursions of 1 cm to 4 cm reported.[62] There are several strategies that can be employed to account for or control tumor motion. The most straightforward technique is the use of 4-dimensional CT (4-DCT) to account for liver motion throughout the respiratory cycle. This creates a larger margin and treats more liver than other techniques but is adequate for most small liver metastases. More advanced respiratory gating techniques include liver immobilization through deep inspiratory breath hold (**Fig. 1**) and end expiratory gating, which limits tumor motion by restricting radiation delivery to the extreme phases of the respiratory cycle.[63,64] Abdominal compression (**Fig. 2**) also can be used to restrict respiratory excursion but may not be optimal if it compresses organs, such as the stomach closer to the left lobe.[65] This generally is much less of a concern for the right lobe. More advanced techniques are able to precisely track tumors throughout treatment.[66] All these techniques have certain advantages and disadvantages and determination of the best technique for motion management for an individual patient is highly dependent on both tumor location as well as the technological expertise of the radiation oncology team. In general, comparisons between these techniques are limited and opinions must be interpreted with the

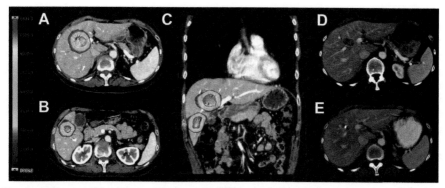

Fig. 1. A 60-year-old woman with stage IV EGFR mutated non–small cell lung adenocarcinoma involving the lung, lymph nodes, liver, and bone currently on osimertinib with oligo-progression in 2 liver lesions in segment 4a/8, measuring 3 cm, and segment 5, measuring 2 cm. Fiducial markers were placed to aid in tumor identification at time of treatment. Patient was simulated in the supine position with IV contrast. Deep inspiratory breath hold was utilized for motion management. The gross tumor with 0.5-cm margin was treated to 50-Gy in 10-Gy fractions. Axial images of (*A*) segment 4a/8 lesion and (*B*) segment 5 lesion, and (*C*) coronal image of both lesions depicting the SABR treatment plan. The pre-SABR tumor is delineated in red (*D*) and on post-treatment imaging at 2 months the patient had a complete response (*E*).

understanding that most centers have extensive experience with 1 or 2 of these techniques and very little experience with the others. The authors prefer deep inspiration breath hold for its reproducibility and reliability for limiting motion during the 40-second to 60-second cone beam CT (CBCT) image acquisition and treatment delivery.

Treatment using traditional alignment is often inadequate to account for day to day (interfraction) motion. Liver position relative to bony anatomy has been shown to change between fractions by up to 1 cm.[67,68] Because metastatic tumors are difficult to visualize on noncontrast CBCT images obtained on the treatment machine, liver shape and/or diaphragmatic shape has been used as surrogates of tumor location.[69]

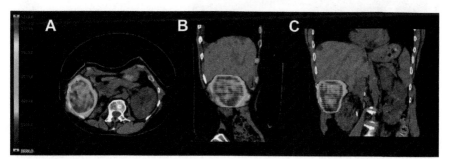

Fig. 2. A 62-year-old woman with chronic obstructive pulmonary disease (COPD) and stage IV urothelial cancer involving the on maintenance nivolumab with oligo-progression in the liver, segment 6, measuring 6 cm. CT simulation in the supine position with no contrast given renal function. Patient was unable to hold breath given her COPD, so abdominal compression was utilized for motion management. Axial (*A*), sagittal (*B*), and coronal (*C*) images of the SABR treatment plan for her segment 6 metastasis. The abdominal compression sleeve is clearly visible on the axial (*A*) and sagittal (*B*) images.

The placement of fiducial markers (see **Fig. 1**) in and around the tumor, or utilization of surgical clips (**Fig. 3**), in the immediate proximity of the tumor, have been shown to aid in localization and improve confidence in daily tumor localization before treatment.[70–72] Fiducial markers also permit real time intrafraction motion assessment because orthogonal radiographs can be obtained periodically throughout treatment to ensure target accuracy within 1 mm to 2 mm.[60] A well-executed motion management strategy permits utilization of smaller treatment margins and thus facilitates ablation of larger tumors and tumors abutting critical serial luminal organs, such as the stomach, small, and large intestine.

Adopting Strategies for Large Tumors or Tumors Close to Critical Organs at Risk

Because the efficacy of surgical metastasectomy and RFA in the treatment of metastatic liver tumors is well established, SABR is most appropriately reserved for unresectable tumors, medically inoperable patients, or for tumors in close proximity to vessels or the biliary tree. The safe delivery of liver SABR can be challenging in patients with large tumors, limiting the volume of healthy normal liver parenchyma or tumors abutting or in close proximity to radiosensitive organs arranged in serial functional subunits (FSUs), such as the small or large intestine.[73] Although many of the initial reports evaluating ablative liver radiation have reported on the efficacy of SABR (ie, BED of 100 Gy in ≤5 fractions), these doses cannot be safely delivered near sensitive organs using these dose. Radiation oncologists have most commonly elected to reduce the dose below an ablative threshold to a palliative level in these situations. Ablative doses can easily be achieved, however, with moderately hypofractionated treatment

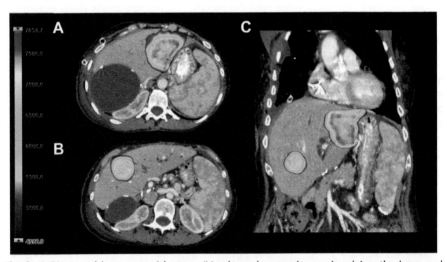

Fig. 3. A 58-year-old woman with stage IV colon adenocarcinoma involving the lung and liver status post–extended right posterior segmentectomy and hepatic arterial pump placement with isolated bilobar liver progression with a 5-cm lesion in the superior left lobe and a 2.5-cm lesion in the inferior right lobe. Patient was simulated in the supine position with IV contrast. Deep inspiratory breath hold was utilized for motion management. Given the proximity of the stomach to the left lobe metastasis, a moderately hypofractionated treatment schedule was selected to treat the tumor to 67.5 Gy in 4.5-Gy fractions. Surgical clips adjacent to the tumor were used as fiducials for target localization. Axial images of (*A*) superior left lobe lesion and (*B*) segment 5 lesion and (*C*) coronal image of both lesions depicting the SABR treatment plan.

schedules of 10, 15, or even 25 fractions. The principle of increasing fractionation to improve the therapeutic index is as old as the field of radiotherapy itself. Sublethal DNA damage is repaired between fractions, thus resulting in greater normal tissue tolerance. Moderately hypofractionated regimens enable prioritization of patient safety by limiting the risk of RILD, biliary stricture, gastrointestinal bleeding, and chest wall pain while maintaining ablative doses.[72] If liver or bowel dose constraints cannot be met for a 5-fraction SABR treatment during the planning process, the options are (1) to proceed with treatment and accept a greater risk of RILD, (2) to reduce the dose to the tumor to minimize the risk of RILD but compromising on likelihood of tumor control, or (3) to fractionate treatment to maintain ablative dose to the tumor (BED >100 Gy) while minimizing risk of RILD and gastrointestinal toxicity. Although the majority of radiation oncologists simply would accept a lower dose and, thereafter, lower tumor control, the authors favor increasing the number of fractions to facilitate ablative treatment to maximize tumor control while maintaining a low risk of toxicity (see **Fig. 3**). Large liver tumors are among the most challenging cases to treat because of the proximity of the duodenum, colon, stomach, and main bile ducts; the sensitivity of the liver parenchyma to radiation; the potential for underlying liver disease; and the respiratory and interfraction motion of the upper abdomen. These challenges may be overcome while delivering ablative doses by fractionating radiation to improve the therapeutic index and using heterogenous dose distribution when the tumor is in direct abutment with sensitive luminal organs. By intentionally underdosing at the interface of critical organs, such as the large and small intestine, safety is ensured. Controlling respiratory motion with gating techniques helps to decrease treatment margins and facilitate adequate daily CBCT imaging that can be used to assess day-to-day changes in normal tissue anatomy. This provides adequate image guidance to assess when a change in the radiation plan (adaptive planning) is necessary.[72]

ROLE OF PROTON THERAPY FOR ABLATIVE LIVER RADIATION

In patients with large tumors or underlying liver dysfunction, proton beam radiotherapy should be considered. Proton beam radiotherapy utilizes charged particles, or protons, which come to rest within the patient and deposit their energy at a prespecified range, the characteristic Bragg peak. A dosimetric advantage for protons exists because beyond the Bragg peak there is minimal exit dose, unlike photon-based therapy. Given this discrete dose deposition, protons have the advantage of sparing more normal tissues, including the liver, lung, esophagus, kidney, and spinal cord, than photon-based IMRT for ablative radiation to liver metastases.[74] In carefully selected patients with large tumors or bilobar tumors, where the liver dose constraints are unable to be met, it is prudent to consider ablative proton therapy in lieu of compromising on the dose and accepting a less effective or palliative treatment (**Fig. 4**).[75] The techniques for motion management and image guidance not always are available at all proton facilities, but the same principles described previously should be used when they are. In hepatocellular carcinoma, patients treated with proton therapy had less liver decompensation and improved survival compared with patients treated with photon-based IMRT with no differences appreciated in locoregional recurrence.[76] This improvement in survival likely was secondary to a decreased risk of nonclassic RILD resulting from a significantly lower mean liver dose with protons compared with IMRT-based plans.[76] The most notable disadvantage to proton therapy is when luminal organs are in close proximity to the tumor. The lateral penumbra is wider with protons than with photons, and in these cases the relative merits of sparing the liver with protons must be balanced with the sacrifice in tumor coverage. Early-

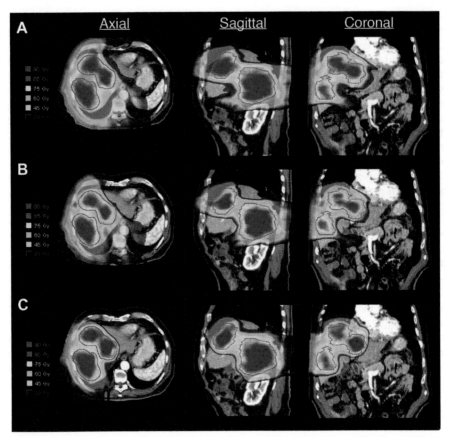

Fig. 4. A 77-year-old man with newly diagnosed stage IV colon adenocarcinoma metastatic to the liver with 13cm posterior right and 7 c-m segment 4a liver metastases. Patient was simulated in the supine position with abdominal compression and 4-DCT. Liver SABR photon-proton comparison plans to deliver 67.5 Gy in 4.5-Gy fractions with a central hotspot of 90 Gy in 6-Gy fractions for colorectal liver metastases. Initial photon plan prioritized tumor coverage (99% coverage) but significantly exceeded liver dose constraints (A). Because this treatment was deemed unsafe, photon replanning to prioritize liver dose constraints was performed but resulted in significant underdosing with approximately 10% of tumor under covered (B). Proton replanning was able to meet acceptable liver dose constraints to ensure safety, while maintaining a tumor target coverage of approximately 100% (C).

phase clinical trials have demonstrated the safety and efficacy of proton stereotactic body radiation therapy for liver metastases.[77,78] In fact, the dosimetric advantage of protons is greater for larger tumors and larger doses per fraction.

SUMMARY AND FUTURE DIRECTIONS FOR ABLATIVE LIVER RADIATION

Modern radiotherapy techniques permit the safe delivery of high-dose radiation to partial liver volumes. Locoregional control rates of 85% or greater can be achieved in appropriately selected patients treated with ablative radiation. The safe delivery of ablative liver radiation can be challenging in patients with large tumors, which increases the volume of healthy normal liver parenchyma that must be treated and in tumors abutting or in close proximity to radiosensitive organs arranged in serial FSUs, such as the small or large intestine. In patients with underlying liver disease, limited liver reserve, or exceptionally large liver tumors, proton beam radiation should be considered. For definitive ablative treatment, utilization of fractionation, heterogenous dose distribution, and appropriate respiratory motion control are important tools to effectively and safely ablate liver metastases. Recent studies have suggested that local ablation of all metastatic lesions in patients with oligometastatic disease is safe and associated with prolongation of PFS in patients across a range of tumor histologies.[79–81] Although confirmatory phase III studies are ongoing, interest in local metastatic ablation has increased significantly and it is important to prioritize patient safety while maintaining ablative doses for the treatment of liver metastases.

DISCLOSURE

P.B. Romesser reports research funding from and is a consultant for EMD Serono and has received travel support from Elekta.

CLINCS CARE POINTS

- External beam radiation is a complementary modality to other modalities for liver directed therapy.
- There is an ablative threshold dose which should be achieved.
- Respiratory motion needs to be accounted for.
- Key organs such as the normal healthy liver and the luminal GI organs need to be protected.

REFERENCES

1. Costi R, Leonardi F, Zanoni D, et al. Palliative care and end-stage colorectal cancer management: the surgeon meets the oncologist. World J Gastroenterol 2014; 20(24):7602–21.
2. Aitken KL, Hawkins MA. Stereotactic body radiotherapy for liver metastases. Clin Oncol (R Coll Radiol) 2015;27(5):307–15.
3. Goodman KA, Kavanagh BD. Stereotactic body radiotherapy for liver metastases. Semin Radiat Oncol 2017;27(3):240–6.
4. Hellman S, Weichselbaum RR. Oligometastases. J Clin Oncol 1995;13(1):8–10.
5. Riihimaki M, Hemminki A, Sundquist J, et al. Patterns of metastasis in colon and rectal cancer. Sci Rep 2016;6:29765.
6. Moertel CG, Fleming TR, Macdonald JS, et al. Fluorouracil plus levamisole as effective adjuvant therapy after resection of stage III colon carcinoma: a final report. Ann Intern Med 1995;122(5):321–6.
7. Fong Y, Fortner J, Sun RL, et al. Clinical score for predicting recurrence after hepatic resection for metastatic colorectal cancer: analysis of 1001 consecutive cases. Ann Surg 1999;230(3):309–18 [discussion: 318–21].
8. Morris EJ, Forman D, Thomas JD, et al. Surgical management and outcomes of colorectal cancer liver metastases. Br J Surg 2010;97(7):1110–8.
9. Nordlinger B, Guiguet M, Vaillant JC, et al. Surgical resection of colorectal carcinoma metastases to the liver. A prognostic scoring system to improve case selection, based on 1568 patients. Assoc Francaise de Chirurgie. Cancer 1996;77(7): 1254–62.

10. Onaitis MW, Petersen RP, Haney JC, et al. Prognostic factors for recurrence after pulmonary resection of colorectal cancer metastases. Ann Thorac Surg 2009; 87(6):1684–8.

11. Choti MA, Sitzmann JV, Tiburi MF, et al. Trends in long-term survival following liver resection for hepatic colorectal metastases. Ann Surg 2002;235(6):759–66.

12. Lehnert T, Knaebel HP, Duck M, et al. Sequential hepatic and pulmonary resections for metastatic colorectal cancer. Br J Surg 1999;86(2):241–3.

13. Shah SA, Haddad R, Al-Sukhni W, et al. Surgical resection of hepatic and pulmonary metastases from colorectal carcinoma. J Am Coll Surg 2006;202(3):468–75.

14. McCormack PM, Burt ME, Bains MS, et al. Lung resection for colorectal metastases. 10-year results. Arch Surg 1992;127(12):1403–6.

15. Adam R, Chiche L, Aloia T, et al. Hepatic resection for noncolorectal nonendocrine liver metastases: analysis of 1,452 patients and development of a prognostic model. Ann Surg 2006;244(4):524–35.

16. Hewish M, Cunningham D. First-line treatment of advanced colorectal cancer. Lancet 2011;377(9783):2060–2.

17. Jawed I, Wilkerson J, Prasad V, et al. Colorectal cancer survival gains and novel treatment regimens: a systematic review and analysis. JAMA Oncol 2015;1(6): 787–95.

18. Kruger S, Ilmer M, Kobold S, et al. Advances in cancer immunotherapy 2019 - latest trends. J Exp Clin Cancer Res 2019;38(1):268.

19. Fan Y, Zhang C, Jin S, et al. Progress of immune checkpoint therapy in the clinic (Review). Oncol Rep 2019;41(1):3–14.

20. Heinemann V, von Weikersthal LF, Decker T, et al. FOLFIRI plus cetuximab versus FOLFIRI plus bevacizumab as first-line treatment for patients with metastatic colorectal cancer (FIRE-3): a randomised, open-label, phase 3 trial. Lancet Oncol 2014;15(10):1065–75.

21. Garcea G, Lloyd TD, Aylott C, et al. The emergent role of focal liver ablation techniques in the treatment of primary and secondary liver tumours. Eur J Cancer 2003;39(15):2150–64.

22. Ruers T, Van Coevorden F, Punt CJ, et al. Local treatment of unresectable colorectal liver metastases: results of a randomized phase II trial. J Natl Cancer Inst 2017;109(9).

23. Ruers T, Punt C, Van Coevorden F, et al. Radiofrequency ablation combined with systemic treatment versus systemic treatment alone in patients with non-resectable colorectal liver metastases: a randomized EORTC Intergroup phase II study (EORTC 40004). Ann Oncol 2012;23(10):2619–26.

24. Wong SL, Mangu PB, Choti MA, et al. American Society of Clinical Oncology 2009 clinical evidence review on radiofrequency ablation of hepatic metastases from colorectal cancer. J Clin Oncol 2010;28(3):493–508.

25. Hoyer M, Swaminath A, Bydder S, et al. Radiotherapy for liver metastases: a review of evidence. Int J Radiat Oncol Biol Phys 2012;82(3):1047–57.

26. Bydder S, Spry NA, Christie DR, et al. A prospective trial of short-fractionation radiotherapy for the palliation of liver metastases. Australas Radiol 2003;47(3): 284–8.

27. Borgelt BB, Gelber R, Brady LW, et al. The palliation of hepatic metastases: results of the Radiation Therapy Oncology Group pilot study. Int J Radiat Oncol Biol Phys 1981;7(5):587–91.

28. Soliman H, Ringash J, Jiang H, et al. Phase II trial of palliative radiotherapy for hepatocellular carcinoma and liver metastases. J Clin Oncol 2013;31(31):3980–6.

29. Reed GB Jr, Cox AJ Jr. The human liver after radiation injury. A form of veno-occlusive disease. Am J Pathol 1966;48(4):597–611.
30. Ingold JA, Reed GB, Kaplan HS, et al. Radiation Hepatitis. Am J Roentgenol Radium Ther Nucl Med 1965;93:200–8.
31. Lawrence TS, Robertson JM, Anscher MS, et al. Hepatic toxicity resulting from cancer treatment. Int J Radiat Oncol Biol Phys 1995;31(5):1237–48.
32. Toesca DAS, Ibragimov B, Koong AJ, et al. Strategies for prediction and mitigation of radiation-induced liver toxicity. J Radiat Res 2018;59(suppl_1):i40–9.
33. Pan CC, Kavanagh BD, Dawson LA, et al. Radiation-associated liver injury. Int J Radiat Oncol Biol Phys 2010;76(3 Suppl):S94–100.
34. Robertson JM, Lawrence TS, Dworzanin LM, et al. Treatment of primary hepatobiliary cancers with conformal radiation therapy and regional chemotherapy. J Clin Oncol 1993;11(7):1286–93.
35. Jackson A, Ten Haken RK, Robertson JM, et al. Analysis of clinical complication data for radiation hepatitis using a parallel architecture model. Int J Radiat Oncol Biol Phys 1995;31(4):883–91.
36. Robertson JM, Lawrence TS, Andrews JC, et al. Long-term results of hepatic artery fluorodeoxyuridine and conformal radiation therapy for primary hepatobiliary cancers. Int J Radiat Oncol Biol Phys 1997;37(2):325–30.
37. Dawson LA, McGinn CJ, Normolle D, et al. Escalated focal liver radiation and concurrent hepatic artery fluorodeoxyuridine for unresectable intrahepatic malignancies. J Clin Oncol 2000;18(11):2210–8.
38. Lawrence TS, Ten Haken RK, Kessler ML, et al. The use of 3-D dose volume analysis to predict radiation hepatitis. Int J Radiat Oncol Biol Phys 1992;23(4):781–8.
39. Dawson LA, Normolle D, Balter JM, et al. Analysis of radiation-induced liver disease using the Lyman NTCP model. Int J Radiat Oncol Biol Phys 2002;53(4):810–21.
40. Ben-Josef E, Normolle D, Ensminger WD, et al. Phase II trial of high-dose conformal radiation therapy with concurrent hepatic artery floxuridine for unresectable intrahepatic malignancies. J Clin Oncol 2005;23(34):8739–47.
41. Cheng JC, Wu JK, Huang CM, et al. Radiation-induced liver disease after radiotherapy for hepatocellular carcinoma: clinical manifestation and dosimetric description. Radiother Oncol 2002;63(1):41–5.
42. Cheng JC, Wu JK, Lee PC, et al. Biologic susceptibility of hepatocellular carcinoma patients treated with radiotherapy to radiation-induced liver disease. Int J Radiat Oncol Biol Phys 2004;60(5):1502–9.
43. Liang SX, Zhu XD, Xu ZY, et al. Radiation-induced liver disease in three-dimensional conformal radiation therapy for primary liver carcinoma: the risk factors and hepatic radiation tolerance. Int J Radiat Oncol Biol Phys 2006;65(2):426–34.
44. Blomgren H, Lax I, Naslund I, et al. Stereotactic high dose fraction radiation therapy of extracranial tumors using an accelerator. Clinical experience of the first thirty-one patients. Acta Oncol 1995;34(6):861–70.
45. Herfarth KK, Debus J, Lohr F, et al. Stereotactic single-dose radiation therapy of liver tumors: results of a phase I/II trial. J Clin Oncol 2001;19(1):164–70.
46. Méndez Romero A, Wunderink W, Hussain SM, et al. Stereotactic body radiation therapy for primary and metastatic liver tumors: a single institution phase i-ii study. Acta Oncol 2006;45(7):831–7.
47. Rusthoven KE, Kavanagh BD, Cardenes H, et al. Multi-institutional phase I/II trial of stereotactic body radiation therapy for liver metastases. J Clin Oncol 2009;27(10):1572–8.

48. Lee MT, Kim JJ, Dinniwell R, et al. Phase I study of individualized stereotactic body radiotherapy of liver metastases. J Clin Oncol 2009;27(10):1585–91.

49. Rule W, Timmerman R, Tong L, et al. Phase I dose-escalation study of stereotactic body radiotherapy in patients with hepatic metastases. Ann Surg Oncol 2011; 18(4):1081–7.

50. Comito T, Cozzi L, Clerici E, et al. Stereotactic Ablative Radiotherapy (SABR) in inoperable oligometastatic disease from colorectal cancer: a safe and effective approach. BMC Cancer 2014;14:619.

51. Scorsetti M, Comito T, Tozzi A, et al. Final results of a phase II trial for stereotactic body radiation therapy for patients with inoperable liver metastases from colorectal cancer. J Cancer Res Clin Oncol 2015;141(3):543–53.

52. Goodman KA, Wiegner EA, Maturen KE, et al. Dose-escalation study of single-fraction stereotactic body radiotherapy for liver malignancies. Int J Radiat Oncol Biol Phys 2010;78(2):486–93.

53. Meyer JJ, Foster RD, Lev-Cohain N, et al. A phase I dose-escalation trial of single-fraction stereotactic radiation therapy for liver metastases. Ann Surg Oncol 2016;23(1):218–24.

54. Scorsetti M, Comito T, Clerici E, et al. Phase II trial on SBRT for unresectable liver metastases: long-term outcome and prognostic factors of survival after 5 years of follow-up. Radiat Oncol 2018;13(1):234.

55. Dawson LA, Winter KA, Katz AW, et al. NRG oncology/RTOG 0438: a phase 1 trial of highly conformal radiation therapy for liver metastases. Pract Radiat Oncol 2019;9(4):e386–93.

56. Schefter TE, Kavanagh BD, Timmerman RD, et al. A phase I trial of stereotactic body radiation therapy (SBRT) for liver metastases. Int J Radiat Oncol Biol Phys 2005;62(5):1371–8.

57. Chmura SJ, Winter KA, Salama JK, et al. Phase I trial of Stereotactic Body Radiation Therapy (SBRT) to multiple metastatic sites: a NRG oncology study. Int J Radiat Oncol Biol Phys 2018;102(3):S68–9.

58. Klement RJ. Radiobiological parameters of liver and lung metastases derived from tumor control data of 3719 metastases. Radiother Oncol 2017;123(2): 218–26.

59. Rusthoven KE, Kavanagh BD, Burri SH, et al. Multi-institutional phase I/II trial of stereotactic body radiation therapy for lung metastases. J Clin Oncol 2009; 27(10):1579–84.

60. Wurm RE, Gum F, Erbel S, et al. Image guided respiratory gated hypofractionated Stereotactic Body Radiation Therapy (H-SBRT) for liver and lung tumors: initial experience. Acta Oncol 2006;45(7):881–9.

61. Kirilova A, Lockwood G, Choi P, et al. Three-dimensional motion of liver tumors using cine-magnetic resonance imaging. Int J Radiat Oncol Biol Phys 2008; 71(4):1189–95.

62. Worm ES, Hoyer M, Fledelius W, et al. Three-dimensional, time-resolved, intra-fraction motion monitoring throughout stereotactic liver radiation therapy on a conventional linear accelerator. Int J Radiat Oncol Biol Phys 2013;86(1):190–7.

63. Vogel L, Sihono DSK, Weiss C, et al. Intra-breath-hold residual motion of image-guided DIBH liver-SBRT: an estimation by ultrasound-based monitoring correlated with diaphragm position in CBCT. Radiother Oncol 2018;129(3):441–8.

64. Briere TM, Beddar S, Balter P, et al. Respiratory gating with EPID-based verification: the MDACC experience. Phys Med Biol 2009;54(11):3379–91.

65. Heinzerling JH, Anderson JF, Papiez L, et al. Four-dimensional computed tomography scan analysis of tumor and organ motion at varying levels of abdominal

compression during stereotactic treatment of lung and liver. Int J Radiat Oncol Biol Phys 2008;70(5):1571–8.

66. Iizuka Y, Matsuo Y, Ishihara Y, et al. Dynamic tumor-tracking radiotherapy with real-time monitoring for liver tumors using a gimbal mounted linac. Radiother Oncol 2015;117(3):496–500.

67. Case RB, Moseley DJ, Sonke JJ, et al. Interfraction and intrafraction changes in amplitude of breathing motion in stereotactic liver radiotherapy. Int J Radiat Oncol Biol Phys 2010;77(3):918–25.

68. Case RB, Sonke JJ, Moseley DJ, et al. Inter- and intrafraction variability in liver position in non-breath-hold stereotactic body radiotherapy. Int J Radiat Oncol Biol Phys 2009;75(1):302–8.

69. Yang J, Cai J, Wang H, et al. Is diaphragm motion a good surrogate for liver tumor motion? Int J Radiat Oncol Biol Phys 2014;90(4):952–8.

70. Wunderink W, Mendez Romero A, Seppenwoolde Y, et al. Potentials and limitations of guiding liver stereotactic body radiation therapy set-up on liver-implanted fiducial markers. Int J Radiat Oncol Biol Phys 2010;77(5):1573–83.

71. Seppenwoolde Y, Wunderink W, Wunderink-van Veen SR, et al. Treatment precision of image-guided liver SBRT using implanted fiducial markers depends on marker-tumour distance. Phys Med Biol 2011;56(17):5445–68.

72. Crane CH, Koay EJ. Solutions that enable ablative radiotherapy for large liver tumors: fractionated dose painting, simultaneous integrated protection, motion management, and computed tomography image guidance. Cancer 2016; 122(13):1974–86.

73. Bujold A, Massey CA, Kim JJ, et al. Sequential phase I and II trials of stereotactic body radiotherapy for locally advanced hepatocellular carcinoma. J Clin Oncol 2013;31(13):1631–9.

74. Mondlane G, Gubanski M, Lind PA, et al. Dosimetric comparison of plans for photon- or proton-beam based radiosurgery of liver metastases. Int J Part Ther 2016;3(2):277–84.

75. Colbert LE, Cloyd JM, Koay EJ, et al. Proton beam radiation as salvage therapy for bilateral colorectal liver metastases not amenable to second-stage hepatectomy. Surgery 2017;161(6):1543–8.

76. Sanford NN, Pursley J, Noe B, et al. Protons versus photons for unresectable hepatocellular carcinoma: liver decompensation and overall survival. Int J Radiat Oncol Biol Phys 2019;105(1):64–72.

77. Kang JI, Sufficool DC, Hsueh CT, et al. A phase I trial of proton stereotactic body radiation therapy for liver metastases. J Gastrointest Oncol 2019;10(1):112–7.

78. Hong TS, Wo JY, Borger DR, et al. Phase II study of proton-based stereotactic body radiation therapy for liver metastases: importance of tumor genotype. J Natl Cancer Inst 2017;109(9).

79. Palma DA, Olson R, Harrow S, et al. Stereotactic ablative radiotherapy versus standard of care palliative treatment in patients with oligometastatic cancers (SABR-COMET): a randomised, phase 2, open-label trial. Lancet 2019; 393(10185):2051–8.

80. Gomez DR, Tang C, Zhang J, et al. Local consolidative therapy vs. maintenance therapy or observation for patients with oligometastatic non-small-cell lung cancer: long-term results of a multi-institutional, phase II, randomized study. J Clin Oncol 2019;37(18):1558–65.

81. Iyengar P, Wardak Z, Gerber DE, et al. Consolidative radiotherapy for limited metastatic non-small-cell lung cancer: a phase 2 randomized clinical trial. JAMA Oncol 2018;4(1):e173501.

Hepatic Perfusion for Diffuse Metastatic Cancer to the Liver: Open and Percutaneous Techniques

H. Richard Alexander Jr, MD[a],*, Virginia Devi-Chou, BA, MA[b]

KEYWORDS

- IHP • PHP • Hepatic perfusion • Metastatic cancer • Diffuse liver • Liver metastases
- Metachronous disease

KEY POINTS

- In many cancer patients, metastatic disease may be isolated to the liver or the liver may be the dominant site of progressive metastatic cancer.
- In this setting, progression of disease in the liver is generally the most significant cause of morbidity and mortality.
- Isolated Hepatic Perfusion is a surgical technique that delivers targeted chemotherapy to treat colorectal cancer liver metastases.
- Percutaneous Hepatic Perfusion is a less invasive alternative to IHP.

INTRODUCTION

In 2020, it is estimated that approximately 20% to 25% of the 148,000 people in the United States diagnosed with colorectal cancer (CRC) will present with synchronous liver metastases, and an additional 20% to 30% of patients will develop metachronous disease.[1,2] Unfortunately, a majority of patients with CRC liver metastases harbor unresectable disease and systemic chemotherapy usually is the first therapeutic intervention for these patients. Although various chemotherapy regimens combining 5-fluorouracil, oxaliplatin, and irinotecan, with or without biological agents, have response rates ranging from 35% to 60% and median survival times ranging from 15 months to 27 months, disease progression is common, highlighting the need for additional therapeutic options.[3–12]

Other malignancies, such as ocular melanoma and neuroendocrine cancers, also have a propensity to metastasize selectively to the liver. In patients with ocular melanoma, the liver is the most common site of metastatic disease. Systemic therapy

---

[a] Department of Surgery, Division of Surgical Oncology, Rutgers Cancer Institute of New Jersey, Rutgers Robert Wood Johnson Medical School, 195 Little Albany Street, Room 2009, New Brunswick, NJ 08901, USA; [b] Division of Surgical Oncology, Rutgers Cancer Institute of New Jersey, Rutgers Robert Wood Johnson Medical School, New Brunswick, NJ, USA
* Corresponding author.
E-mail address: Richard.Alexander@Rutgers.edu

Surg Oncol Clin N Am 30 (2021) 175–188
https://doi.org/10.1016/j.soc.2020.08.007
1055-3207/21/© 2020 Elsevier Inc. All rights reserved.

options for these patients are limited in number and efficacy[13–15] and, although resection of limited disease in highly selected patients may improve survival, recurrence rates are high and 5-year survival rates are less than or equal to 20%.[16–18] In cases of neuroendocrine cancers, although prolonged survival may be observed in patients with diffuse liver metastases, significant systemic symptoms may develop due to disease burden and/or hormone production.[19,20] Therefore, for both malignancies, treatments that target the liver may be of substantial clinical benefit.

Liver-directed treatments, also known as regional hepatic therapies, have the advantages of delivering dose intensive therapy to the cancer-burdened organ while limiting unnecessary systemic toxicities; these therapies have an increasing important role in the management of patients with unresectable liver metastases. The pathophysiologic basis for the use of hepatic perfusion or hepatic artery infusion (HAI) comes from the landmark study of 2 pathologists at the University of Pennsylvania, Breedis and Young,[21] who demonstrated that in contrast to the dual blood supply of hepatic parenchyma (hepatic artery and portal vein), hepatic metastases derive their blood supply almost exclusively from the hepatic artery (vs the portal vein). Both open isolated hepatic perfusion (IHP) and percutaneous hepatic perfusion (PHP) use the hepatic artery to selectively deliver therapy and have demonstrated efficacy in patients who are refractory to other therapies.

Development of Isolated Hepatic Perfusion and Percutaneous Hepatic Perfusion

Historically, 3 critical advances made the development of isolation perfusion techniques possible. In 1935, Dr Alexis Carrel, who won the Nobel Prize for his description of anastomosing blood vessels, and his collaborator, Charles Lindbergh, who developed fame a few years earlier for being the first to fly solo across the Atlantic Ocean, described a technique to maintain organs ex vivo using a perfusion circuit consisting of a pump, reservoir, and oxygenator.[22] Further refinement of their discovery led to the application of cardiopulmonary bypass machines in the early 1950s.[23] The second advance was the description of chemicals in the 1940s that had potent anticancer properties, one of the first of which, L-phenylalanine mustard, or melphalan, was a derivative of nitrogen mustard used as a poisonous gas during World War I.[24] Then in 1958, 2 cardiac surgeons from Tulane, Creech and colleagues, reported the initial human experience with isolated limb perfusion (ILP) for melanoma and sarcoma.[25] In that seminal report, they stated, "as a result of experiences with a heart-lung apparatus in the treatment of intracardiac defects, it occurred to us that this extracorporeal circuit might provide a means of temporarily isolating and maintaining a tumor-bearing area while it was being perfused with maximal amounts of an alkylating agent." In 1969, Stehlin[26] demonstrated that hyperthermia augmented the effects of chemotherapy in ILP and the combination of hyperthermia and chemotherapy become the standard approach for decades.

The modern era of isolation perfusion probably started in the early 1990s when tumor necrosis factor (TNF-α), a biological agent with antitumor activity, was used in ILP[27] (**Table 1**). Because humans experience severe toxicity with even low doses or exposures to TNF-α, its use in isolation perfusion resulted in marked refinement and standardization in perfusion techniques to minimize leak of dangerous amounts of perfusate into the systemic circulation.

In 1961, Dr Robert Ausman,[28] at the Roswell Park Memorial Institute (now known as the Roswell Park Comprehensive Cancer Center), published an article describing the technique for IHP. The technique first was refined in a canine model and then was tested in 5 patients with various hepatic malignancies. Although there was no long-term follow-up and the morbidity was significant, therapeutic effect likely was observed in 2 patients.[29]

Table 1
Summary of outcomes with isolated hepatic perfusion and percutaneous hepatic perfusion in selected series

Study	Histology	Modality	n	Radiographic Response	Overall Survival (mo)
van Iersel et al,[39] 2008	CRC	IHP	105	50%	24.8
Alexander et al,[40] 2009	CRC	IHP ± HAI Rx[a]	120	61%	17.4
Alexander et al,[41] 2005	CRC	IHP second-line Rx	25	60%	12
de Leede et al,[42] 2016	Melanoma	IHP	30	-	10
Alexander et al,[43] 2000	Melanoma	IHP	22	62%	11
Hughes et al,[48] 2016	Melanoma	PHP	40	36.4%	10.6
Karydis et al,[49] 2018	Melanoma	PHP	51	47%	15.3
Grover and Alexander,[51] 2004	Neuroendocrine tumor	IHP	12	50%	48

[a] Rx: treatment.
Data from Refs.[39–43,48,49,51]

Because of the significant morbidity and potential mortality associated with IHP, this technique did not gain widespread acceptance over the following 3 decades. Several small, single-institution series, however, were published during this time, but patient selection criteria and perfusion parameters were variable, limiting the interpretation of these studies.[30–32] The early clinical reports showing marked antitumor activity in melanoma and sarcoma using chemotherapy and TNF-α in ILP suggested that the regimen may have efficacy across several histologies.[27,33] A patient with extensive and regionally metastatic eccrine gland adenocarcinoma treated at the National Cancer Institute with ILP using TNF-α and melphalan had a rapid and complete response (**Fig. 1**), suggesting the possibility that IHP perfusion with the same agents might produce similar results for patients with metastatic adenocarcinoma in the liver.

During the 1990s, several groups in the United States and Europe developed protocols to evaluate the safety and efficacy of IHP in patients with unresectable liver malignancies.[34–37] A phase II study from the National Cancer Institute evaluated the efficacy of high-dose melphalan, TNF-α, and moderate hyperthermia for the management of unresectable malignancies confined to the liver.[34] The maximum tolerated doses of melphalan and TNF-α were established from a previously conducted phase I study. Complete vascular isolation was confirmed using continuous intraoperative leak monitoring with I-131 human serum albumin34, 34 patients were treated and 33 were assessable for response (1 treatment mortality). A majority of patients (76%) had CRC liver metastases and 60% had received prior systemic or regional treatment. The overall radiographic response rate was 75% and was observed in patients with advanced disease or those who had prior treatment (**Fig. 2**). Transient grade III or greater hepatic toxicity was experienced by most patients (75%). This study, therefore, established IHP as a viable treatment option for patients with unresectable liver metastases, although it was clear that refinements in the technique and delivery of therapeutic agents needed to be explored.

TECHNIQUE FOR OPEN ISOLATED HEPATIC PERFUSION

IHP is a complex surgical procedure; access to the liver and the porta hepatis is obtained using a subcostal incision. Although peritoneal metastases encountered at

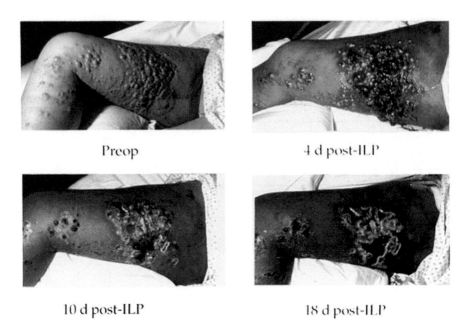

Preop   4 d post-ILP

10 d post-ILP   18 d post-ILP

Fig. 1. Images of a patient's leg showing extensive in transit metastases from a primary eccrine gland adenocarcinoma of the foot. The patient underwent a 90-minute hyperthermic ILP using TNF-α and melphalan. The patient experienced rapid tumor response with necrosis and eschar formation within days of treatment. This was the first observation of this regimen having clinical efficacy against an adenocarcinoma. *Panels*: Upper left, preoperative stage; Upper right, 4 days post ILP; Bottom left, 10 days post ILP; Bottom right, 18 days post ILP.

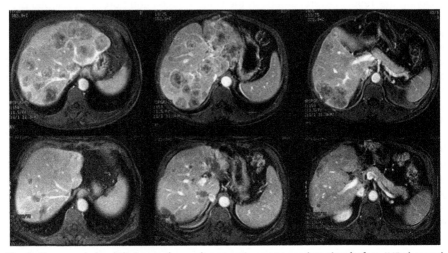

Fig. 2. Top panels (gadolinium-enhanced magnetic resonance imaging before IHP therapy) show extensive hepatic metastases from CRC in a patent who had been previously treated with systemic and hepatic artery infusion chemotherapy. Bottom panels show corresponding liver cuts 1 year after IHP.

operation would be a contraindication to the procedure, involvement of resectable lymph nodes limited to the porta hepatis does not adversely affect outcomes. The right and left lobes of the liver are extensively mobilized and a Kocher maneuver is performed to expose the inferior vena cava (IVC). The entire retrohepatic vena cava is dissected and all retroperitoneal venous tributaries, including the right adrenal vein and phrenic veins, are ligated. The structures of the porta hepatis, including the proper hepatic artery, portal vein, and common bile duct are completely exposed. The gastroduodenal artery is identified and serves as the cannulation site for the perfusion. The IHP circuit is depicted in **Fig. 3**.

The patient is systemically anticoagulated using heparin and a venovenous bypass circuit then is placed from the saphenous vein to the axillary vein to maintain systemic venous return while the IVC is temporarily occluded with vascular clamps during the perfusion. The saphenous vein is cannulated with a catheter positioned just below the renal veins. Another catheter is placed into the central venous system via the axillary vein. These 2 cannulas then are attached to a centrifugal pump and form the venous bypass circuit.

To create the perfusion circuit, a vascular clamp is placed across the IVC just above the renal veins and a catheter is inserted in the retrohepatic vena cava that serves as the venous outflow for the hepatic perfusion circuit. The portal vein and common hepatic artery are occluded with vascular clamps, and arterial inflow to the proper

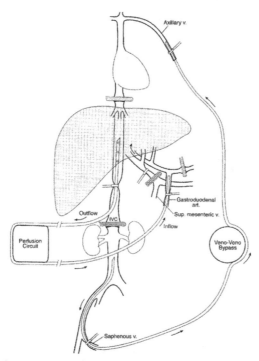

Fig. 3. Drawing of the IHP circuit. The extracorporeal perfusion circuits is on the patient's right. It shows the inflow cannula positioned in the gastroduodenal artery and an outflow cannula in an isolated segment of the retrohepatic IVC. There are vascular occlusion clamps on the common hepatic artery and portal vein. A second venous bypass circuit is shown on the patient's left to shunt IVC blood flow back to the heart during perfusion. Axillary V, axillary vein; Gastroduodenal art, gastroduodenal artery; Sup. mesenteric V, superior mesenteric vein; Saphenous V, saphenous vein; Veno-Veno Bypass, venovenous bypass.

hepatic artery is created via a catheter placed retrograde into the gastroduodenal artery. Complete isolation of the liver is achieved by placing a vascular clamp across the suprahepatic vena cava.

The perfusion circuit for the open technique consists of a roller pump, membrane oxygenator, and a heat exchanger. The 1-L perfusate consists of a balanced salt solution and 1 unit of packed red blood cells. Arterial and venous blood gases are monitored throughout the perfusion to maintain a perfusate pH between 7.2 and 7.3. The heat exchanger is utilized to warm the perfusate to maintain hepatic parenchymal temperatures between 38.5°C and 40°C. Flow rates of greater than 400 mL per minute should be achieved and optimal flow rates are 600 mL/min to 800 mL/min. The perfusion continues for 60 minutes and then the liver is flushed with crystalloid and colloid. The vascular structures are decannulated and repaired and normal liver perfusion is restored. Because complete vascular isolation can be consistently achieved in IHP, a leak monitoring system is not necessary.

Technique of Percutaneous Hepatic Perfusion

PHP has particular advantages because it requires only percutaneous access and treatments can be repeated. In contrast to IHP, PHP does not achieve complete vascular isolation of the organ and some leak of therapeutic agent into the systemic circulations occurs. With PHP, the therapeutic agent is administered into the proper hepatic artery via a percutaneously placed catheter and the chemotherapy containing hepatic venous effluent collected, filtered, and then returned to systemic circulation. PHP usually is administered with the patient under general anesthesia in an interventional radiology suite or an operating room that has fluoroscopic imaging ability. A right subclavian vein or jugular venous catheter serves as the site for return of blood to the systemic circulation from the extracorporeal filtration system. A femoral artery cannulation is performed and a catheter is advanced into the proper hepatic artery for infusion of chemotherapy. At the initial procedure a visceral angiogram is performed and the gastroduodenal artery and other nearby accessory vessels are embolized. On occasion, aberrant hepatic arterial anatomy is encountered that requires infusion of melphalan into 2 feeding arteries sequentially by repositioning the inflow catheter midway through treatment. A double-balloon catheter is advanced into the retrohepatic vena cava from the femoral vein (**Fig. 4**). The PHP venous catheter has several unique design features that allow the hepatic venous effluent to be isolated, collected, and filtered through an extracorporeal filtration system before being returned to the systemic circulation.

The cephalad balloon is inflated with dilute contrast containing saline and seated under fluoroscopic control at the atrial-caval junction and the caudal balloon is inflated just above the renal veins to isolate the retrohepatic IVC (see **Fig. 4**). A venovenous centrifugal pump is used to obtain flow rates of approximately 500 mL/min to 600 mL/min. Once this is accomplished, the filtration system is brought on-line.

A melphalan dose of 3 mg/kg of ideal body weight (maximum dose of 200 mg) is delivered over 30 minutes. After the melphalan infusion is completed, filtration of hepatic venous effluent continues for an additional 30 minutes. Then the filtration system is stopped, the balloons are deflated, and the venous catheters are removed.

PHP is a complex procedure that has some potential risks associated with it. During the PHP procedure, when the venous balloons are inflated and when the filters in the bypass circuit are activated, hypotension occurs and is treated with cardiopressor support, such as norepinephrine, phenylephrine, or both. The anesthetic management of the hemodynamic and metabolic alterations that occur during PHP has been

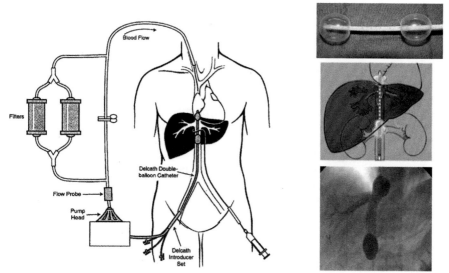

Fig. 4. Diagram of PHP circuit (Delcath). Melphalan is administered into the proper hepatic artery through a catheter placed via the femoral artery. Hepatic venous outflow is isolated via a double-balloon catheter in the retrohepatic IVC (*right panels*). Blood is drawn out of the retro hepatic IVC through multiple fenestrations located along the length of the catheter between the cranial and caudal balloons. Effluent blood then is pumped through a pair of activated charcoal filters prior to return to the systemic circulation via an internal jugular vein catheter. *Right Panels:* Upper right, double balloon catheter; Middle Right, diagram of double balloon catheter in retrohepatic IVC; Bottom right, radiographic Image of Double Balloon Catheter in IVC.

described.[38] During the first 24 hours, a resuscitation pathway is followed for correction of coagulopathy with fresh frozen plasma and platelets.

RESULTS OF HEPATIC PERFUSION FOR PATIENTS WITH COLORECTAL CANCER

Most data related to treatment of patients with CRC metastases surround IHP. In a Dutch study conducted at the Leiden University Medical Center, a retrospective analysis of 154 eligible patients was performed with 105 patients ultimately undergoing IHP.[39] The hepatic response rate was 50% and median duration of response was 11.4 months in 97 assessable patients. Ultimately, almost all 97 patients, save 4, did experience disease progression. Median overall survival was 24.8 months. In a 2009 study at the National Cancer Institute, similar results were reported[40]; 120 patients with unresectable isolated CRC liver metastases were treated with a 60-minute hyperthermic IHP with melphalan, TNF-α, or both. Median overall survival in the cohort was 17.4 months. Overall radiographic response was observed in 61% of patients and median time to in-liver hepatic progression-free survival was 7 months.

There are 2 important similarities between the 2 studies, both of which report outcomes in large patient cohorts. First, both reported longer duration of hepatic progression-free survival when patients were treated with some form of post-IHP therapy. Patients who received HAI postoperatively had a significantly longer hepatic progression-free survival of 13 months versus 5.8 months. There also was a significant difference in progression-free survival between patients receiving adjuvant systemic chemotherapy (13.6 months) and those not (6.8 months). These findings suggest that postperfusion treatment should be considered after IHP.

There are data that support the use of IHP as second-line therapy (see **Table 1**). Analysis of a 25 patient cohort at the National Cancer Institute reported no significant difference in response rates when IHP was administered in chemotherapy naïve patients versus in those receiving IHP as second-line therapy.[41] van Iersel and colleagues,[39] reported, however, that absence of systemic chemotherapy before IHP was a positive prognostic factor for progression-free survival. Certainly, the data show that IHP has meaningful clinical activity when used as initial or second-line treatment. Results of IHP using melphalan and hyperthermia administered to the 25 patients who experienced tumor progression after second-line therapy with irinotecan reported a 60% radiographic response and a median response duration of 13.2 months (see **Fig. 2**).[41]

Common post-IHP toxicities included transient hyperbilirubinemia, elevated transaminases, and coagulopathy. Complications included bleeding, pleural effusion, atrial fibrillation, ascites, sepsis, and splenic rupture. Mortality after IHP ranges from 4% to 7%.[39–41]

RESULTS OF ISOLATED HEPATIC PERFUSION IN PATIENTS WITH LIVER METASTASES FROM OCULAR MELANOMA

A retrospective analysis of outcomes in 31 patients with liver metastases from uveal melanoma treated with IHP recently has been reported.[42] Median progression-free survival was only 6 months and median overall survival was 10 months. The investigators suggested that IHP may prolong overall survival because previously reported studies using other treatment methods have demonstrated overall survival of 3.6 months to 15 months. In a phase I–II study, 22 ocular melanoma patients with liver metastases were treated with IHP using melphalan with or without TNF-α.[43] A 62% response rate was observed with a median response duration of 14 months. Median overall survival was 11 months. A follow-up report with 7 additional patients showed similar response rates.[41] Finally, in an 8-patient cohort, Noter and colleagues[44] observed a median time to progression of 6.7 months and median survival of 9.9 months after treatment with IHP. Together, these results demonstrate that IHP results in high initial response rates that generally are of short duration in patients with ocular melanoma. Response rates and overall survival seem better than historical controls of patients undergoing other forms of systemic therapy but are similar to outcomes seen with other regional hepatic treatments.[45]

PERCUTANEOUS HEPATIC PERFUSION

Although IHP has high response rates against various histologies, the technical demands and duration of procedure are substantial. Moreover, it has the potential for morbidity and mortality.[46] PHP is a less invasive alternative to IHP that takes advantage of endovascular techniques to deliver targeted chemotherapy to the liver. In contrast to IHP, PHP can be repeated. It does not, however, completely isolate the blood flow to the liver so that systemic toxicities from therapy can be clinically significant. In a 2005 report, Pingpank and colleagues[47] analyzed the safety and efficacy of PHP in 28 patients with a range of primary histologies, including ocular melanoma, CRC, neuroendocrine tumor, and pancreatic adenocarcinoma. The study determined that PHP can be safely performed with a maximum safe tolerated dose of 3 mg/kg of melphalan based on ideal body weight. Furthermore, the average filtration efficiency of hepatic effluent was determined to be 75.8% resulting in dramatically reduced systemic chemotherapy concentrations. The investigators observed a "10 fold increase in the hepatic versus systemic Cmax of melphalan at the maximum tolerated dose."

The results of a multicenter prospective random assignment trial comparing PHP to best alternative care (BAC) in patients with diffuse ocular melanoma liver metastases has been reported.[48]; 40 patients were treated with PHP and 49 were treated with BAC, which included systemic chemotherapy, chemoembolization, radioembolization, or supportive care. The study design allowed crossover of patients in the BAC arm with disease progression to undergo PHP. Median hepatic progression-free survival was significantly longer in the PHP versus BAC groups (7 months vs 1.6 months, respectively) (Fig. 5). Although the median time to liver progression in the BAC group was 1.6 months, the 25 patients who crossed over into the PHP group demonstrated a median time to liver progression of 8.4 months after PHP and a median overall survival of 13.1 months. Karydis and colleagues[49] reported the safety and efficacy of PHP in 51 patients with uveal melanoma and showed an overall response rate of 47%, a median overall survival rate of 15.3 months, and progression-free survival of 8.1 months. Taken together, these studies indicate that PHP is a viable, less invasive alternative to IHP that can be used to manage hepatic metastases in select patients (see **Table 1**). Common toxicities from PHP include included anemia, thrombocytopenia, elevated transaminases, hypoalbuminemia, and neutropenia.[47–49]

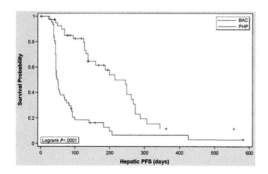

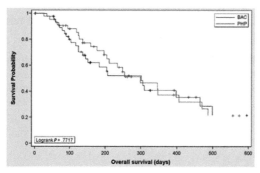

Fig. 5. Actuarial hepatic progression-free survival (PFS) (*top panel*) and overall survival (*bottom panel*) in patients with diffuse liver metastases from melanoma randomly assigned to receive PHP versus BAC. Patients who underwent PHP had significantly longer hepatic PFS, the primary endpoint of the study. (*Adapted from* Hughes MS, Zager J, Faries M, et al. Results of a Randomized Controlled Multicenter Phase III Trial of Percutaneous Hepatic Perfusion Compared with Best Available Care for Patients with Melanoma Liver Metastases. Ann Surg Oncol. 2016;23(4):1309-1319.)

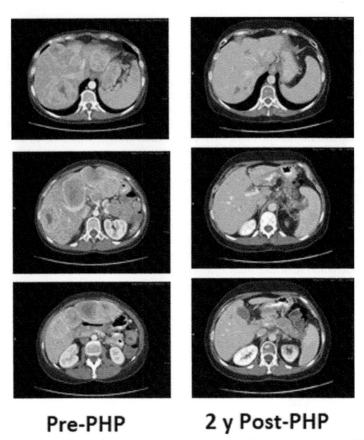

Pre-PHP   2 y Post-PHP

Fig. 6. Gadolinium-enhanced magnetic resonance images from a patient with diffuse liver metastases from neuroendocrine cancer before (*left panels*) and corresponding images taken 24 months after 2 PHP treatments (*right panels*).

RESULTS OF HEPATIC PERFUSION FOR PATIENTS WITH LIVER METASTASES FROM NEUROENDOCRINE TUMOR

In a 2004 article by Grover and colleagues,[50] 13 patients were enrolled in a study analyzing the effects of IHP with melphalan only or melphalan with TNF-α. The investigators found an overall response rate of 50% with a median hepatic progression-free survival of 9 months and median actuarial overall survival of 48 months (**Fig. 6**). Common toxicities and morbidities were like previous studies and included elevated transaminases, elevated creatinine, pleural effusion, thrombocytopenia, and arrhythmia.

SUMMARY

In summary, IHP and PHP have shown promising results in patients with liver metastases from varying histologies. The main advantage of these regional therapies is the ability to deliver targeted chemotherapy to the liver while limiting systemic toxicity. For select patients where systemic chemotherapy fails to significantly alter the trajectory of illness, regional therapies can prolong progression-free survival and improve quality of life. The authors recommend that IHP and PHP be considered in the treatment options for patients with unresectable liver metastases that prove challenging to manage medically.

CLINICS CARE POINTS

- Dual blood supply to the liver and liver metastases' almost exclusive blood supply from the hepatic artery, allows for targeted delivery of chemotherapeutic agents and avoidance of systemic toxicities.
- While Percutaneous Hepatic Perfusion does not achieve complete isolation and some leak of the chemotherapeutic agent occurs, it can be performed several times and may be associated with fewer adverse effects than IHP.
- Intrahepatic arterial perfusion has shown promising results in both the initial and second-line treatment of CRC liver metastases.

DISCLOSURE

The authors have nothing to disclose.

REFERENCES

1. Leporrier J, Maurel J, Chiche L, et al. A population-based study of the incidence, management and prognosis of hepatic metastases from colorectal cancer. Br J Surg 2006;93(4):465–74.
2. Scheele J, Stangl R, Altendorf-Hofmann A. Hepatic metastases from colorectal carcinoma: impact of surgical resection on the natural history. Br J Surg 1990; 77:1241–6.
3. Fuchs CS, Marshall J, Mitchell E, et al. Randomized, controlled trial of irinotecan plus infusional, bolus, or oral fluoropyrimidines in first-line treatment of metastatic colorectal cancer: results from the BICC-C Study. J Clin Oncol 2007;25(30): 4779–86.
4. Goldberg RM, Sargent DJ, Morton RF, et al. A randomized controlled trial of fluorouracil plus leucovorin, irinotecan, and oxaliplatin combinations in patients with previously untreated metastatic colorectal cancer. J Clin Oncol 2004;22(1):23–30.
5. Hurwitz H, Fehrenbacher L, Novotny W, et al. Bevacizumab plus irinotecan, fluorouracil, and leucovorin for metastatic colorectal cancer. N Engl J Med 2004; 350(23):2335–42.
6. Saltz LB, Clarke S, az-Rubio E, et al. Bevacizumab in combination with oxaliplatin-based chemotherapy as first-line therapy in metastatic colorectal cancer: a randomized phase III study. J Clin Oncol 2008;26(12):2013–9.
7. Tournigand C, Andre T, Achille E, et al. FOLFIRI followed by FOLFOX6 or the reverse sequence in advanced colorectal cancer: a randomized GERCOR study. J Clin Oncol 2004;22(2):229–37.
8. Tournigand C, Cervantes A, Figer A, et al. OPTIMOX1: a randomized study of FOLFOX4 or FOLFOX7 with oxaliplatin in a stop-and-Go fashion in advanced colorectal cancer–a GERCOR study. J Clin Oncol 2006;24(3):394–400.
9. van CE, Kohne CH, Hitre E, et al. Cetuximab and chemotherapy as initial treatment for metastatic colorectal cancer. N Engl J Med 2009;360(14):1408–17.
10. Cunningham D, Humblet Y, Siena S, et al. Cetuximab monotherapy and cetuximab plus irinotecan in irinotecan-refractory metastatic colorectal cancer. N Engl J Med 2004;351(4):337–45.

11. Oki E, Kato T, Bando H, et al. A multicenter clinical phase II Study of FOLFOXIRI plus bevacizumab as first-line therapy in patients with metastatic colorectal cancer: QUATTRO Study. Clin Colorectal Cancer 2018;17(2):147–55.
12. Loupakis F, Cremolini C, Masi G, et al. Initial therapy with FOLFOXIRI and bevacizumab for metastatic colorectal cancer. N Engl J Med 2014;371(17):1609–18.
13. Bedikian AY, Legha SS, Mavligit G, et al. Treatment of uveal melanoma metastatic to the liver: a review of the M. D. Anderson Cancer Center experience and prognostic factors. Cancer 1995;76(9):1665–70.
14. Bedikian AY, Papadopoulos N, Plager C, et al. Phase II evaluation of temozolomide in metastatic choroidal melanoma. Melanoma Res 2003;13(3):303–6.
15. Pyrhonen S, Hahka-Kemppinen M, Muhonen T, et al. Chemoimmunotherapy with bleomycin, vincristine, lomustine, dacarbazine (BOLD), and human leukocyte interferon for metastatic uveal melanoma. Cancer 2002;95(11):2366–72.
16. Mariani P, Piperno-Neumann S, Servois V, et al. Surgical management of liver metastases from uveal melanoma: 16 years' experience at the Institut Curie. Eur J Surg Oncol 2009;35(11):1192–7.
17. Pawlik TM, Zorzi D, Abdalla EK, et al. Hepatic resection for metastatic melanoma: distinct patterns of recurrence and prognosis for ocular versus cutaneous disease. Ann Surg Oncol 2006;13(5):712–20.
18. Rivoire M, Kodjikian L, Baldo S, et al. Treatment of liver metastases from uveal melanoma. Ann Surg Oncol 2005;12(6):422–8.
19. Chamberlain RS, Canes D, Brown KT, et al. Hepatic neuroendocrine metastases: does intervention alter outcomes? J Am Coll Surg 2000;190(4):432–45.
20. Kvols LK, Moertel CG, O'Connell MJ, Schutt AJ, Rubin J, Hahn RG. Treatment of the malignant carcinoid syndrome. Evaluation of a long-acting somatostatin analogue. N Engl J Med 1986;315(11):663–6.
21. Breedis C, Young G. Blood supply of neoplasms of the liver. Am J Pathol 1954;30:969–85.
22. Carrel A, Lindbergh CA. THE CULTURE OF WHOLE ORGANS. Science 1935;81(2112):621–3. https://doi.org/10.1126/science.81.2112.621. PMID: 17733174.
23. Gibbon JH. Development of Artificial Heart and Lung Extracorporeal Blood Circuit. J Am Med Assoc 1968;206(9):1983.
24. Goodman LS, Wintrobe MM, Dameshek W, et al. Nitrogen Mustard Therapy - Use of Methyl-Bis(Beta-Chloroethyl)Amine Hydrochloride and Tris(Beta-Chloroethyl) Amine Hydrochloride for Hodgkins Disease, Lymphosarcoma, Leukemia and Certain Allied and Miscellaneous Disorders. JAMA 1946;132(3):126–32.
25. Creech O, Krementz ET, Ryan RF, et al. Chemotherapy of cancer: regional perfusion utilizing an extracorporeal circuit. Ann Surg 1958;148:616–32.
26. Stehlin JS. Hyperthermic perfusion with chemotherapy for cancers of the extremities. Surg Gynecol Obstet 1969;129:305–8.
27. Lienard D, Ewalenko P, Delmotte JJ, et al. High dose recombinant tumor necrosis factor alpha in combination with interferon gamma and melphalan in isolation perfusion of the limbs for melanoma and sarcoma. J Clin Oncol 1992;10:52–60.
28. Ausman RK. Development of a technic for isolated perfusion of the liver. N Y State J Med 1961;61:3393–7.
29. Ausman RK, Aust JB. Studies in isolated perfusion chemotherapy. I. Nitrogen mustard. Ann Surg 1961;153:527–32.
30. Aigner K, Walther H, Tonn J, et al. First experimental and clinical results of isolated liver perfusion with cytotoxics in metastases from colorectal primary. Recent Results Cancer Res 1983;86:99–102.

31. Schwemmle K, Link KH, Rieck B. Rationale and indications for perfusion in liver tumors: current data. World J Surg 1987;11(4):534–40.

32. Skibba JL, Quebbeman EJ. Tumoricidal effects and patient survival after hyperthermic liver perfusion. Arch Surg 1986;121:1266–71.

33. Fraker DL, Alexander HR. Isolated limb perfusion with high-dose tumor necrosis factor for extremity melanoma and sarcoma. In: DeVita VTJ, Hellman S, Rosenberg SA, editors. Important advances in oncology. Philadelphia: J.B. Lippincott; 1994. p. 179–92.

34. Alexander HR, Bartlett DL, Libutti SK, et al. Isolated hepatic perfusion with tumor necrosis factor and melphalan for unresectable cancers confined to the liver. J Clin Oncol 1998;16:1479–89.

35. Hafström LR, Holmberg SB, Naredi PLJ, et al. Isolated hyperthermic liver perfusion with chemotherapy for liver malignancy. Surg Oncol 1994;3:103–8.

36. Lindnér P, Fjälling M, Hafström L, et al. Isolated hepatic perfusion with extracorporeal oxygenation using hyperthermia, tumour necrosis factor alpha and melphalan. Eur J Surg Oncol 1999;25:179–85.

37. Marinelli A, Vahrmeijer AL, van de Velde CJ. Phase I/II studies of isolated hepatic perfusion with mitomycin C or melphalan in patients with colorectal cancer hepatic metastases. Recent Results Cancer Res 1998;147:83–94.

38. Miao N, Pingpank JF, Alexander HR, et al. Percutaneous hepatic perfusion in patients with metastatic liver cancer: anesthetic, hemodynamic, and metabolic considerations. Ann Surg Oncol 2008;15(3):815–23.

39. van Iersel LB, Gelderblom H, Vahrmeijer AL, et al. Isolated hepatic melphalan perfusion of colorectal liver metastases: outcome and prognostic factors in 154 patients. Ann Oncol 2008;19(6):1127–34.

40. Alexander HR Jr, Bartlett DL, Libutti SK, et al. Analysis of factors associated with outcome in patients undergoing isolated hepatic perfusion for unresectable liver metastases from colorectal center. Ann Surg Oncol 2009;16(7):1852–9.

41. Alexander HR Jr, Libutti SK, Pingpank JF, et al. Isolated hepatic perfusion for the treatment of patients with colorectal cancer liver metastases after irinotecan-based therapy. Ann Surg Oncol 2005;12(2):138–44.

42. de Leede EM, Burgmans MC, Kapiteijn E, et al. Isolated (hypoxic) hepatic perfusion with high-dose chemotherapy in patients with unresectable liver metastases of uveal melanoma: results from two experienced centres. Melanoma Res 2016; 26(6):588–94.

43. Alexander HR, Libutti SK, Bartlett DL, et al. A Phase I-II study of isolated hepatic perfusion using melphalan with or without tumor necrosis factor for patients with ocular melanoma metastatic to liver. Clin Cancer Res 2000;6:3062–70.

44. Noter SL, Rothbarth J, Pijl ME, et al. Isolated hepatic perfusion with high-dose melphalan for the treatment of uveal melanoma metastases confined to the liver. Melanoma Res 2004;14(1):67–72.

45. Reddy SK, Kesmodel SB, Alexander HR Jr. Isolated hepatic perfusion for patients with liver metastases. Ther Adv Med Oncol 2014;6(4):180–94.

46. Burgmans MC, de Leede EM, Martini CH, et al. Percutaneous Isolated Hepatic Perfusion for the Treatment of Unresectable Liver Malignancies. Cardiovasc Intervent Radiol 2016;39(6):801–14.

47. Pingpank JF, Libutti SK, Chang R, et al. Phase I study of hepatic arterial melphalan infusion and hepatic venous hemofiltration using percutaneously placed catheters in patients with unresectable hepatic malignancies. J Clin Oncol 2005;23(15):3465–74.

48. Hughes MS, Zager J, Faries M, et al. Results of a Randomized Controlled Multicenter Phase III Trial of Percutaneous Hepatic Perfusion Compared with Best Available Care for Patients with Melanoma Liver Metastases. Ann Surg Oncol 2016;23(4):1309–19.
49. Karydis I, Gangi A, Wheater MJ, et al. Percutaneous hepatic perfusion with melphalan in uveal melanoma: A safe and effective treatment modality in an orphan disease. J Surg Oncol 2018;117:1170–8.
50. Grover AC, Libutti SK, Pingpank JF, et al. Isolated hepatic perfusion for the treatment of patients with advanced liver metastases from pancreatic and gastrointestinal neuroendocrine neoplasms. Surgery 2004;136(6):1176–82.
51. Grover A, Alexander HR Jr. The past decade of experience with isolated hepatic perfusion. Oncologist 2004;9(6):653–64.

Systemic Therapy Improvements Will Render Locoregional Treatments Obsolete for Patients with Cancer with Liver Metastases

Satya Das, MD, MSCI*, Jordan Berlin, MD

KEYWORDS

- Systemic therapy • Immunotherapy • Chemoembolization • Radioembolization
- Hepatic debulking • Liver metastases

KEY POINTS

- Outside of curative resection of hepatic metastases, locoregional therapy for liver metastases has not demonstrated benefit over systemic therapy in patients with neuroendocrine tumor, hepatobiliary, or colorectal cancer.
- Although studies reporting on patients with neuroendocrine tumor treated with hepatic debulking (even incomplete resections) present impressive survival data, these analyses do not include patients treated with newer systemic standards such as peptide receptor radionuclide therapy.
- In diseases such as hepatocellular carcinoma or colorectal cancer, embolization therapy has not added any survival benefit for patients when combined with standard-of-care systemic therapies. In other diseases such as cholangiocarcinoma, the survival benefit of embolization therapy in combination with systemic therapy, is approximated by novel systemic therapy combinations.
- Advances in systemic therapy for gastrointestinal and indeed all patients with cancer have been driven by the identification of targetable biological subgroups, the development of more potent therapeutics, and the widespread adoption of immunotherapy.

BACKGROUND

Systemic therapies across the spectrum of cancer have improved dramatically over the last decade, largely driven by the development of more potent therapeutics and a greater understanding of molecular drivers of disease. Still, liver metastases and

Department of Medicine, Division of Hematology Oncology, Vanderbilt University Medical Center, 777 Preston Research Building, 2220 Pierce Avenue, Nashville, TN 37232, USA
* Corresponding author.
E-mail address: Satya.das@vumc.org
Twitter: @nanudasmd (S.D.); @jordanberlin5 (J.B.)

Surg Oncol Clin N Am 30 (2021) 189–204
https://doi.org/10.1016/j.soc.2020.08.008
surgonc.theclinics.com

downstream complications of hepatic infiltration remain a major driver of mortality in this patient cohort. In rare circumstances, such as oligometastatic disease in colorectal cancer (CRC), a defined role for resection (metastasectomy) exists, whereas in most other circumstances, practice patterns pertaining to management of hepatic disease vary dramatically. Locoregional treatments, or liver-directed therapies and debulking surgery, are used routinely in patients without clear evidence of any survival benefit. Herein, using gastrointestinal malignancies as their backdrop, the authors argue that systemic treatment advances will render locoregional hepatic therapies obsolete within the next decade. In the following paragraphs, the authors canvass the evidence used to justify locoregional approaches in neuroendocrine tumors (NETs), hepatobiliary cancer, and CRC; discuss the landmark studies that define the current state of systemic therapy for these diseases; and highlight pending advances that build the case for systemic treatment being the preferred approach over locoregional treatment in patients with liver metastases in the near future.

NEUROENDOCRINE TUMORS

Hepatic debulking has been thought to be most optimal in patients with NET with liver-limited metastatic disease.[1,2] Its role in patients with unresectable extrahepatic disease is more controversial. The authors describe briefly the primary studies that have been cited as justification for hepatic debulking before providing perspective on more recent studies, which suggest systemic treatment approaches may be equally effective. In a 15-year single-center experience from Gustave-Roussy, 47 patients with well-differentiated NETs underwent hepatectomies for liver metastases.[3] Of these patients, 51% had nonpancreatic NETs, whereas 49% had pancreatic NETs. In addition to undergoing hepatic tumor resections, 77% also underwent extrahepatic disease resection. An R0 resection was achieved in 53% of patients, although 97% of tumors were removed in each patient. Median survival was 91 months with a 5-year survival rate of 71%. At 10 years, 75% of patients had recurred in the liver. A retrospective analysis of cases collected from a multicenter database compared outcomes in patients with well-differentiated NET with hepatic metastases who underwent surgical cytoreduction versus hepatic embolization.[4] Of the 120 patients, 61 underwent surgical cytoreduction, whereas 59 underwent embolization. The patients who underwent surgery experienced a mean survival of 43 ± 26 months compared with 24 ± 16 months in patients who underwent embolization (P<.001). Of the surgical patients, 62% were able to undergo R0 resections, whereas the remaining patients had incomplete resections. When separating outcomes by completeness of resection, patients with both R0 and incomplete resections demonstrated improved survival compared with patients undergoing embolization; patients with R0 resections demonstrated the best overall survival (OS) (50 ± 28 months) followed by patients who underwent incomplete resections (32 ± 19 months).

In another large multicenter retrospective analysis, outcomes in 339 patients with NET who underwent hepatic resection between 1985 and 2009 were analyzed.[5] Of these patients, 52.2% had low- or intermediate-grade tumors, 15% had high-grade tumors, and 32.7% had tumors of unknown grade. Most patients (83.8%) had liver-limited disease, whereas the remainder had extrahepatic disease. Among all patients who underwent initial resections, 53.7% achieved R0 resections. The median time to first recurrence postresection was 15.2 months in the entire cohort. The 1-, 3-, and 5-year progression-free survival (PFS) of included cases were 56.9%, 24.2%, and 5.9%, respectively. No difference in recurrence rates were identified between patients who did and did not undergo R0 resections. Median OS of patients with extrahepatic disease was 85.1 months compared with 148 months in patients with liver limited disease ($P<.001$). On multivariate analysis, extrahepatic disease presence was the strongest negative prognostic influence for patients.

Focusing solely on embolization in patients with hepatic metastases from NETs, only one small randomized study comparing between modalities (chemo-, bland-) has been reported to date.[6] In this study, 26 patients with well-differentiated G1 or G2 small intestinal NET with progressive disease were randomized to bland embolization or chemoembolization. No differences in PFS were seen between the 2 arms (23.6 months vs 19.2 months; $P = .9$). A larger prospective study comparing between embolization modalities is ongoing; however, it will not report findings until at least 2023 [NCT02724540].

An important caveat of all these studies was they occurred before the regular utilization of the 2 most potent cytoreductive systemic options available to patients with well-differentiated NET: peptide receptor radionuclide therapy (PRRT) and capecitabine plus temozolomide (CAPTEM). Furthermore, most of the previously discussed studies do not mention the number of patients at baseline with progressive disease, making it difficult to discern the true benefit of the locoregional therapy used. PRRT has been a transformative therapy for patients with metastatic or unresectable somatostatin receptor-avid neuroendocrine tumors. In a post-hoc analysis from the NETTER-1 study, which garnered ^{177}Lu-DOTATATE its Food and Drug Administration (FDA) approval, the hazard ratio (HR) for disease progression in patients with small intestinal NET, regardless of hepatic tumor burden (<25%, 25%–50%, >50%), was 19.[7,8] The 30-month PFS rate was greater than 75%. From a large Dutch registry study of 443 patients with gastroenteropancreatic, bronchial, and unknown primary NET treated with ^{177}Lu-DOTATATE, median OS was 63 months.[9] Of the patients included in the analysis, 53.9% had progressive disease at baseline. In patients with pancreatic NETs, median OS was the longest at 71 months, whereas in small intestinal NETs, median OS was 60 months. Patients with liver or bone metastases had an inferior median OS of 57 months. The median PFS in the entire cohort was 29 months.

^{177}Lu-DOTATATE uses a beta-emitting radionuclide that elicits objective response in 18% to 39% of patients with NET. Although its biggest benefit is in preventing tumor progression, the extent of cytoreduction it can generate is modest. Newer generation PRRT agents using alpha particles or somatostatin receptor antagonists have demonstrated the potential to create greater tumor death in preclinical studies.[10] Alpha particles such as actinium-225 (^{225}Ac) and bismuth-213 (^{213}Bi) possess a higher linear energy transfer than beta-emitting particles and have a shorter range of action, suggesting they can generate greater amounts of double strand breaks and irreversible DNA damage.[11] Clinical experience with ^{225}Ac was reported in 32 patients with stable (44%) or progressive disease (56%) posttreatment with ^{177}Lu-DOTATATE.[12] Of the treated patients, 62.5% achieved a partial response and 100% achieved disease control. Somatostatin antagonists such as ^{177}Lu-satoreotide tetraxetan have demonstrated increased uptake and retention in NET cells compared with agonists, suggesting the possibility that they could lead to greater cell kill.[13] This preclinical rationale has led to a phase I study with ^{177}Lu-satoreotide tetraxetan, with initial results suggesting a response rate of 45% in treated patients.[14]

CAPTEM has become another cornerstone systemic cytoreductive therapy for patients with NET. In a randomized trial in patients with well-differentiated pancreatic NET with progressive disease within 12 months of study enrollment, PFS in patients who received the combination was 22.7 months.[15] Median OS was not reached in the combination arm; however, greater than 80% of patients were alive at 50 months. In smaller series, CAPTEM demonstrated activity in patients with small bowel NET with median PFS times greater than 22 months.[16] Beyond CAPTEM and PRRT, novel cyto-reductive tyrosine kinase inhibitors such as cabozantinib and lenvatinib have demonstrated sustained PFS benefit in patients with metastatic well-differentiated NET along with promising cytoreductive potential. In a multicohort phase II study of patients with well-differentiated NET with baseline progressive disease, patients with pancreatic NET, and small intestinal NET treated with lenvatinib experienced a PFS of 15.5 months and 15.4 months, respectively.[17] Similarly, in a phase II study of cabozantinib in patients with progressive well-differentiated NET, patients with pancreatic NETs and small intestinal NETs achieved PFS times of 21.8 months and 31.4 months, respectively.[18]

Although in general, surgical debulking and embolization seem to elicit greater response rates in patients with NETs than systemic therapies, there do not seem to be differences in the more relevant endpoints of PFS and OS between the modalities (**Table 1**). Furthermore, recent systemic treatments such as ^{177}Lu-DOTATATE prolong disease progression and survival in patients to a greater extent than has previously been observed with locoregional treatments. Newer iterations of PRRT (alpha-emitting particles, somatostatin receptor antagonists) and emerging combinations with the more cytoreductive tyrosine kinase inhibitors offer the potential for even greater benefit and should replace locoregional therapy for NET patients with liver metastases within the next decade.

HEPATOBILIARY CANCERS

In hepatocellular carcinoma (HCC), locoregional therapies currently have a defined role for a small subset of patients. Apart from patients who are able to undergo resection (patients with liver-limited disease, no vascular invasion, and adequate hepatic reserve), in whom there is potential for long-term survival, the benefit from liver-directed therapies seems to be more modest.[19] In an early study comparing chemoembolization to bland embolization, 112 patients with Child-Pugh A and B HCC were randomized between the 2 treatments.[20] The study was stopped early when a definitive survival benefit emerged in the chemoembolization arm (HR: 0.47, $P = .025$). The survival probabilities at 1 and 2 years were 82% and 63%, respectively. Other subsequent studies suggested a similar benefit of radioembolization with selective internal radiation therapy (SIRT) in HCC.[21] Based on these findings, both modalities were combined with sorafenib and compared against sorafenib monotherapy in randomized trials.

In the phase III SORAMIC study, 424 patients were randomized to sorafenib plus SIRT versus sorafenib alone.[22] No difference in OS was appreciated between the 2 arms (12.1 months for the combination arm vs 11.4 months for the monotherapy arm, $P = .953$). Based on these data, there is no proven role for SIRT off a clinical trial in this disease. Grade 3/4 adverse events were reported in 64.8% of patients in the combination arm compared with 53.8% of patients in the sorafenib arm ($P = .04$). In the phase III STAH trial, 339 patients were randomized to chemoembolization plus sorafenib versus sorafenib monotherapy.[23] No difference in OS was appreciated between the 2 arms (12.8 months for the combination arm vs 10.6 months for the monotherapy arm, $P = .29$). Serious adverse events ($\geq$grade 3) occurred in 33.3% of the combination-treated patients compared with 19.8% of patients in the sorafenib monotherapy arm ($P = .006$).

The systemic treatment armamentarium for HCC has changed dramatically over the last 5 years, with multiple FDA drug approvals and others pending. Sorafenib, which had been the gold standard of systemic therapy in this disease for several years,

Table 1
Outcomes in patients with neuroendocrine tumor treated with systemic therapy and liver-directed therapy

Treatment	Patient Population	Sample Size	Study Type	Endpoint (OS and PFS Median Unless Otherwise Specified)
¹⁷⁷Lu-DOTATATE Plus Octreotide vs High-Dose Octreotide[7]	Midgut NETs	229	Randomized Trial	OS: NR vs 27.4 mo; PFS: HR: 0.21 (95% CI .14–.33)
¹⁷⁷Lu-DOTATATE[9]	Pancreatic NETs Midgut NETs	133 181	Cohort Analysis	OS: 71 mo OS: 60 mo
CAPTEM vs Temozolomide[15]	Pancreatic NETs	144	Randomized Trial	PFS: 22.7 mo vs 14.4 mo (HR: 0.58, P = .023); OS: NR vs 38 mo (HR: 0.41, P = .012)
Cabozantinib[18]	Pancreatic NETs Midgut NETs	20 41	Single-Arm Prospective Trial	PFS: 21.8 mo (95% CI 8.5–32) PFS: 31.4 mo (95% CI 8.5-NR)
Lenvatinib[17]	Pancreatic NETs Midgut NETs	55 56	Single-Arm Prospective Trial	PFS: 15.5 mo (95% CI, 11.3-NR) PFS: 15.4 mo (95% CI, 11.5–19.4)
Chemoembolization vs Bland Embolization[6]	Progressive small intestinal NETs	26	Randomized Trial	PFS: 23.6 mo vs 19.2 mo (P = .9)
Hepatic Debulking vs Bland Embolization[4]	Well-differentiated NETs	120	Retrospective Analysis	Mean OS: 43 ± 26 mo vs 24 ± 15.8 mo (P<.001)

Abbreviations: 95% CI, 95% confidence interval; ¹⁷⁷Lu-DOTATATE, lutetium-177 DOTATATE; CAPTEM, capecitabine plus temozolomide; NR, not reached.

now faces significant competition from immunotherapy combinations and more potent tyrosine kinase inhibitors[24] (**Table 2**). Most recently, in the IMBrave150 randomized phase III study, atezolizumab plus bevacizumab demonstrated OS superiority compared with sorafenib in patients with treatment-naïve metastatic HCC.[25] In this 501-patient study, patients who received atezolizumab plus bevacizumab had an HR of 0.58 (P = .0006) for OS compared with patients treated with sorafenib. No significant difference in grade 3/4 adverse events occurred between the 2 arms (57% vs 55%). Lenvatinib was shown to be noninferior to sorafenib in a randomized phase III study (13.6 months vs 12.3 months) and demonstrated a greater objective response rate.[26] In the second-line setting, nivolumab plus ipilimumab has garnered accelerated approval for patients with HCC with progressive disease on sorafenib. From 49 patients in the cohort from Checkmate-040 treated with the combination, 33% achieved a partial response.[27] Duration of response ranged from 4.6 to 30.5 months with 31% lasting 24 months.

Many of these systemic therapies have only been trialed in patients with a significant burden of hepatic disease. It is plausible to believe that if used in lower volume settings, such as where embolization is routinely used, they would be even more effective. Furthermore, in the studies where embolization was added to the previous systemic standard-of-care sorafenib, it did not add any survival benefit. Now, with improved systemic therapies, it does not seem to be illogical to presume that these therapies would also be superior to embolization.

Based on case reports of efficacy in intrahepatic cholangiocarcinoma (CCA), a prospective single-arm phase II study of SIRT in combination with gemcitabine plus cisplatin was recently reported.[28] In this trial, 46 treatment-naïve patients with

Table 2
Comparison of reported first-line studies in patients with hepatocellular carcinoma and cholangiocarcinoma

Treatment	Patient Population	PFS (Median)	OS (Median)
Atezolizumab Plus Bevacizumab vs Sorafenib[25]	Treatment-naïve unresectable HCC patients	6.8 mo vs 4.5 mo (HR: 0.59, 95% CI 0.47–0.76)	NR vs 13.2 mo (HR: 0.58, 95% CI 0.42–0.79)
Lenvatinib vs Sorafenib[26]	Treatment-naïve unresectable HCC patients	7.4 mo vs 3.7 mo (HR: 0.66, 95% CI 0.57–0.77)	13.6 mo vs 12.3 mo (HR: 0.92, 95% CI 0.79–1.06)
Sorafenib Plus SIRT vs Sorafenib[22]	Treatment-naïve advanced HCC patients	5.2 mo vs 3.6 mo (HR: 0.73, 95% CI 0.59–.91)	12.8 vs 10.8 mo (HR: 0.91, 95% CI 0.69–1.21)
Sorafenib Plus Chemoembolization vs Sorafenib[23]	Systemic treatment-naïve advanced HCC patients	Not provided	12.1 mo vs 11.4 mo (HR: 1.01, 95% CI 0.81–1.25)
Gemcitabine Plus Cisplatin Plus SIRT[28]	Unresectable treatment-naïve CCA patients	14 mo (95% CI 8–17)	22 mo (95% CI 14–52)
Gemcitabine Plus Cisplatin Plus Nab-Paclitaxel[30]	Unresectable treatment-naïve CCA patients	11.8 mo (95% CI 6–15.6)	19.2 mo (95% CI 13.2 –NR)

Abbreviations: 95% CI, 95% confidence interval; CCA, cholangiocarcinoma; NR, not reached.

unresectable intrahepatic CCA were treated with SIRT (to either one or both liver lobes) plus gemcitabine plus cisplatin. The median OS of treated patients was 22 months with a 1-year OS rate of 75%. Of these patients, 9% were also able to be converted to surgical candidates. Although the absolute survival benefit seems to be an improvement over gemcitabine plus cisplatin (11.7 months in the ABC-02 trial), systemic therapy efficacy has not been reported in patients with cholangiocarcinoma specifically with liver-limited disease.[29] It is possible that the favorable disease biology of these patients was what led to the survival benefit compared with historical controls. Furthermore, novel systemic therapies in CCA may create the same degree of benefit as locoregional treatment combinations. A phase II study of gemcitabine, cisplatin, and nab-paclitaxel in patients with treatment-naïve CCA (38% with intrahepatic) elicited median OS times of 19.2 months.[30] A randomized phase III study of gemcitabine, cisplatin ± nab-paclitaxel is ongoing, and if the study is positive, this will establish a new first-line standard of care in patients with metastatic or unresectable biliary cancer [NCT02392637].

Broad molecular profiling efforts in CCA have revealed a significant proportion of actionable mutations, particularly in patients with intrahepatic CCA.[31] *IDH1* mutations and *FGFR2* fusions have been found in 30% and 15% of tumors, respectively, and targeted therapies directed toward both have demonstrated tremendous promise in refractory settings. In the randomized phase III study CLARIDHY, which enabled crossover, patients with *IDH1*-mutant CCA who received the IDH1 inhibitor ivosidenib had an HR of 0.37 (P<.001) for PFS.[32] In a phase I/II study, the FGFR2 inhibitor derazantinib elicited a PFS of 5.7 months and response rate of 20.7% in patients with treatment-refractory CCA with *FGFR2* fusions.[33] In another phase II study, the pan-FGFR inhibitor pemigatinib elicited a PFS of 6.9 months and response rate of 35.5% in patients with unresectable CCA with *FGFR2* fusions or rearrangements.[34] Both approaches suggest meaningful disease progression can be achieved in patients with CCA (with targetable mutations) with progression on first-line chemotherapy. In the unresectable setting for patients with CCA, it seems that improvements in systemic therapy already trump the potential of locoregional treatment. Furthermore, currently available agents targeting IDH1 and FGFR2 are first-generation drugs and the spectrum of resistance mechanisms are still being identified. Gatekeeper mutations that create acquired resistance to FGFR inhibitors have already begun to be identified. In a patient who progressed on pemigatinib, rapid autopsy revealed the presence of a *FGFR2* N549H tumor mutation.[35] It is conceivable within the next decade that newer generation FGFR2 inhibitors will be able to overcome such gatekeeper mutations akin to osimertinib in *EGFR*-mutant non–small cell lung adenocarcinoma.

COLORECTAL CANCER

Apart from resection of oligometastatic disease to the liver, which offers patients with CRC an opportunity for prolonged survival and cure, several other liver-directed approaches such as radioembolization, chemoembolization, hepatic arterial infusions (HAI), and stereotactic ablative radiation therapy (SABR) have been used, with varying degrees of evidence. A small 21-patient study that compared ^{90}Y-radioembolization plus systemic fluorouracil versus systemic fluorouracil in patients with metastatic CRC (86% who possessed liver-limited disease) found that patients treated with the combination experienced both time to progressive disease (18.6 months vs 3.6 months, P<.0005) and response rate benefit.[36] Other large nonrandomized prospective series have suggested a greater benefit from SIRT in patients with metastatic

CRC who are less pretreated.[37] Based on these signals, a series of phase III trials (FOXFIRE, SIRFLOX, and FOXFIRI-Global), designed to be analyzed in aggregate, randomized patients with treatment-naive metastatic CRC to FOLFOX plus SIRT (concurrent with cycle 1 or 2) or FOLFOX[38] Of the included patients, 65% had liver-limited disease. Median OS was no different between the 2 arms (22.6 months in the combination arm vs 23 months in the FOLFOX arm, $P = .61$). This study definitively proved there was no benefit to upfront addition of radioembolization to chemotherapy in treatment-naïve patients with metastatic CRC. As with HCC, there is no established role for this liver-directed therapy in CRC outside the auspices of a clinical trial.

In a large pooled analysis from Memorial Sloan Kettering Cancer Center (MSKCC), outcomes between 948 patients with metastatic CRC with liver involvement treated with HAI, chemoembolization, and SIRT were compared.[39] The HR for HAI compared with chemoembolization was 0.37, and the HR for HAI compared with SIRT was 0.45; this was consistent across patients with both liver-limited and extrahepatic disease. Further provocative data suggest the largest benefit of HAI may be in the perioperative setting for patients with CRC with resectable liver metastases. A 20-year single-center database analysis of patients with CRC with resectable liver metastases from MSKCC suggested that the median OS of patients treated with HAI was 67 months compared with 44 months in patients who were not treated with HAI.[40] Most patients (74%–97%) who were treated with HAI also received systemic chemotherapy. Although the OS observed in patients in this analysis was striking, a randomized phase II study of FOLFOXIRI $\pm$ panitumumab in patients with *RAS* wild-type treatment-naïve CRC produced similar outcomes.[41] In the cohort of patients with resectable liver metastases, patients treated with FOLFOXIRI and the biological agent experienced an OS of 52 months. HAI has never been compared in a randomized phase III trial against systemic chemotherapy in either patients with resectable or unresectable CRC liver metastases.

The randomized phase II trial SABR-COMET included 18 patients with metastatic CRC.[42] In this 99-patient study, patients were randomized to systemic therapy plus SABR to each metastatic site (up to 5) or systemic therapy alone. Patients in the experimental arm achieved OS times of 41 months compared with 28 months in the standard treatment arm (HR: 0.57, $P = .09$). By the prespecified statistical design, the study met statistical significance. The specific location of metastases in patients with primary tumor site was not provided in the original manuscript, thus it is unclear whether the findings are applicable to patients with liver-predominant CRC.

Some of the most profound advances in systemic therapy for CRC have occurred in molecular subsets previously considered to be poorly prognostic (microsatellite instability-high [MSI-H], *NTRK* fusions, BRAFV600E) (**Table 3**).[43] Pembrolizumab and nivolumab are FDA approved for patients with refractory MSI-H CRC who have progressed on prior therapy. Nivolumab elicited a response rate of 31.1%, 24-month PFS rate of just under 50%, and a median duration of response that had not yet been reached in treated patients.[44] Pembrolizumab produced a response rate of 33%, median OS of 31.4 months, and median duration of response that had not yet been reached in treated patients.[45] A recent press release from the Keynote-177 study, where pembrolizumab is being compared against FOLFOX-based chemotherapy in the first-line setting for patients with metastatic MSI-H CRC, suggests the immunotherapy-treated patients achieved a statistically significant improvement in PFS compared with chemotherapy-treated patients; the final OS data are still pending.[46] Beyond checkpoint inhibitor monotherapy, combining the checkpoint inhibitors nivolumab and ipilimumab has also been shown to be effective in refractory MSI-H CRC.[47] Nivolumab plus ipilimumab has also been tested in patients with

Table 3
Outcomes in patients with colorectal cancer with actionable mutations

Study Population	Treatment	Sample Size	Study Type	Endpoint (OS and PFS Median Unless Otherwise Specified)
Pretreated MSI-H CRC patients[44]	Nivolumab	74	Multicohort Prospective Trial	12-mo OS: 73.4%; 12-mo PFS: 50.4%
Pretreated MSI-H CRC patients[47]	Nivolumab Plus Ipilimumab	119	Multicohort Prospective Trial	12-mo OS: 85%; 12-mo PFS: 71%
MSI-H Treatment Naïve CRC patients[48]	Nivolumab Plus Ipilimumab	45	Multicohort Prospective Trial	12-mo OS: 83%; 12-mo PFS: 77%
Pretreated patients with *NTRK* fusions[50]	Larotrectinib	55	Prospective Basket Trial	PFS: NR; ORR: 75%
Pretreated patients with *NTRK* fusions[51]	Entrectinib	54	Prospective Basket Trial	PFS: 11 mo; ORR: 57%
Pretreated *BRAFV600 E* CRC patients[57]	Encorafenib Plus Cetuximab ± Binimetinib vs Chemotherapy	665	Randomized Trial	Triplet OS: 9 mo vs 5.4 mo (HR: 0.52, 95% CI 0.39–0.7); Doublet OS: 8.4 mo vs 5.4 mo (HR: 0.6, 95% CI 0.45–0.79)

Abbreviations: 95% CI, 95% confidence interval; MSI-H, microsatellite instability-high, NR, not reached; ORR, objective response rate.

treatment-naïve metastatic CRC. In a single cohort of 45 patients who received treatment with the combination in the Checkmate-142 trial, response rate was 60%, 12-month survival was 83%, and median duration of response had not yet been reached.[48] Despite the striking duration of response of checkpoint inhibitors, currently, they are only available for the 5% of patients with metastatic CRC with MSI-H tumors.

During the widespread adoption of genomic profiling in order to capture MSI-H CRC tumors, other colocalizing mutations such as NTRK fusions were identified. Although these fusions are found in only 1% of patients with CRC, they represent a truly actionable mutation.[49] In an aggregate analysis of 55 patients with mixed tumor types pooled from early phase I/II studies, the TRK inhibitor larotrectinib elicited a response rate of 75%.[50] Of the 4 CRC patients included, 2 achieved a partial response and 1 achieved stable disease. At 1 year, 71% of responses remained ongoing and median duration of response and PFS had not yet been reached. In a subsequently reported aggregate analysis of 54 patients with mixed tumor types treated with the TRK inhibitor entrectinib, response rate was 57% and median duration of response was 10.9 months.[51] Of the 4 CRC patients included, 2 achieved a partial response and 1 achieved stable disease. It is anticipated that there will be ongoing discovery of new biological CRC subsets defined by highly actionable targets in the next several years.

Massive ongoing research efforts are exploring methods to sensitize microsatellite stable (MSS) CRC to checkpoint inhibitors. One promising strategy involves combining nivolumab with the antiangiogenic regorafenib; the latter is thought to reduce feedback expression of immune suppressive markers programmed death ligand-1 (PD-L1) and indoleamine 2,3-dioxygenase (IDO) on tumor cells in response to checkpoint inhibitors.[52] In the phase I study of the combination in 25 patients with metastatic MSS CRC, 29% of patients achieved an objective response.[53] In the past, nivolumab or other checkpoint inhibitor monotherapy elicited response rates of 0% in this patient group.[54] A single-arm phase II study of nivolumab plus regorafenib in patients with MSS CRC is ongoing [NCT04126733]. Beyond regorafenib, a staggering array of molecules are being tested in combination with checkpoint inhibitors in MSS CRC to try to unlock the efficacy of the agents. Some of these include other immune modulators, chemotherapeutics, and biological agents.[55] The authors believe that within the next decade the puzzle of unlocking the immunosuppressive tumor microenvironment of MSS CRC will be achieved. Once immunotherapy becomes a cornerstone therapy in most patients with CRC, given the likelihood of durable response in patients deriving benefit from the treatments, there will be much less need for locoregional therapies, including resection, in patients with CRC with hepatic metastases.

BRAFV600E mutations are found in 5% to 15% of patients with CRC and carry an extremely poor prognosis.[56] The median OS of patients with metastatic CRC with the mutation is close to 1 year, whereas the median OS for patients with metastatic CRC is greater than 30 months. A recent phase III study that compared nonchemotherapy triplet (cetuximab, encorafenib, and binimetinib) and doublet combinations (cetuximab, encorafenib) with standard second-line chemotherapy demonstrated significant improvements in both experimental arms compared with the chemotherapy arm.[57] This trial established cetuximab plus encorafenib as the second-line treatment standard for patients with BRAFV600E and backbone upon which future experimental agents may be added. Outcomes in patients with BRAFV600E have in large part not been reported from studies of patients undergoing liver-directed therapies. It is likely these patients were excluded from such studies by not being candidates due to fulminant disease. The authors anticipate that with subsequent additions to the encor-afenib plus cetuximab backbone over the next 10 years, the OS in patients with BRAFV600E CRC will approach the OS in other patients with CRC.

RAS mutant CRC tumors remain a subgroup in need of further drug development. RAS mutations are found in 40% to 45% of metastatic CRC and, beyond predicting a lack of benefit from frontline therapy with anti-EGFR agents, tend to predict a more aggressive disease course.[58] Many agents have been developed for this target but have failed in clinical testing; initial treatment approaches targeted posttransla-tional RAS modifications including MEK and farnesyltransferase inhibitors.[59] Preclini-cal work suggests the promise of novel agents such as the engineered pan-RAS monoclonal antibody inRAS37 as monotherapy or in combination with inhibitors of downstream effectors.[60] It is anticipated that in the coming decade a successful RAS inhibitor will be developed for patients with CRC. Whether the agent is added to first-line chemotherapy or perhaps used in the maintenance setting postresponse to initial chemotherapy, it will add to the armamentarium of active therapies available for patients with CRC.

OTHER GASTROINTESTINAL MALIGNANCIES

The authors have discussed the data for locoregional therapy for hepatic metastases in gastrointestinal cancers where the practice is routinely used. In several others, such as pancreatic adenocarcinoma and gastroesophageal adenocarcinoma, liver-directed therapy, including complete resection of synchronous metastases, is not often attempted due to the lack of prospective data about the practice changing dis-ease outcomes for patients.[61,62] Systemic treatments for patients with pancreatic can-cer and gastroesophageal adenocarcinoma have improved steadily over the last decade with the development of therapeutics targeting DNA damage repair, HER2 amplifications, and PD-L1 overexpression. Recent data on patients with pancreatic adenocarcinoma suggest patients with actionable mutations who are matched to appropriate targeted therapies demonstrate significant survival benefit over patients who receive standardized therapies.[63] Given the emergence of novel targets and ongoing preclinical drug development efforts, we anticipate breakthroughs, as the landscape of systemic therapy continues to evolve in these diseases.

SUMMARY

Although liver metastases are an important cause of morbidity and mortality in patients with cancer, the authors demonstrate, using a backdrop of gastrointestinal cancer, that current evidence for locoregional therapy, outside of curative resection, is not su-perior to the current evidence for systemic therapies in patients. In fact, few studies have shown survival benefit for any liver-directed therapy in cancer aside from poten-tially curative resection, and the continued use of liver-directed therapies is usually based on retrospective data or single-arm phase II studies with highly selected patient cohorts. The use of many of these unproven therapies off clinical trials impedes the advancement of novel therapies in patients who may not be receiving benefit and are getting toxicities. Further, the authors contend that pending developments in the field, such as the widespread adoption of immunotherapy, identification of new targetable biological disease subsets through comprehensive genomic profiling, and development of increasingly potent therapeutics will produce more durable re-sponses and render liver-directed therapies obsolete over time. The last decade has seen an unparalleled series of advances in most cancers. In fact, many diseases such as lung cancer, breast cancer, and melanoma have seen more advances than the gastrointestinal cancers opted to discuss in this article. The promise of immuno-therapy, targeted therapy, and other agents such as antibody-drug conjugates is encouraging and at some point will hopefully reduce the need for surgical resection as well. Although this may seem controversial, the authors believe the preceding paragraphs fortify their position.

DISCLOSURE

S. Das receives Speakers' Bureau fees from Ipsen and has received honoraria in the past from Targeted Oncology and Medsphere; J. Berlin participates in a consulting or advisory role for Abbvie, Arno Therapeutics, AstraZeneca, Bayer Health, BeiGene, Celgene, Cornerstone Pharmaceuticals, Eisai, EMD Serono, Erytech Pharma, Exelixis, Five Prime Therapeutics, Genentech/Roche, Gritstone Oncology, Karyopharm Therapeutics, LSK Biopharma and Seattle Genetics. He has received honoraria in the past from Nestle Health Science.

REFERENCES

1. Glazer E, Tseng J, Al-Refaie W, et al. Long-term survival after surgical management of neuroendocrine hepatic metastases. HPB (Oxford) 2010;12(6):427–33.
2. Maxwell JE, Sherman SK, O'Dorisio TM, et al. Liver-directed surgery of neuroendocrine metastases: What is the optimal strategy? Surgery 2016;159:320–33.
3. Elias D, Lasser P, Ducreux M, et al. Liver resection (and associated extrahepatic resections) for metastatic well-differentiated endocrine tumors: a 15-year single center prospective study. Surgery 2003;133(4):375–82.
4. Osborne D, Zervos E, Strosberg J, et al. Improved outcome with cytoreduction versus embolization for symptomatic hepatic metastases of carcinoid and neuroendocrine tumors. Ann Surg Oncol 2006;13(4):572–81.
5. Mayo S, de Jong M, Pulitano C, et al. Surgical management of hepatic neuroendocrine tumor metastasis: results from an international multi-institutional analysis. Ann Surg Oncol 2010;17(12):3129–36.
6. Maire F, Lombard-Bohas C, O'Toole D, et al. Hepatic arterial embolization versus chemoembolization in the treatment of liver metastases from well-differentiated midgut endocrine tumors: a prospective randomized study. Neuroendocrinology 2012;96(4):294–300.
7. Strosberg J, El-Haddad G, Wolin E, et al. Phase 3 Trial of 177Lu-dotatate for midgut neuroendocrine tumors. N Engl J Med 2017;376:125–35.
8. Strosberg J, Kunz P, Hendifar A, et al. Impact of liver tumour burden, alkaline phosphatase elevation, and target lesion size on treatment outcomes with 177Lu-Dotatate: an analysis of the NETTER-1 study. Eur J Nucl Med Mol Imaging 2020. https://doi.org/10.1007/s00259-020-04709-x.
9. Brabander T, Van der Zwan W, Teunissen J, et al. Long-term efficacy, survival and safety of [177Lu-DOTA0,Tyr3]octreotate in patients with gastroenteropancreatic and bronchial neuroendocrine tumors. Clin Cancer Res 2017;23(16):4617–24.
10. Miederer M, Henriksen G, Alke A, et al. Preclinical evaluation of the α-particle generator nuclide 225Ac for somatostatin receptor radiotherapy of neuroendocrine tumors. Clin Cancer Res 2008;14(11):3555–61.
11. Goodhead DT, Thacker J, Cox R. Effects of radiations of different qualities on cells: molecular mechanisms of damage and repair. Int J Radiat Biol 1993; 63(5):543–56.
12. Ballal S, Yadav M, Bal C, et al. Broadening Horizons With 225 Ac-DOTATATE Targeted Alpha Therapy for gastroenteropancreatic neuroendocrine tumour patients

stable or refractory to 177 Lu-DOTATATE PRRT: First clinical experience on the efficacy and safety. Eur J Nucl Med Mol Imaging 2020;47(4):934–46.

13. Wild D, Fani M, Behe M, et al. First clinical evidence that imaging with somatostatin receptor antagonists is feasible. J Nucl Med 2011;52(9):1412–7.

14. Reidy-Lagunes D, Pandit-Taskar N, O'Donoghue J, et al. Phase I Trial of Well-Differentiated Neuroendocrine Tumors (NETs) with Radiolabeled Somatostatin Antagonist 177 Lu-Satoreotide Tetraxetan. Clin Cancer Res 2019;25(23):6939–47.

15. Kunz P, Catalano P, Nimieri H, et al. A randomized study of temozolomide or temozolomide and capecitabine in patients with advanced pancreatic neuroendocrine tumors: A trial of the ECOG-ACRIN Cancer Research Group (E2211). J Clin Oncol 2018;36(15):S4004.

16. Fine RL, Gulati A, Tsushima D, et al. Prospective phase II study of capecitabine and temozolomide (CAPTEM) for progressive, moderately, and well-differentiated metastatic neuroendocrine tumors. J Clin Oncol 2014;32(3):S179.

17. Capdevila J, Fazio N, Lopez C, et al. Final results of the TALENT trial (GETNE1509): a prospective multicohort phase II study of lenvatinib in patients (pts) with G1/G2 advanced pancreatic (panNETs) and gastrointestinal (giNETs) neuroendocrine tumors (NETs). J Clin Oncol 2019;37(15):S4106.

18. Chan J, Faris J, Murphy J, et al. Phase II trial of cabozantinib in patients with carcinoid and pancreatic neuroendocrine tumors (pNET). J Clin Oncol 2017;35(4):S228.

19. Yang T, Tabrizian P, Zhang H, et al. Comparison of Patterns and Outcomes of Liver Resection for Hepatocellular Carcinoma: East vs West. Clin Gatroenterol Hepatol 2017;15(12):1972–4.

20. Llovet J, Real M, Montana X, et al. Arterial Embolisation or Chemoembolisation Versus Symptomatic Treatment in Patients With Unresectable Hepatocellular Carcinoma: A Randomised Controlled Trial. Lancet 2002;359(9319):1734–9.

21. Salem R, Lewandowski R, Kulik L, et al. Radioembolization results in longer time-to-progression and reduced toxicity compared with chemoembolization in patients with hepatocellular carcinoma. Gastroenterology 2011;140(2):497–507.e2.

22. Ricke J, Klumpen H, Amthauer H, et al. Impact of combined selective internal radiation therapy and sorafenib on survival in advanced hepatocellular carcinoma. J Hepatol 2019;71(6):1164–74.

23. Park J, Kim Y, Kim D, et al. Sorafenib with or without concurrent transarterial chemoembolization in patients with advanced hepatocellular carcinoma: the phase III STAH trial. J Hepatol 2019;70(4):684–91.

24. Llovet J, Ricci S, Mazzaferro V, et al. Sorafenib in Advanced Hepatocellular Carcinoma. N Engl J Med 2008;359:378–90.

25. Cheng A, Quin S, Ikeda M, et al. LBA3IMbrave150: Efficacy and safety results from a ph III study evaluating atezolizumab (atezo) + bevacizumab (bev) vs sorafenib (Sor) as first treatment (tx) for patients (pts) with unresectable hepatocellular carcinoma (HCC). Ann Oncol 2019;30(suppl_9):ix183–202.

26. Kudo M, Finn R, Qin S, et al. Lenvatinib versus sorafenib in first-line treatment of patients with unresectable hepatocellular carcinoma: a randomised phase 3 non-inferiority trial. Lancet 2018;391(10126):1163–73.

27. Yau T, Kang Y, Kim Y, et al. Nivolumab (NIVO) + ipilimumab (IPI) combination therapy in patients (pts) with advanced hepatocellular carcinoma (aHCC): Results from CheckMate 040. J Clin Oncol 2019;37(15):S4012.

28. Edeline J, Touchefu Y, Guiu B, et al. Radioembolization plus chemotherapy for first-line treatment of locally advanced intrahepatic cholangiocarcinoma: a phase 2 clinical trial. JAMA Oncol 2019;6(1):51–9.

29. Valle J, Wasan H, Palmer D, et al. Cisplatin plus gemcitabine versus gemcitabine for biliary tract cancer. N Engl J Med 2010;362:1273–81.

30. Shroff R, Javle M, Xiao L, et al. Gemcitabine, cisplatin, and nab-paclitaxel for the treatment of advanced biliary tract cancers: a phase ii clinical trial. JAMA Oncol 2019;5(6):824–30.

31. Lowery M, Ptashkin R, Jordan E, et al. Comprehensive molecular profiling of intra- and extrahepatic cholangiocarcinomas: potential targets for intervention. Clin Cancer Res 2018. https://doi.org/10.1158/1078-0432.CCR-18-0078.

32. Abou-Alfa G, Mercade T, Javle M, et al. CLARIDHY: A Global, Phase 3, Randomized, Double-Blind Study of Ivosidenib (IVO) vs Placebo in Patients with Advanced Cholangiocarcinoma (CC) with an Isocitrate Dehydrogenase 1 (IDH1) Mutation. Ann Oncol 2019;30(suppl_5):v851–934.

33. Mazzaferro V, El-Rayes B, Busset M, et al. Derazantinib (ARQ 087) in advanced or Inoperable FGFR2 Gene fusion-positive intrahepatic cholangiocarcinoma. Br J Cancer 2019;120(2):165–71.

34. Abou-Alfa G, Sahai V, Hollebecque A, et al. Pemigatinib for previously treated, locally advanced or metastatic cholangiocarcinoma: a multicentre, open-label, phase 2 study. Lancet Oncol 2020. https://doi.org/10.1016/S1470-2045(20)30109-1.

35. Krook M, Bonneville R, Chen H, et al. Tumor heterogeneity and acquired drug resistance in FGFR2-fusion-positive cholangiocarcinoma through rapid research autopsy. Cold Spring Harb Mol Case Stud 2019;5(4):a004002.

36. Van Hazel G, Blackwell A, Anderson J, et al. Randomised Phase 2 Trial of SIR-spheres plus fluorouracil/leucovorin chemotherapy versus fluorouracil/leucovorin chemotherapy alone in advanced colorectal cancer. J Surg Oncol 2004;88(2):78–85.

37. Lewandowski R, Memon K, Mulcahy M, et al. Twelve-year experience of radioembolization for colorectal hepatic metastases in 214 patients: survival by era and chemotherapy. Eur J Nucl Med Mol Imaging 2014;41(10):1861–9.

38. Wasan H, Gibbs P, Sharma N, et al. First-line selective internal radiotherapy plus chemotherapy versus chemotherapy alone in patients with liver metastases from colorectal cancer (FOXFIRE, SIRFLOX, and FOXFIRE-Global): a combined analysis of three multicentre, randomised, phase 3 trials. Lancet Oncol 2017;18(9):1159–71.

39. Moutinho V, Connell L, D'Angelica M, et al. Hepatic artery therapies for unresectable colorectal liver metastases: Pooled survival analysis of 968 patients from TACE, yttrium-90, and HAI studies. J Clin Oncol 2017;35(4):S747.

40. Koerkamp B, Sadot E, Kemeny N, et al. Perioperative hepatic arterial infusion pump chemotherapy is associated with longer survival after resection of colorectal liver metastases: a propensity score analysis. J Clin Oncol 2017;35(17):1938–44.

41. Modest D, Martens U, Riera-Knorrenschild J, et al. FOLFOXIRI plus panitumumab as first-line treatment of RAS wild-type metastatic colorectal cancer: the randomized, open-label, phase II VOLFI Study (AIO KRK0109). J Clin Oncol 2019;37(35):3401–11.

42. Palma D, Olson R, Harrow S, et al. Stereotactic ablative radiotherapy versus standard of care palliative treatment in patients with oligometastatic cancers

(SABR-COMET): a randomised, phase 2, open-label trial. Lancet 2019; 393(10185):2051–8.

43. Manthravadi S, Sun W, Saeed A, et al. Prognostic impact of BRAF V600E mutation in patients with non-metastatic colorectal cancer with microsatellite instability: A systematic review and meta-analysis. J Clin Oncol 2018;36(15):S3587.

44. Overman M, McDermott R, Leach J, et al. Nivolumab in patients with metastatic DNA mismatch repair-deficient or microsatellite instability-high colorectal cancer (CheckMate 142): an open-label, multicentre, phase 2 study. Lancet Oncol 2017; 18(9):1182–91.

45. Le D, Kim T, Van Cutsem E, et al. Phase II open-label study of pembrolizumab in treatment-refractory, microsatellite instability–high/mismatch repair–deficient metastatic colorectal cancer: KEYNOTE-164. J Clin Oncol 2019;38(1):11–9.

46. Broderick J. Pembrolizumab Improves PFS in Frontline MSI-H/dMMR Colorectal Cancer. Available at: https://www.onclive.com/web-exclusives/pembrolizumab-improves-pfs-in-msihdmmr-colorectal-cancer. Accessed April 4, 2020.

47. Overman M, Lonardi S, Wong K, et al. Durable clinical benefit with nivolumab plus ipilimumab in DNA mismatch repair-deficient/microsatellite instability-high metastatic colorectal cancer. J Clin Oncol 2018;36(8):773–9.

48. Lenz H, Lonardi S, Zagonel V, et al. Nivolumab (NIVO) + low-dose ipilimumab (IPI) as first-line (1L) therapy in microsatellite instability-high/DNA mismatch repair deficient (MSI-H/dMMR) metastatic colorectal cancer (mCRC): Clinical update. J Clin Oncol 2019;37(15):S3521.

49. Okamura R, Boichard A, Kato S, et al. Analysis of NTRK Alterations in Pan-Cancer Adult and Pediatric Malignancies: Implications for NTRK-Targeted Therapeutics. JCO Precis Oncol 2018. https://doi.org/10.1200/PO.18.00183.

50. Drilon A, Laetsch T, Kummar S, et al. Efficacy of Larotrectinib in TRK Fusion–Positive Cancers in Adults and Children. N Engl J Med 2018;378:731–9.

51. Doebele R, Drilon A, Paz-Ares L, et al. Entrectinib in patients with advanced or metastatic NTRK fusion-positive solid tumours: integrated analysis of three phase 1–2 trials. Lancet Oncol 2020;21(2):271–82.

52. Wu R, Kong P, Xia L, et al. Regorafenib Promotes Antitumor Immunity via Inhibiting PD-L1 and IDO1 Expression in Melanoma. Clin Cancer Res 2019. https://doi.org/10.1158/1078-0432.CCR-18-2840.

53. Fukuoka S, Hara H, Takahashi N, et al. Regorafenib plus nivolumab in patients with advanced gastric (GC) or colorectal cancer (CRC): An open-label, dose-finding, and dose-expansion phase 1b trial (REGONIVO, EPOC1603). J Clin Oncol 2019;37(15):S2522.

54. Le D, Uram J, Wang H, et al. PD-1 Blockade in Tumors with Mismatch-Repair Deficiency. N Engl J Med 2015;372:2509–20.

55. Huyghe N, Baldwin P, den Eynde M. Immunotherapy with immune checkpoint inhibitors in colorectal cancer: what is the future beyond deficient mismatch-repair tumours? Gastroenterol Rep 2020;8(1):11–24.

56. Ducreux M, Chamseddine A, Laurent-Puig P, et al. Molecular targeted therapy of BRAF-mutant colorectal cancer. Ther Adv Med Oncol 2019;11:1–15.

57. Kopetz S, Grothey A, Yaeger R, et al. Encorafenib, Binimetinib, and Cetuximab in BRAF V600E–Mutated Colorectal Cancer. N Engl J Med 2019;381:1632–43.

58. Serebriiskii I, Connelly C, Frampton G, et al. Comprehensive characterization of RAS mutations in colon and rectal cancers in old and young patients. Nat Commun 2019;10(1):3722.

59. Dienstmann R, Connor K, Byrne A, et al. Precision Therapy in RAS Mutant Colorectal Cancer. Gastroenterology 2020;158(4):806–11.

60. Shin S, Kim J, Park S, et al. Direct targeting of oncogenic RAS mutants with a tumor-specific cytosol-penetrating antibody inhibits RAS mutant–driven tumor growth. Sci Adv 2020;6(3):eaay2174.

61. Voss N, Izbicki J, Nentwich M. Oligometastases in pancreatic cancer (Synchronous resections of hepatic oligometastatic pancreatic cancer: Disputing a principle in a time of safe pancreatic operations in a retrospective multicenter analysis). Ann Gastroenterol Surg 2019;3(4):373-7.

62. MacCormick S, Chong KC, Sullivan HO, et al. Benefits of Metastasectomy in Esophagogastric Cancer. Clin Oncol 2017;2(1250):1-4.

63. Pishvaian M, Blais E, Brody J, et al. Overall survival in patients with pancreatic cancer receiving matched therapies following molecular profiling: a retrospective analysis of the Know Your Tumor registry trial. Lancet Oncol 2020;21(4):508-18.

Debate

Improvements in Systemic Therapies for Liver Metastases Will Increase the Role of Locoregional Treatments

Yoshikuni Kawaguchi, MD, PhD[a,b], Mario De Bellis, MD[a],
Elena Panettieri, MD[a], Gregor Duwe, MD[a],
Jean-Nicolas Vauthey, MD[a],*

KEYWORDS

- Colorectal liver metastasis • Resection • Chemotherapy
- Molecular-targeted therapy • Conversion therapy • Two-stage hepatectomy
- Neuroendocrine liver metastasis • Gastric liver metastasis

KEY POINTS

- The oncologic benefit of resection of liver metastases depends on the primary disease. Resection of colorectal and neuroendocrine liver metastases are effective, whereas resection of gastric liver metastases should be limited.
- For resectable colorectal liver metastases (CLMs), postoperative adjuvant medical therapy and perioperative medical therapy have not been shown to improve overall survival.
- For unresectable and borderline resectable CLM, improvement in medical therapy facilitates conversion therapy, increasing the rate of complete resection.
- For bilateral CLMs, 2-stage hepatectomy, which combines liver resection, chemotherapy, and portal vein embolization (PVE), improves resectability.
- New technical refinements in 2-stage hepatectomy with PVE include fast-track 2-stage hepatectomy using a hybrid room and combined hepatic vein embolization.

INTRODUCTION

Resection is one of the treatment options for liver metastases. Advancements in surgical technique and perioperative management, and improved understanding

Grant support: This research was supported in part by the National Institutes of Health (T32 CA 009599) and the MD Anderson Cancer Center Support Grant, CA016672.
[a] Department of Surgical Oncology, The University of Texas, MD Anderson Cancer Center, Houston, TX, USA; [b] Hepato-Biliary-Pancreatic Surgery Division, Department of Surgery, Graduate School of Medicine, the University of Tokyo, Tokyo, Japan
* Corresponding author. 1515 Holcombe Boulevard, Unit 1484, Houston, TX 77030.
E-mail address: jvauthey@mdanderson.org

of surgical complexity, have decreased postoperative complication rates and facilitated complex surgical procedures.[1–3] Therefore, an increasing number of liver resection procedures are feasible. However, it is important to understand which liver metastases should be resected and how liver metastases should be managed in the context of a multidisciplinary approach. The oncologic benefit of resection of liver metastases depends on the primary disease. This article details the outcome of resection of colorectal liver metastases (CLMs), neuroendocrine liver metastases (NLMs), and gastric liver metastases (GLM), and particularly focuses on updates of CLM management.

RESECTION OF LIVER METASTASES
Resection of Colorectal Liver Metastases

The liver is the most common site of metastases from colorectal cancer. Approximately 15% to 30% of patients with colorectal cancer have CLM.[4] **Fig. 1** shows the impact of liver resection on survival. For patients who were alive 12 months after diagnosis, patients who had undergone CLM resection were associated with better survival than patients with unresectable metastatic colorectal cancer; the 5-year overall survival (OS) was 55.2% versus 19.5%.[5] The 5-year OS rates in patients undergoing CLM resection range from 40% to 59%.[6–9] Recent studies showed that the 5-year OS rates of patients with favorable genetic tumor biology (eg, wild-types of BRAF, RAS, TP53, and SMAD4) were close to 70%.[10–12] For patients undergoing curative CLM resection, patients with wild-types of RAS, TP53, and SMAD4 were associated with significantly better OS than patients with alterations of RAS, TP53, and SMAD4: the 5-year OS was 74% versus 10%; hazard ratio (95% confidence interval), 0.12 (0.05–0.26), P<.001.[12] The oncologic benefit and curative potential of liver resection is well established in patients with CLM.

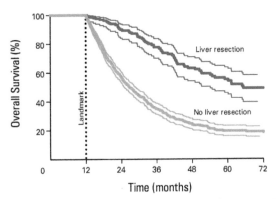

Fig. 1. Overall survival by landmark analysis of patients with metastatic colorectal cancer. Of those patients alive at 12 months, median overall survival was 65 months in the population of patients who underwent liver resection during the first year. Error bars represent 95% confidence intervals. (*From* Kopetz S, Chang GJ, Overman MJ, et al. Improved survival in metastatic colorectal cancer is associated with adoption of hepatic resection and improved chemotherapy. Journal of clinical oncology: official journal of the American Society of Clinical Oncology. Aug 1 2009;27(22):3677-3683; with permission.)

Resection of Neuroendocrine Tumor

Resection of NLM is recognized to have oncologic benefit (**Table 1**). The 5-year OS in patients undergoing R0 resection is high, approximately 75%,[13–15] compared with the 5-year OS in patients undergoing medical therapy alone, ranging from 30% to 50%. Studies have reported that cytoreductive and debulking surgery of NLM is also effective,[16–21] relieving symptoms[16] and providing long-term survival similar to patients undergoing R0 resection of NLM.[17–20] A 70% cytoreduction has been used as a useful cutoff for ensuring favorable survival after NLM resection.[19,20] The consensus guidelines of the North American Neuroendocrine Tumor Society in 2017 recommended that a 70% cytoreduction can be achieved and a parenchyma-sparing approach may be used.[22] A recent study confirmed this recommendation and showed that the 5-year OS was similar between patients undergoing more than a 90% cytoreduction and patients undergoing a 70% to 90% cytoreduction: 79% versus 78%.[21] In contrast, the 5-year OS in patients undergoing a less than 70% cytoreduction was 43%. Liver resection is recommended in patients with NLM whenever it is feasible and a 70% cytoreduction can be achieved.

Resection of Gastric Liver Metastases

Gastric cancer is regarded as having worse tumor biology than colorectal cancer and neuroendocrine tumor. The liver is also a common target of metastases from gastric cancer.[23] However, resection of GLM remains controversial because extrahepatic metastases, including peritoneal dissemination and lymph node metastases, are common, which limits the oncologic benefit of GLM resection. Studies reported that the median OS was approximately 30 months in patients undergoing GLM resection (**Table 2**), compared with approximately 10 months in patients undergoing medical therapy.[24] Although systemic medical therapy is currently the first choice of treatment of GLM, the selection of patients for GLM resection is important. The following risk factors associated with worse survival after GLM resection were reported: large diameter of GLM, multiple tumors, primary T factor, primary N factor, and the differentiation type of primary tumor.

Table 1
Overall survival in patients with neuroendocrine liver metastases: data from retrospective studies

Study, Year	Regions	N	Treatment	Median OS (mo)	5-y OS (%)
Chamberlain et al,[13] 2000	United States	34	Liver resection	Not reached	76
		33	Embolization	Not reached	50
		18	Medical therapy	24	0
Osborne et al,[14] 2006	United States	38	Liver resection	50	79[a]
		23	Cytoreduction	32	63[a]
		59	Embolization	24	35[a]
Mayo et al,[15] 2011	United States and Europe	339	Liver resection	123	74
		414	Intra-arterial therapy	34	30
Scott et al,[21] 2019	United States	36	<70% cytoreduction	38	43[a]
		82	70%–90% cytoreduction	134	78[a]
		54	>90% cytoreduction	Not reached	79[a]

[a] Estimated by Kaplan-Meier curve.
Data from Refs.[13–15,21]

Table 2
Median overall survival in patients undergoing resection of gastric liver metastases

Study, Year	Regions	N	Surgical Indication	Median OS (mo)	Risk Factors for Survival
Takemura et al,[61] 2012	Asia	64	Number of tumors ≤3	34	≥5 cm in diameter pT4 of primary tumor
Kinoshita et al,[62] 2014	Asia	256	NS	31	pT4 of primary tumor ≥5 cm in diameter Number of tumors ≥3
Tiberio et al,[63] 2014	Europe	53	No extrahepatic metastases	34	≥6 cm in diameter D2 dissection
Guner et al,[64] 2015	Asia	68	No extrahepatic metastases	24	≥3 cm in diameter
Oki et al,[65] 2015	Asia	94	No extrahepatic metastases	34	≥3 cm in diameter Multiple tumors primary LN status ≥N2
Ito et al, 2018	Asia	31	Number of tumors ≤3 Chemotherapy response	38	Diffuse/other type R1/R2 resection

Abbreviations: LN, lymph node; NS, nonsignificant.
Data from Refs.[61–65]

IMPROVEMENTS IN SYSTEMIC THERAPIES AND RESECTION OF COLORECTAL LIVER METASTASES

Over the last 2 decades, systemic medical therapies for colorectal cancer have improved. First, irinotecan and oxaliplatin proved to be effective for the treatment of patients with colorectal cancer and became key drugs for this patient group. Another important advancement in medical therapy is the use of molecular-targeted therapy, including anti–vascular endothelial growth factor (VEGF) and anti–epidermal growth factor receptor (EGFR) agents. To further improve the oncologic benefit of CLM resection, randomized control trials for perioperative medical therapy and postoperative adjuvant therapy have been conducted (**Table 3**). Previous studies have suggested a disease-free survival or progression-free survival benefit of perioperative medical therapy and postoperative adjuvant therapy but no benefit on OS in patients with resectable CLM.[25–29] For patients with resectable CLM, a recent clinical trial compared patients who received preoperative chemotherapy including oxaliplatin-containing or irinotecan-containing regimens plus cetuximab with patients who received preoperative chemotherapy alone (the New Epoc Trial). Importantly, the study showed that the OS was significantly worse in patients who received chemotherapy plus cetuximab than in patients who received chemotherapy alone. The clear evidence supporting perioperative medical therapy and postoperative adjuvant therapy is limited. However, given the high recurrence rates after CLM resection,[9–12] the National Comprehensive Cancer Network Clinical Practice Guidelines in Oncology: Colon Cancer and Rectal Cancer recommends consideration of perioperative chemotherapy or postoperative adjuvant chemotherapy in patients with resectable CLM.[30,31] The recommended regimens of this patient group are folinic acid, fluorouracil, and oxaliplatin (FOLFOX); capecitabine and oxaliplatin (CAPEOX); folinic acid, fluorouracil, and irinotecan (FOLFIRI); or folinic acid, fluorouracil, oxaliplatin, and irinotecan (FOLFOXIRI).[30,31]

Table 3
Median overall survival after resection of colorectal liver metastases: data from randomized control trials and our recent retrospective cohort study

Study, Year	Regions	N	Assignment	Median OS (mo)
Randomized Controlled Trials				
Postoperative Adjuvant Chemotherapy				
Portier et al,[25] 2006	Europe	87	Surgery alone	46
		86	Fluorouracil and folinic acid	62
Perioperative Chemotherapy				
Nordlinger et al,[26] 2013 Epoc Trial	Europe	182	Surgery alone	54
		182	Perioperative FOLFOX4	61
Bridgewater et al,[27] 2020 New Epoc Trial	Europe	128	Perioperative chemotherapy[a] alone	81
		129	Perioperative chemotherapy[a] alone plus cetuximab	55
Our Retrospective Cohort Study				
Kawaguchi et al,[12] 2019	United States	507	Perioperative chemotherapy, 90% Oxaliplatin-containing regimen, 74% Anti-VEGF agent– containing regimen, 70%	*RAS* Status Wild-type 88 Mutation 54

Abbreviation: FOLFOX, folinic acid, fluorouracil, and oxaliplatin.
[a] Including regimens using oxaliplatin and irinotecan.
Data from Refs.[12,25–27]

At present, our clinical practice for patients with resectable CLM is to use 4 courses of preoperative FOLFOX plus bevacizumab followed by liver resection and 8 courses of postoperative FOLFOX. According to our recent study including patients undergoing CLM resection during 2000 to 2016, 91% of patients received perioperative chemotherapy.[9] Oxaliplatin-containing regimens and anti-VEGF agent–containing regimens were used in approximately 70% of patients (see **Table 3**). After CLM resection, the median OS was 88 months in patients with *RAS* wild-type and 54 months in patients with *RAS* mutation.

SYSTEMIC THERAPIES FOR IMPROVING RESECTABILITY OF COLORECTAL LIVER METASTASES

Most patients with CLM are initially resectable. Given the better survival and potential chance of cure after R0 resection, the strategy to improve resectability is important. Two strategies are discussed here: conversion therapy and 2-stage hepatectomy.

Conversion Therapy

Conversion therapy is a strategy to improve initially unresectable and borderline resectable disease to resectable condition. In patients who achieved successful conversion, the OS was better than in patients who received medical therapy alone, although it was worse than in patients who underwent resection of initially resectable

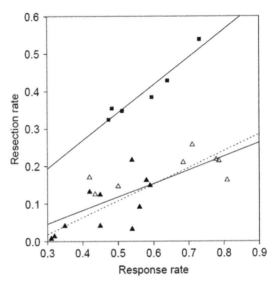

Fig. 2. Rate of liver resection following chemotherapy. The squares represent patients in studies/retrospective analyses with nonresectable metastases confined to the liver (selected patients, $r = 0.96$, $P = .002$). Studies with nonselected patients with colorectal cancer are shown as triangles. Because of the high heterogeneity of these studies, the observed correlation is less strong ($r = 0.74$, $P<.001$, *solid line*). A similar correlation was observed when the phase III trials (*filled triangles*) were separately analyzed ($r = 0.67$, $P = .024$, *dashed line*). (*From* Folprecht G, Grothey A, Alberts S, Raab HR, Kohne CH. Neoadjuvant treatment of unresectable colorectal liver metastases: correlation between tumour response and resection rates. Annals of oncology: official journal of the European Society for Medical Oncology / ESMO. Aug 2005;16(8):1311-1319; with permission.)

CLM.[5,32,33] **Fig. 2** shows the relation between CLM resection rate and chemotherapy response in patients with initially unresectable disease. This study clearly showed that the CLM resection rate (ie, conversion rate) increased with an increase of chemotherapy response rate.[34] As such, for patients with unresectable CLM, it is important to increase chemotherapy response rate. Two phase II studies including patients with unresectable liver-limited disease[35,36] showed that the chemotherapy response rate and the conversion rate were similar between patients receiving FOLFOX and patients receiving FOLFIRI (**Table 4**). In both studies, the conversion rate was 33%. The addition of anti-VEGF and anti-EGFR therapies to chemotherapy is generally associated with improved survival and response rate (see **Table 4**). The PRIME study showed that, for patients with *RAS* or *KRAS* wild-type, median OS and response rate was better in patients who received FOLFOX plus panitumumab than in patients who received FOLFOX alone: median OS, 26 months versus 20 months; response rate, 57% versus 48%. In addition, the PRIME study showed that, in patients with liver-limited disease, the rate of conversion to resection was higher in patients receiving FOLFOX plus panitumumab than in patients receiving FOLFOX alone: 28% versus 18%.

Two randomized controlled trials tested a FOLFOXIRI regimen versus FOLFIRI regimen in patients with unresectable colorectal cancer and showed that the FOLFOXIRI regimen was associated with better response rate than the FOLFIRI regimen (**Table 5**).[37,38] The oncologic benefit of the addition of bevacizumab to FOLFOXIRI

Table 4
Survival and response rate in patients with unresectable liver-limited disease: data from phase II and III studies

Study, Year	Regions	N	Treatment or Assignment	Median OS (mo)	Response Rate (%)	Conversion Rate (%)
Chemotherapy						
Alberts et al,[35] 2005	United States	42	FOLFOX4	26	60	33
Barone et al,[36] 2007	Europe	40	FOLFIRI	32	48	33
Okines et al,[66] 2009 (First Beat)	Europe and United States	949 (350[a]) 662 (230[a])	Oxaliplatin-containing regimen Irinotecan-containing regimen	NA NA	NA NA	20 (71 out of 350) 14 (33 out of 230)
Chemotherapy Plus Molecular-targeted Therapy						
Wong et al,67 2011 (Boxer)	Europe	46 (30[a])	CAPOX + bevacizumab	NA	78	40 (12 out of 30)
Folprecht et al,[57,60] 2010 and 2014 (CELIM)	Europe	56 55	FOLFOX + cetuximab FOLFIRI + cetuximab	36 29	68 57	38 30
Douillard et al,[58,59] 2013 and 2014 (PRIME)	Europe	540 (253[b]) 546 (259[b])	FOLFOX FOLFOX + panitumumab	20 (of 253 patients) 26 (of 259 patients)	48 of 317 patients[c] 57 of 324 patients[c]	18[d] 28[d]

Abbreviations: CAPOX, capecitabine and oxaliplatin; NA, not available.
[a] Initially unresectable CLM.
[b] Patients without *RAS* mutation.
[c] Patients with *KRAS* wild-type.
[d] Of 118 patients with liver-limited disease in both groups.
Data from Refs.[57–60,67]

Table 5
Median overall survival in patients with unresectable colorectal cancer: data from randomized control trials testing the folinic acid, fluorouracil, oxaliplatin, and irinotecan regimen

Study, Year	Regions	N	Assignment	Median OS mo	Median OS HR 95% CI	Response Rate (%)
Souglakos et al,[37] 2006	Europe	146	FOLFIRI	20	NA	34
		137	FOLFOXIRI	22		43
Falcone et al,[38] 2007	Europe	122	FOLFIRI	17	Reference	34
		122	FOLFOXIRI	23	0.70 0.50–0.96	60
Loupakis et al,[39] 2014 TRIBE	Europe	256	FOLFIRI plus bevacizumab	26	Reference	53
		252	FOLFOXIRI plus bevacizumab	31	0.79 0.63–1.00	65

Abbreviations: CI, confidence interval; HR, hazard ratio.
   Data from Refs.[37–39]

was shown in the TRIBE study.[39] The response rate was higher in patients receiving FOLFOXIRI plus bevacizumab than in patients receiving FOLFIRI plus bevacizumab: 65% versus 53%, $P<.006$. From this evidence, our current clinical practice for patients with unresectable and borderline resectable CLM is to use FOLFOXIRI plus bevacizumab and aim for conversion to resectable disease in patients who can tolerate this regimen.

Two-Stage Hepatectomy

Another strategy to improve resectability is 2-stage hepatectomy. Two-stage hepatectomy is a sequential treatment approach for bilateral CLMs that combines liver resection, chemotherapy, and portal vein embolization (PVE).[40–42] Typically, after chemotherapy, first-stage hepatectomy is to remove CLMs in the future liver remnant (generally, the left liver) followed by PVE. A second-stage hepatectomy (generally, right hepatectomy or extended right hepatectomy) is performed 5 to 8 weeks after PVE. This strategy has been adopted in clinical practice as a safe and potentially curative procedure. The reported 5-year OS ranges widely, from 30% to 60%, in patients who completed the sequential treatment.[43–46] Two-stage hepatectomy is generally performed in patients with high tumor burden. As such, recurrence after 2-stage hepatectomy is frequent. Studies have reported that repeat surgery for recurrence after 2-stage hepatectomy is feasible, safe, and associated with better survival, compared with patients who did not undergo repeat surgery.[47,48] The 5-year OS rate was 46% to 67% in patients who underwent repeat surgery for recurrence and 10% to 26% in patients who did not.[47,48] New technical refinements of 2-stage hepatectomy and PVE have recently been reported. One is a fast-track 2-stage hepatectomy that performs removal of tumors in the future liver remnant and PVE at the same time in the hybrid room followed by a second-stage hepatectomy (**Fig. 3**). This refined approach shortens the completion of the planned sequential treatment by 2–4 months compared with the traditional 2-stage hepatectomy and may contribute to early return to intended oncologic treatment.[49] Another technical refinement is combined hepatic vein embolization (HVE) and PVE.[50–56] A recent large series including 21 patients who underwent HVE and PVE showed that combined HVE and PVE was associated with better degree of hypertrophy (8.5% vs 5.6%) and kinetic growth rate (2.9% vs 1.4%) compared with patients undergoing PVE alone.[55]

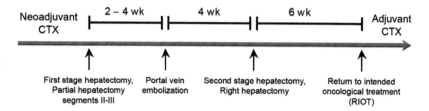

A Traditional two-stage hepatectomy

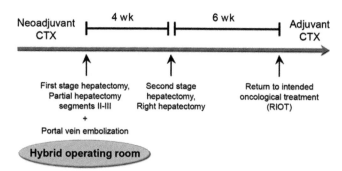

B Fast-track two-stage hepatectomy

Fig. 3. (A) Treatment sequence and timeline of traditional 2-stage hepatectomy and (B) fast-track 2-stage hepatectomy. CTX, chemotherapy. (*From* Odisio BC, Simoneau E, Holmes AA, Conrad CH, Vauthey JN. Fast-Track Two-Stage Hepatectomy Using a Hybrid Interventional Radiology/Operating Suite as Alternative Option to Associated Liver Partition and Portal Vein Ligation for Staged Hepatectomy Procedure. Journal of the American College of Surgeons. Aug 2018;227(2): e5-e10.)

DISCUSSION

The oncologic benefit of resection for liver metastases depends on the primary disease. NLM has favorable tumor biology. Prolonged survival is expected in patients who are able to undergo not only R0 resection but also greater than 70% cytoreduction. The resection of GLM remains controversial because it is associated with aggressive tumor biology. Patients with advanced gastric cancer frequently develop peritoneal dissemination and lymph node metastases. At present, a multidisciplinary approach is well established for the treatment of CLM. Although effective chemotherapy regimens and molecular-targeted therapy have advanced, resection of CLM still has an important role in the management of CLM. To achieve a cure from CLM, clinicians should be familiar with the knowledge and strategy required to convert patients with unresectable disease into candidates for curative-intent surgery. The median OS in patients undergoing CLM resection is 40 to 80 months,[9,25-27] which is better than that of patients who had initially unresectable CLM and received medical therapy (median OS, 15–36 months).[35,36,57-60] Chemotherapy regimens for patients with resectable CLM have improved disease-free or progression-free survival but not OS. For patients with initially unresectable CLM, medical therapy improves the resectability of CLM. The FOLFOXIRI regimen is currently the most effective chemotherapy regimen for patients with colorectal cancer. The addition of bevacizumab to

FOLFOXIRI is also effective and associated with better OS and response rate than FOLFOXIRI alone.[39] The appropriate selection and use of medical therapy and resection contribute to increasing the chance of cure.

DISCLOSURES

The authors have nothing to disclose.

REFERENCES

1. Cloyd JM, Mizuno T, Kawaguchi Y, et al. Comprehensive complication index validates improved outcomes over time despite increased complexity in 3707 consecutive hepatectomies. Ann Surg 2020;271(4):724–31.
2. Kawaguchi Y, Fuks D, Kokudo N, et al. Difficulty of laparoscopic liver resection: proposal for a new classification. Ann Surg 2018;267(1):13–7.
3. Kawaguchi Y, Hasegawa K, Tzeng CD, et al. Performance of a modified three-level classification in stratifying open liver resection procedures in terms of complexity and postoperative morbidity. Br J Surg 2020;107(3):258–67.
4. Manfredi S, Lepage C, Hatem C, et al. Epidemiology and management of liver metastases from colorectal cancer. Ann Surg 2006;244(2):254–9.
5. Kopetz S, Chang GJ, Overman MJ, et al. Improved survival in metastatic colorectal cancer is associated with adoption of hepatic resection and improved chemotherapy. J Clin Oncol 2009;27(22):3677–83.
6. Choti MA, Sitzmann JV, Tiburi MF, et al. Trends in long-term survival following liver resection for hepatic colorectal metastases. Ann Surg 2002;235(6):759–66.
7. Abdalla EK, Vauthey J-N, Ellis LM, et al. Recurrence and outcomes following hepatic resection, radiofrequency ablation, and combined resection/ablation for colorectal liver metastases. Ann Surg 2004;239(6):818–27.
8. Fernandez FG, Drebin JA, Linehan DC, et al. Five-year survival after resection of hepatic metastases from colorectal cancer in patients screened by positron emission tomography with F-18 fluorodeoxyglucose (FDG-PET). Ann Surg 2004;240(3):438–50.
9. Kawaguchi Y, Lillemoe HA, Panettieri E, et al. Conditional recurrence-free survival after resection of colorectal liver metastases: persistent deleterious association with RAS and TP53 co-mutation. J Am Coll Surg 2019;229(3):286–294 e1.
10. Mizuno T, Cloyd JM, Vicente D, et al. SMAD4 gene mutation predicts poor prognosis in patients undergoing resection for colorectal liver metastases. Eur J Surg Oncol 2018;44(5):684–92.
11. Chun YS, Passot G, Yamashita S, et al. Deleterious effect of RAS and evolutionary high-risk TP53 double mutation in colorectal liver metastases. Ann Surg 2019;269(5):917–23.
12. Kawaguchi Y, Kopetz S, Newhook TE, et al. Mutation status of RAS, TP53, and SMAD4 is superior to mutation status of ras alone for predicting prognosis after resection of colorectal liver metastases. Clin Cancer Res 2019;25(19):5843–51.
13. Chamberlain RS, Canes D, Brown KT, et al. Hepatic neuroendocrine metastases: does intervention alter outcomes? J Am Coll Surg 2000;190(4):432–45.
14. Osborne DA, Zervos EE, Strosberg J, et al. Improved outcome with cytoreduction versus embolization for symptomatic hepatic metastases of carcinoid and neuroendocrine tumors. Ann Surg Oncol 2006;13(4):572–81.
15. Mayo SC, de Jong MC, Bloomston M, et al. Surgery versus intra-arterial therapy for neuroendocrine liver metastasis: a multicenter international analysis. Ann Surg Oncol 2011;18(13):3657–65.

16. Chambers AJ, Pasieka JL, Dixon E, et al. The palliative benefit of aggressive surgical intervention for both hepatic and mesenteric metastases from neuroendocrine tumors. Surgery 2008;144(4):645–51 [discussion 651–43].
17. Elias D, Lasser P, Ducreux M, et al. Liver resection (and associated extrahepatic resections) for metastatic well-differentiated endocrine tumors: a 15-year single center prospective study. Surgery 2003;133(4):375–82.
18. Sarmiento JM, Heywood G, Rubin J, et al. Surgical treatment of neuroendocrine metastases to the liver: a plea for resection to increase survival. J Am Coll Surg 2003;197(1):29–37.
19. Graff-Baker AN, Sauer DA, Pommier SJ, et al. Expanded criteria for carcinoid liver debulking: Maintaining survival and increasing the number of eligible patients. Surgery 2014;156(6):1369–76 [discussion 1376–67].
20. Maxwell JE, Sherman SK, O'Dorisio TM, et al. Liver-directed surgery of neuroendocrine metastases: What is the optimal strategy? Surgery 2016;159(1):320–33.
21. Scott AT, Breheny PJ, Keck KJ, et al. Effective cytoreduction can be achieved in patients with numerous neuroendocrine tumor liver metastases (NETLMs). Surgery 2019;165(1):166–75.
22. Howe JR, Cardona K, Fraker DL, et al. The surgical management of small bowel neuroendocrine tumors: consensus guidelines of the north american neuroendocrine tumor society. Pancreas 2017;46(6):715–31.
23. Sakamoto Y, Ohyama S, Yamamoto J, et al. Surgical resection of liver metastases of gastric cancer: an analysis of a 17-year experience with 22 patients. Surgery 2003;133(5):507–11.
24. Boku N, Yamamoto S, Fukuda H, et al. Fluorouracil versus combination of irinotecan plus cisplatin versus S-1 in metastatic gastric cancer: a randomised phase 3 study. Lancet Oncol 2009;10(11):1063–9.
25. Portier G, Elias D, Bouche O, et al. Multicenter randomized trial of adjuvant fluorouracil and folinic acid compared with surgery alone after resection of colorectal liver metastases: FFCD ACHBTH AURC 9002 trial. J Clin Oncol 2006;24(31):4976–82.
26. Nordlinger B, Sorbye H, Glimelius B, et al. Perioperative FOLFOX4 chemotherapy and surgery versus surgery alone for resectable liver metastases from colorectal cancer (EORTC 40983): long-term results of a randomised, controlled, phase 3 trial. Lancet Oncol 2013;14(12):1208–15.
27. Bridgewater JA, Pugh SA, Maishman T, et al. Systemic chemotherapy with or without cetuximab in patients with resectable colorectal liver metastasis (New EPOC): long-term results of a multicentre, randomised, controlled, phase 3 trial. Lancet Oncol 2020;21(3):398–411.
28. Ychou M, Hohenberger W, Thezenas S, et al. A randomized phase III study comparing adjuvant 5-fluorouracil/folinic acid with FOLFIRI in patients following complete resection of liver metastases from colorectal cancer. Ann Oncol 2009;20(12):1964–70.
29. Hasegawa K, Saiura A, Takayama T, et al. Adjuvant oral uracil-tegafur with leucovorin for colorectal cancer liver metastases: a randomized controlled trial. PloS one 2016;11(9):e0162400.
30. Benson AB 3rd, Venook AP, Al-Hawary MM, et al. NCCN clinical practice guidelines in oncology: rectal cancer. version 2.2020. Available at: NCCN.org. Accessed May 20, 2020.
31. Benson AB, Venook AP, Al-Hawary MM, et al. NCCN clinical practice guidelines in oncology: colon cancer. version 2.2020. Available at: NCCN.org. Accessed May 20, 2020.

32. Morris EJ, Forman D, Thomas JD, et al. Surgical management and outcomes of colorectal cancer liver metastases. Br J Surg 2010;97(7):1110–8.

33. Adam R, Delvart V, Pascal G, et al. Rescue surgery for unresectable colorectal liver metastases downstaged by chemotherapy: a model to predict long-term survival. Ann Surg 2004;240(4):644–57 [discussion 657–648].

34. Folprecht G, Grothey A, Alberts S, et al. Neoadjuvant treatment of unresectable colorectal liver metastases: correlation between tumour response and resection rates. Ann Oncol 2005;16(8):1311–9.

35. Alberts SR, Horvath WL, Sternfeld WC, et al. Oxaliplatin, fluorouracil, and leucovorin for patients with unresectable liver-only metastases from colorectal cancer: a north central cancer treatment group phase II study. J Clin Oncol 2005;23(36): 9243–9.

36. Barone C, Nuzzo G, Cassano A, et al. Final analysis of colorectal cancer patients treated with irinotecan and 5-fluorouracil plus folinic acid neoadjuvant chemotherapy for unresectable liver metastases. Br J Cancer 2007;97(8):1035–9.

37. Souglakos J, Androulakis N, Syrigos K, et al. FOLFOXIRI (folinic acid, 5-fluorouracil, oxaliplatin and irinotecan) vs FOLFIRI (folinic acid, 5-fluorouracil and irinotecan) as first-line treatment in metastatic colorectal cancer (MCC): a multicentre randomised phase III trial from the Hellenic oncology research group (HORG). Br J Cancer 2006;94(6):798–805.

38. Falcone A, Ricci S, Brunetti I, et al. Phase III trial of infusional fluorouracil, leucovorin, oxaliplatin, and irinotecan (FOLFOXIRI) compared with infusional fluorouracil, leucovorin, and irinotecan (FOLFIRI) as first-line treatment for metastatic colorectal cancer: the gruppo oncologico nord ovest. J Clin Oncol 2007;25(13): 1670–6.

39. Loupakis F, Cremolini C, Masi G, et al. Initial therapy with FOLFOXIRI and bevacizumab for metastatic colorectal cancer. N Engl J Med 2014;371(17):1609–18.

40. Adam R, Laurent A, Azoulay D, et al. Two-stage hepatectomy: a planned strategy to treat irresectable liver tumors. Ann Surg 2000;232(6):777–85.

41. Jaeck D, Bachellier P, Nakano H, et al. One or two-stage hepatectomy combined with portal vein embolization for initially nonresectable colorectal liver metastases. Am J Surg 2003;185(3):221–9.

42. Kawaguchi Y, Lillemoe HA, Vauthey JN. Dealing with an insufficient future liver remnant: portal vein embolization and two-stage hepatectomy. J Surg Oncol 2019;119(5):594–603.

43. Wicherts DA, Miller R, de Haas RJ, et al. Long-term results of two-stage hepatectomy for irresectable colorectal cancer liver metastases. Ann Surg 2008;248(6): 994–1005.

44. Brouquet A, Abdalla EK, Kopetz S, et al. High survival rate after two-stage resection of advanced colorectal liver metastases: response-based selection and complete resection define outcome. J Clin Oncol 2011;29(8):1083–90.

45. Narita M, Oussoultzoglou E, Jaeck D, et al. Two-stage hepatectomy for multiple bilobar colorectal liver metastases. Br J Surg 2011;98(10):1463–75.

46. Turrini O, Ewald J, Viret F, et al. Two-stage hepatectomy: who will not jump over the second hurdle? Eur J Surg Oncol 2012;38(3):266–73.

47. Imai K, Benitez CC, Allard MA, et al. Impact of Surgical treatment for recurrence after 2-stage hepatectomy for colorectal liver metastases, on patient outcome. Ann Surg 2017;269(2):322–30.

48. Lillemoe HA, Kawaguchi Y, Passot G, et al. Surgical resection for recurrence after two-stage hepatectomy for colorectal liver metastases is feasible, is safe, and improves survival. J Gastrointest Surg 2018;23(1):84–92.

49. Odisio BC, Simoneau E, Holmes AA, et al. Fast-track two-stage hepatectomy using a hybrid interventional radiology/operating suite as alternative option to associated liver partition and portal vein ligation for staged hepatectomy procedure. J Am Coll Surg 2018;227(2):e5–10.

50. Hwang S, Lee SG, Ko GY, et al. Sequential preoperative ipsilateral hepatic vein embolization after portal vein embolization to induce further liver regeneration in patients with hepatobiliary malignancy. Ann Surg 2009;249(4):608–16.

51. Hwang S, Ha TY, Ko GY, et al. Preoperative sequential portal and hepatic vein embolization in patients with hepatobiliary malignancy. World J Surg 2015; 39(12):2990–8.

52. Guiu B, Chevallier P, Denys A, et al. Simultaneous trans-hepatic portal and hepatic vein embolization before major hepatectomy: the liver venous deprivation technique. Eur Radiol 2016;26(12):4259–67.

53. Le Roy B, Perrey A, Fontarensky M, et al. Combined preoperative portal and hepatic vein embolization (biembolization) to improve liver regeneration before major liver resection: a preliminary report. World J Surg 2017;41(7):1848–56.

54. Niekamp AS, Huang SY, Mahvash A, et al. Hepatic vein embolization after portal vein embolization to induce additional liver hypertrophy in patients with metastatic colorectal carcinoma. Eur Radiol 2020;30(7):3862–8.

55. Kobayashi K, Yamaguchi T, Denys A, et al. Liver venous deprivation compared to portal vein embolization to induce hypertrophy of the future liver remnant before major hepatectomy: a single center experience. Surgery 2020;167(6):917–23.

56. Vauthey JN. Commentary: liver venous deprivation: optimizing liver regeneration with combined inflow and outflow venous occlusion of the liver. Surgery 2020; 167(6):924–5.

57. Folprecht G, Gruenberger T, Bechstein W, et al. Survival of patients with initially unresectable colorectal liver metastases treated with FOLFOX/cetuximab or FOLFIRI/cetuximab in a multidisciplinary concept (CELIM study). Ann Oncol 2014; 25(5):1018–25.

58. Douillard JY, Siena S, Cassidy J, et al. Final results from PRIME: randomized phase III study of panitumumab with FOLFOX4 for first-line treatment of metastatic colorectal cancer. Ann Oncol 2014;25(7):1346–55.

59. Douillard JY, Oliner KS, Siena S, et al. Panitumumab-FOLFOX4 treatment and RAS mutations in colorectal cancer. N Engl J Med 2013;369(11):1023–34.

60. Folprecht G, Gruenberger T, Bechstein WO, et al. Tumour response and secondary resectability of colorectal liver metastases following neoadjuvant chemotherapy with cetuximab: the CELIM randomised phase 2 trial. Lancet Oncol 2010;11(1):38–47.

61. Takemura N, Saiura A, Koga R, et al. Long-term outcomes after surgical resection for gastric cancer liver metastasis: an analysis of 64 macroscopically complete resections. Langenbecks Arch Surg 2012;397(6):951–7.

62. Kinoshita T, Kinoshita T, Saiura A, et al. Multicentre analysis of long-term outcome after surgical resection for gastric cancer liver metastases. Br J Surg 2015; 102(1):102–7.

63. Tiberio GA, Baiocchi GL, Morgagni P, et al. Gastric cancer and synchronous hepatic metastases: is it possible to recognize candidates to R0 resection? Ann Surg Oncol 2015;22(2):589–96.

64. Guner A, Son T, Cho I, et al. Liver-directed treatments for liver metastasis from gastric adenocarcinoma: comparison between liver resection and radiofrequency ablation. Gastric cancer 2015;19(3):951–60.

65. Oki E, Tokunaga S, Emi Y, et al. Surgical treatment of liver metastasis of gastric cancer: a retrospective multicenter cohort study (KSCC1302). Gastric cancer 2015;19(3):968–76.

66. Okines A, Puerto OD, Cunningham D, et al. Surgery with curative-intent in patients treated with first-line chemotherapy plus bevacizumab for metastatic colorectal cancer First BEAT and the randomised phase-III NO16966 trial. Br J Cancer 2009;101(7):1033–8.

67. Wong R, Cunningham D, Barbachano Y, et al. A multicentre study of capecitabine, oxaliplatin plus bevacizumab as perioperative treatment of patients with poor-risk colorectal liver-only metastases not selected for upfront resection. Ann Oncol 2011;22(9):2042–8.

Moving?

Make sure your subscription moves with you!

To notify us of your new address, find your **Clinics Account Number** (located on your mailing label above your name), and contact customer service at:

Email: journalscustomerservice-usa@elsevier.com

800-654-2452 (subscribers in the U.S. & Canada)
314-447-8871 (subscribers outside of the U.S. & Canada)

Fax number: 314-447-8029

Elsevier Health Sciences Division
Subscription Customer Service
3251 Riverport Lane
Maryland Heights, MO 63043

*To ensure uninterrupted delivery of your subscription, please notify us at least 4 weeks in advance of move.